Safety and Improvement in Primary Care: The Essential Guide

Edited by

PAUL BOWIE

PhD FRCPE

Programme Director for Safety and Improvement
NHS Education for Scotland, Glasgow, Scotland, UK

and

CARL DE WET

MBChB DRCOG MRCGP MMed(Fam)

General Practitioner
Associate Adviser in Postgraduate GP Education
NHS Education for Scotland, Glasgow, Scotland, UK

Foreword by

ANEEZ ESMAIL

Director, Greater Manchester Primary Care
Patient Safety Translational Research Centre
University of Manchester, UK

Epilogue by

PHILIP CACHIA

Professor and Postgraduate Dean, NHS Education for Scotland, Scotland, UK

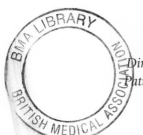

Radcliffe Publishing
London • New York

Radcliffe Publishing Ltd
St Mark's House
Shepherdess Walk
London N1 7BQ
United Kingdom

www.radcliffehealth.com

© 2014 Paul Bowie and Carl de Wet

Paul Bowie and Carl de Wet have asserted their right under the Copyright, Designs and Patents Act 1988 to be identified as the authors of this work.

Every effort has been made to ensure that the information in this book is accurate. This does not diminish the requirement to exercise clinical judgement, and neither the publisher nor the authors can accept any responsibility for its use in practice.

British Library Cataloguing in Publication Data

A catalogue record for this book is available from the British Library.

ISBN-13: 978 184619 580 8

The paper used for the text pages of this book
is FSC® certified. FSC (The Forest Stewardship
Council®) is an international network to promote
responsible management of the world's forests.

Typeset by Darkriver Design, Auckland, New Zealand
Manufacturing managed by 21six

Contents

Foreword

Safety has always been integral to the delivery of healthcare and many people quote the Latin translation of the Hippocratic oath *Primum non nocere* as evidence that it is, and always has been, a principal percept of the training of doctors. The fact that discussions around patient safety never became integral to the delivery of modern healthcare until the Institute of Medicine's landmark report in 1999 is not a reflection of the fact that people didn't care, but perhaps the recognition that discussions around patient safety exposed our collective vulnerability. We continue to have to work in an environment where we have to acknowledge the limitations and gaps in medical knowledge and recognise the difficulty in differentiating between personal ignorance and limitations in medical knowledge. The fact that a great deal of clinical practice is provisional and perhaps even experimental is what gives us a collective sense of vulnerability, with the result that we either blame ourselves or our patients when things go wrong. Ultimately we can deal with the ignorance and sometimes ineptitude associated with medical error but we can never overcome the necessary fallibility and permanent uncertainty that is associated with a lot of clinical practice. This fallibility and uncertainty is writ large in primary care and it was Marshall Marinker who made the perceptive comment that the role of general practice is to accept uncertainty, explore probability and marginalise danger. So anyone who wants to talk about safety and improvement in primary care is already going to make a huge contribution to marginalising the danger inherent in the practice of primary care.

I have always understood my own vulnerability and my first experience of something going terribly wrong was when I was a young trainee just completing my vocational training in general practice in 1985. I had accidentally placed a 30 mg vial of diamorphine in my visit bag because the pharmacist had run out of 10 mg vials. In an emergency situation at a patient's home, when I was required to give someone with a likely myocardial infarction some intravenous analgesia, I accidentally injected a much larger amount of diamorphine than I should have. Luckily, I recognised my mistake promptly and was able to take remedial action which caused the patient no harm. However, it was an early lesson in learning about the role of systems and processes in the cascade leading to an adverse event and a lesson in humility, having to explain to the patient what went wrong. We have come a long way from those days in the mid-1980s, recognising the importance of training doctors in the human factors associated with adverse events and also acknowledging that primary care has its own specific problems which need to be addressed through targeted and directed research. This is a reason why this book is such an important contribution because it unashamedly focuses on primary care and the specifics of patient safety in this context.

Anyone reading this book will, I'm sure, approach it with a view to finding out more about what is happening in relation to patient safety in primary care. A recent review of research on patient safety between 2000 and 2010 which looked at published literature, private initiatives, government grants and regulatory and legislative initiatives in the USA, concluded that major gaps persist in our understanding of patient safety in the ambulatory setting with virtually no credible studies on how to improve safety. An analysis of citations shows that the vast majority of research focusing on patient safety, whether it be on issues of epidemiology, on psychology or sociology or much rarer on interventions, has focused almost exclusively on hospital/specialist care. There are several reasons for this. Firstly, there is a perception of primary care as a low technology environment where safety is not a problem and which therefore engenders a lower profile than the acute sector. Secondly, primary care is much more heterogeneous in its organisational arrangements. In virtually all European countries, the organisational arrangements between primary and secondary care are different and complex, and there is a multiplicity of sites where primary care is carried out (the clinician's office, the telephone and the patient's home). Thirdly, the interfaces between primary and specialist care are hugely important and vary widely between European countries, making the study of patient safety at the interface problematic. Finally, consultation and interpersonal skills are critical to the delivery of primary care and exploring issues related to patient safety in this area raises specific challenges. All of these challenges are addressed in this book.

The relevance of this book is incontrovertible. The fact is that primary care accounts for more than 75 to 80% of the health concerns reported to a physician, whereas hospital care does so for only about 5%. So even if we accept that the risk is lower in primary care, the magnitude makes primary care a significant area of concern. Using the UK as an example, 85% of contacts with the National Health Service take place in primary care and there are 300 million general practice appointments each year. This means that nearly 750 000 patients consult their GP each day. If we assume, based on the best estimate of the literature, that there are between 5 to 80 safety incidents per hundred thousand consultations, this would translate to anything between 37 to 600 incidents per day in the UK. Whilst the vast majority of incidents are of no consequence, the best estimates suggest that between one and two percent of these incidents may result in some harm. Set within the context of a large number of healthcare interactions, this becomes a significant problem. And it is why this book edited by Paul Bowie and Carl de Wet is so timely because for the first time they have brought together the collective experience of over 40 researchers and practitioners from around the world to provide the reader with an essential guide to safety and improvement in primary care.

Amongst clinical academics, books have little currency because they don't count as much in the different research assessment exercises that have become the bane of many academics. The result is that it is very unusual for researchers and practitioners to find in one place the collective knowledge that comes from the huge range of publications in any given area. So it is a credit to Bowie and de Wet that they have used the vast experience gained through their work with NHS Education for Scotland to inform the wider practitioner and research community about practical steps to reduce harm in primary care. From the perspective of patient safety research we are in a much better place than we were 10 years ago. A lot more funding has been directed to patient safety research in primary care and it is a good time, to paraphrase Paulo Freire, to have an overview of where we are, what we need to do and what we can do today so that tomorrow we can do what we are unable to do today.

Aneez Esmail
Director, Greater Manchester Primary Care
Patient Safety Translational Research Centre
University of Manchester
March 2014

Preface

In recent decades most of the international effort given over to studying and improving the safety of patient care has been focused in acute hospital settings. To some extent this was always something of a puzzle to those of us with a direct interest in this important issue, given that there are over 300 million patient consultations in primary care in the United Kingdom (UK) annually and the adverse event rate is estimated at between 1% and 2% of consultations. However, the tide is now slowly turning. Policymakers, healthcare leaders and research grant funders are beginning to recognise that greater evidence is required to understand more about what can and does go wrong in primary care, with increasing attention now being paid to what can be done to minimise avoidable harm to patients in this setting.

The National Health Service (NHS) in Scotland is arguably the first to take a nationwide collaborative approach to addressing some of these concerns, through the creation of the Scottish Patient Safety Programme (www.scottish patientsafetyprogramme.scot.nhs.uk). More recently, NHS England and Wales, the World Health Organization and the European Union have also acknowledged the scale and extent of this problem and the need for concerted action in primary care. NHS Education for Scotland (NES), a special health authority with responsibility for the education, training and lifelong development of the healthcare workforce (www.nes.scot.nhs.uk), has been at the creative forefront of this action for improvement, being a leading force in the fields of patient safety science, education and development in the UK and internationally for over a decade.

This book represents a substantial body of scholarly work – most of it led by NES educators and researchers – which is devoted to learning about and improving the safety of primary healthcare. It is a practical book but it is underpinned, where needed, by related theory and empirical evidence. A broad-based view of what is meant and understood by 'patient safety science', 'quality improvement' and 'improvement science' is adopted throughout. This is contrary to the narrow assumptions made by a minority of healthcare scholars who appear to equate these latter terms with a very specific suite of improvement 'methodologies' (e.g. Plan-Do-Study-Act (PDSA) cycles, Statistical Process Control or Lean) that have their origins in non-healthcare industries.

However, the evidence clearly demonstrates that a more orthodox approach to quality improvement (QI) in primary care is one that involves a broad range of stakeholders in a multi-method endeavour that encompasses education and training (e.g. specialty training); professional approaches to improvement (e.g. peer review, appraisal and clinical audit); regulation (e.g. medical revalidation); the aforementioned industrial or organisational improvement techniques (e.g. PDSA cycles and process mapping); and the implementation of macro-organisational initiatives (e.g. practice accreditation or financial incentivisation).

This book is far from a definitive guide, but it seeks to offer guidance and evidence for a range of related improvement methods, concepts and interventions that were developed and implemented in the recent past by the NES primary care team, or as a direct result of fruitful partnership working with colleagues from academic, professional, public or regulatory institutions across the UK and internationally, as well as other NHS Scotland colleagues.

The primary care front-line service, specialty training, appraisal and continuing professional development (CPD) environments in Scotland are the focus of much of the development and implementation work described in this book. However, to a large extent this is of limited relevance. The topics and ideas that are outlined and debated here are, at a fundamental level, explicitly concerned with *collective learning* to support patient safety and quality improvement – a key issue that resonates strongly in primary care settings worldwide and which we are really only taking the very first steps towards understanding.

The purpose of this book

The book was written with diverse groups of readers in mind, all of whom, regardless of country of origin or professional role, should have a keen interest in improving the quality and safety of primary healthcare. First, for front-line clinicians, managers and administrators, we have included much practical guidance on what different methods and tools can be selected, depending on the problem or issue at hand, to help them to learn and improve collectively as teams and micro-organisations – and ultimately to begin to build or strengthen that all-important, but potentially elusive, 'safety culture'. There is, therefore, a substantial 'how to' aspect in large sections of this book, which contrasts with, but is complementary to, the theoretical and evidential topic considerations in some chapters.

Improvement advisers, patient safety officers, clinical governance leads, risk managers and health services researchers may still be interested in aspects of the 'practical', but perhaps a greater focus will be on critically reviewing the theory and evidence underpinning the implementation of the developments outlined in front-line practice. This is particularly so because many of the methods and approaches described are relatively new to primary care, or are adapted from other settings, potentially sparking interest in the transferability of concepts or tools from one setting or country to another.

For primary care educators, designing and delivering training in safety and improvement concepts – especially safety skills, learning from error and human factors science – is growing in importance. This is particularly so as a means to help trainee doctors, established clinicians, managers and other colleagues meet the related demands and obligations of specialty training, appraisal and revalidation, routine contractual requirements and CPD. Many of the chapter authors are recognised expert leaders in these particular fields. Given their knowledge and experience, we believe ample information and guidance are provided that can be gleaned by educators to help them teach and advise those in training, or in need of professional development support, or who are participating in collaborative improvement programmes. A further consideration for educational policymakers, particularly internationally, is the opportunity to learn about the successful development and implementation of vocational training schemes for general practice nurses and managers, as well as a national GP appraisal system (www.scottishappraisal.scot.nhs.uk/) in support of UK medical revalidation and the aforementioned national patient safety programme for primary care, which are all likely to be unique to the Scottish Health Service.

For healthcare leaders and decision-makers, the book offers varying degrees of implementation evidence on a whole raft of interventions that can be used to improve the quality and safety of primary care at the professional, team and organisational levels. It is now well established that the evidence base underpinning the effectiveness of improvement methods is inconclusive. No single QI approach appears to be any worse or any better than the next: people, systems, context and culture are what really matter. Why, therefore, do we frequently see healthcare systems jumping from one improvement fad to another, at great expense and with predictably limited impact? Why not simply focus on improving, integrating and spreading the learning from the more established professional, organisational and regulatory QI approaches that clinicians and managers are routinely exposed to and are increasingly expected to provide supporting evidence for? Perhaps the best strategy is to narrow attention on the implementation element of improvement and on identifying a broad range of evidence of some of the key determinants of success: Is the approach reliable? Does it have validity? Is it acceptable to the healthcare workforce? Is it feasible to apply in routine practice? Does it positively affect professional and organisational learning? And does it lead to tangible and sustainable improvements in the quality and safety of patient care?

The organisation of this book

This book is organised into five interlinked parts, each with a number of related chapters.

Part I provides an overview of safety and improvement in primary care from an organisational systems perspective. For example, the pressing need for evidence-based improvement initiatives in primary care is considered, and the complex challenge of adapting a one-size-fits-all approach to different organisational contexts is highlighted. The concept of 'safety culture' is also defined and its relevance to, and influence over, the primary care workforce in terms of having an impact on safety-related behaviours is discussed alongside practical guidance on how this concept can be assessed at the care team level. A further chapter argues that data (measurement) alone is insufficient to improve patient safety and that it is only the first of five necessary steps of the 'wisdom hierarchy'. Only once data are transformed into information, information into knowledge, knowledge into understanding and finally into wisdom, does it become possible to take effective and deliberate action to improve the quality and safety of care. Given that data are the foundation of improvement, a prerequisite is that related measurement has to be statistically reliable. Recent development work is described in this section in which the outcome is the proposal of a simple formula to ensure the statistical precision and power of harm rates obtained through clinical record review in primary care settings. Other chapters in this section focus on how the primary care workforce can acquire better knowledge and a deeper understanding of the safety-related intricacies and complexities of workplace systems through application of process mapping, task analysis, systems thinking and the design and implementation of effective policies and protocols.

Part II focuses on the role of people (patients, clinicians and staff) in the context of safety improvement in primary care. The section begins by considering one of the main problems with any improvement project or initiative – actively involving patients and clinicians and overcoming well-known barriers to engagement. The concept of professionalism and the pivotal role it has in inculcating a safety improvement culture at the organisational level is also examined. One of the hallmarks of professionalism is the responsibility of the clinician to self-regulate performance so that minimum safety standards are achieved and opportunities for development are identified. Three of the most important learning activities in this regard are peer review, professional appraisal and multi-source feedback, which are covered in detail in this section. The critical importance of practice managers and practice nurses to the delivery of safe and effective patient care cannot be overstated. These two professions are now so integral to the general practice team that it is difficult to imagine that they did not formally exist when the NHS was founded just over 60 years ago. The final chapters in this section provide a brief history of the evolution of these professions in the Scottish context and describe the creation of a national vocational training scheme and professional development network for practice managers. The learning needs of newly recruited GP nurses are also described alongside recent developments, challenges and opportunities in support of the CPD and appraisal of established GP nurses.

Part III is concerned with the role of learning, education and training in relation to improving the safety of primary care. Within any healthcare system the individual often remains the last barrier between the system and preventable harm to the patient. Therefore, possession of relevant, up-to-date safety skills and knowledge at the individual level is crucial in helping to maintain and promote patient safety. In this section, the qualities and attributes of the safe clinician are explored, together with the use of a safety checklist as a measure to ensure the reliable delivery of 'essential' patient safety education in the GP training environment. Practice-based small group learning is an innovative approach to CPD that is focused on facilitated discussions between peers on the real problems that clinicians encounter and the challenges of integrating evidence-based and patient-centred care to enhance safety improvement. The benefits and challenges of the practice-based small group learning method based on experiences and learning from a well-established system in general practice in Scotland are described, as are plans to adapt this approach by other professional groups, with growing interest also from the rest of the UK and internationally. Also in this section, the benefits of protected learning time in providing valuable opportunities for teams to learn together are outlined, with a clear warning that this approach needs to be carefully managed if the learning needs of all those involved are to be met. Finally, effective communication skills at the clinician–patient interface are often of critical importance from a safety perspective. Two interventions developed specifically to support skill development in this area are described and the potential benefits outlined: a consultation skills course for GPs and a system of peer review of GPs' consultation skills.

Part IV outlines what we know about human error theory and the types and causes of some common patient safety incidents in primary care, while considering how they may be prevented or related risks mitigated or reduced. The two most common sources of patient safety issues in primary care are related to clinical diagnoses and medication. The corresponding chapters describe the range of errors that routinely happen in these areas, explore important contributory factors and suggest potential strategies to reduce such errors. One of these system-based strategies – medication reconciliation – is attracting great interest as a safety improvement intervention and, as such, the findings from a pilot project in a large health authority area are included as a case study in this section. A further source of safety incidents in primary care is the reliability (or otherwise) of practice-based systems for laboratory test ordering and handling investigation results. Therefore, the findings from a recent Pan-European project to build consensus on 'good practice' guidance statements to inform the front-line implementation of safe systems in this important area are presented. Finally, a very specific type of serious but largely preventable patient safety incident – known as a 'Never Event' – is introduced in this section, and the applicability and potential benefit of this concept to primary care is debated alongside discussion of a recently developed preliminary list of potential Never Events for this setting.

Part V focuses on outlining the evidence for, and providing good practice guidance on, a wide selection of improvement methods that can be applied by primary care teams to enhance the safety and reliability of practice systems and care processes. Some, such as significant event analysis and criteria-based audit, are already well established in UK primary care, particularly in general practice, but they can be poorly conducted by care teams. Others, such as the trigger review and care bundle methods, are comparatively new to general practice but evidence of their utility and impact in this setting is starting to accumulate. Guidance on the care bundle method is provided in terms of its practical application and potential value to help improve the reliability of evidence-based care delivery and clinical outcomes, which are a significant source of variation in UK and international general practice. The trigger review method is potentially of great interest, as it can provide care teams with a whole new perspective on patient safety because, unlike other improvement tools, its main focus is on highlighting previously undetected patient safety incidents and latent risks that can lie dormant in the electronic patient record. The potential for this method to inform learning as part of patient safety obligations in specialty training and GP appraisal is also discussed. In the final chapter of this book, a senior healthcare leader shares his personal and philosophical reflections on recent experiences of the deep complexities, challenges and successes linked to primary care improvement processes, with a very specific focus on the application of the Model for Improvement – popularised by the Institute for Healthcare Improvement.

Paul Bowie and Carl de Wet
March 2014

About the editors

Paul Bowie PhD FRCPE is Programme Director for Safety and Improvement with NHS Education for Scotland based in Glasgow, Scotland, UK. He has worked in the National Health Service in Scotland for over 20 years in a range of quality and safety advisory roles. He gained his doctorate in significant event analysis in general medical practice from the University of Glasgow in 2005 and has published over 60 papers on healthcare quality and safety in international peer-reviewed journals. He is Associate Editor of *BMC Family Practice* and a PhD examiner and supervisor with the department of general practice and primary care at the University of Glasgow. In 2011 he was elected honorary Fellow of the Royal College of Physicians (Edinburgh) and is also an affiliated Member of the Institute of Ergonomics and Human Factors.

Email: paul.bowie@nes.scot.nhs.uk

Carl de Wet MBChB DRCOG MRCGP MMed(Fam) has more than 10 years' clinical experience in a wide range of specialties and settings, more recently as a GP partner. After completing a research fellowship in 2008 in the west region of NHS Education for Scotland, he has continued as Associate Adviser in Postgraduate GP Education. In this role he contributes to and leads on the design and development, testing, implementation and evaluation of tools and educational resources to help improve the quality and safety of patient care. The findings have been published in peer-reviewed journals and presented at national and international conferences. He is currently undertaking a PhD on patient safety in general medical practice at the University of Glasgow.

Email: carl.dewet@nes.scot.nhs.uk

List of contributors

Maria Ahmed MBChB MPH PhD is Clinical Research Fellow, Centre for Patient Safety and Service Quality, Imperial College London, London, UK
Email: maria.ahmed@imperial.ac.uk

Dorothy Armstrong Hon DSc BSc RGN MN PgCert RNT is Professional Adviser to the Scottish Public Service Ombudsman, Edinburgh, Scotland, UK
Email: darmstrong@spso.org.uk

Michelle Beattie RN BSc (Hons) MSc is a lecturer in the School of Nursing, Midwifery and Health, University of Stirling, based in Inverness, Scotland, UK
Email: michelle.beattie@stir.ac.uk

David Bruce FRCGP is National Director of Postgraduate GP Education with NHS Education for Scotland, based in Dundee, Scotland, UK
Email: david.bruce@nes.scot.nhs.uk

Rachel Bruce MPharm PhD is Lead Pharmacist for Primary Care Clinical Governance in NHS Greater Glasgow and Clyde, Glasgow, Scotland, UK
Email: rachel.bruce@nhs.net

Philip Cachia MD FRCPE FRCPath is Professor and Postgraduate Dean in the east region of NHS Education for Scotland, and Executive Lead for Patient Safety and Clinical Skills, based in Dundee, Scotland, UK
Email: philip.cachia@nes.scot.nhs.uk

Niall Cameron MPhil FRCGP is a general medical practitioner and National Lead for Medical Appraisal with NHS Education for Scotland, based in Glasgow, Scotland, UK
Email: niall.cameron@nes.scot.nhs.uk

Clare Carolan MBChB MSc MRCP MRCGP is a general medical practitioner and appraiser and Clinical Academic Fellow in the School of Nursing, Midwifery and Health, University of Stirling, Stirling, Scotland, UK
Email: clare.carolan@stir.ac.uk

Andy Crawford MPH Dip Sys Prac(OU) ADN(IC) RMN RGN is Head of Clinical Governance with NHS Greater Glasgow and Clyde, Glasgow, Scotland, UK
Email: andy.crawford@ggc.scot.nhs.uk

David Cunningham PhD FRCGP is a general medical practitioner and Assistant Director of Postgraduate GP Education, based in the west region of NHS Education for Scotland, Glasgow, Scotland, UK
Email: david.cunningham@nes.scot.nhs.uk

Susan Dovey MPH PhD is Professor of General Practice in the Dunedin School of Medicine, University of Otago, New Zealand
Email: susan.dovey@otago.ac.nz

Aneez Esmail PhD LRCP MRCS DTM&H DRCOG MFPHM MRCGP FRCP is Professor of General Practice at the University of Manchester, Manchester, England, UK
Email: aneez.esmail@manchester.ac.uk

Julie Ferguson BSc (Hons) MSc PhD MBPS is a health psychologist and Research & Education Co-ordinator in the west region of NHS Education for Scotland, based in Glasgow, Scotland, UK
Email: julie.ferguson@nes.scot.nhs.uk

Eleanor Forrest BSc MIEHF MBPS is a psychologist and Human Factors Consultant (www.brighthf.co.uk), based in Glasgow, Scotland, UK
Email: eleanor@brighthf.co.uk

Marion Foster PgCert DCRR is a former practice manager in Perthshire, Scotland, UK
Email: mfoster1457@gmail.com

Sander Gaal MD PhD is a general medical practitioner and researcher at the Radboud University Nijmegen Medical Centre, Nijmegen, the Netherlands
Email: s.gaal@iq.umcn.nl

Brian James BA MSc RNMH RGN RCNT RNT is Senior Teaching Fellow and Curriculum Lead for Quality Improvement in the School of Nursing, Midwifery and Health at the University of Stirling, based in Inverness, Scotland, UK
Email: b.l.a.james@stir.ac.uk

Paul Johnson PhD is a statistician and geneticist in the Institute of Biodiversity, Animal Health and Comparative Medicine at the University of Glasgow, Glasgow, Scotland, UK
Email: paul.johnson@glasgow.ac.uk

Moya Kelly MBE PhD FRCGP is Professor of General Practice and Director of Postgraduate GP Education, based in the west region of NHS Education for Scotland, Glasgow, Scotland, UK
Email: moya.kelly@nes.scot.nhs.uk

Susan Kennedy MSc RGN DN is National Co-ordinator for General Practice Nursing with NHS Education for Scotland, based in Glasgow, Scotland, UK
Email: susan.kennedy@nes.scot.nhs.uk

Marion Macleod BA MBA MIHM is National Co-ordinator of the Scottish Practice Management Development Network with NHS Education for Scotland, based in Glasgow, Scotland, UK
Email: marion.macleod@nes.scot.nhs.uk

Ronald MacVicar FRCGP is a general medical practitioner and Director of Postgraduate GP Education in the north region of NHS Education for Scotland, Inverness, Scotland, UK
Email: ronald.macvicar@nes.scot.nhs.uk

John McKay BSc (Hons) MD FRCGP is a general medical practitioner and Assistant Director of Postgraduate GP Education, based in the west region of NHS Education for Scotland, Glasgow, Scotland, UK
Email: john.mckay@nes.scot.nhs.uk

Rhona McMillan DRCOG FRCGP is a general medical practitioner and Training Programme Director in the west region of NHS Education for Scotland, Glasgow, Scotland, UK
Email: rhona.mcmillan@nes.scot.nhs.uk

Elaine McNaughton MBChB FRCGP DRCOG DFSRH is a general medical practitioner and Training Programme Director in the east region of NHS Education for Scotland, Dundee, Scotland, UK
Email: elaine.mcnaughton@nes.scot.nhs.uk

Lucy Mitchell MA MRes PhD is a Research Fellow at the Industrial Psychology Research Centre, University of Aberdeen, Aberdeen, Scotland, UK
Email: l.mitchell@abdn.ac.uk

Jill Murie MBChB MPH DRCOG DFM FRCGP MFFLM is a general medical practitioner and Lead GP Appraisal Adviser in Lanarkshire, Scotland, UK
  Email: jill.murie@aol.com

Margaret Murphy is External Lead Advisor to the World Health Organization Patients for Patient Safety Programme and one of 70 ISQua Global Experts on Healthcare Safety and Improvement
  Email: margaretmurphyireland@gmail.com

Mike Norbury BSc MSc MBChB DRCOG MRCGP is a general medical practitioner and Associate Clinical Director of Lothian Unscheduled Care Service, Edinburgh, Scotland, UK
  Email: michael.norbury@nhs.net

Catherine O'Donnell PhD is Professor of Primary Care Research and Development in the Institute of Health and Wellbeing at the University of Glasgow, Glasgow, Scotland, UK
  Email: kate.o'donnell@glasgow.ac.uk

Julie Price BA RGN is Clinical Risk Programme Manager with the Medical Protection Society (www.medicalprotection.org/uk), based in Leeds, England, UK
  Email: julie.price@mps.org.uk

Brian Robson MBChB MRCGP MPH (Harvard) DRCOG is Executive Clinical Director of Healthcare Improvement Scotland, Edinburgh, Scotland, UK
  Email: brian.robson@nhs.net

Nick Sevdalis PhD is an experimental psychologist and Senior Lecturer in the Department of Surgery and Cancer and the Centre for Patient Safety and Service Quality (www.cpssq.org) of Imperial College London, and Director of the 'Non-Technical Skills and Simulation' Research Group
  Email: n.sevdalis@imperial.ac.uk

Annabel Shepherd MRCGP MBChB DRCOG is a general medical practitioner and former research fellow with NHS Education for Scotland, based in Glasgow, Scotland, UK
  Email: annabel.shepherd@doctors.org.uk

Rachel Spencer MBBS BMedSci is a general medical practitioner and is training as an Academic Clinical Fellow at the University of Nottingham, Nottingham, England, UK
  Email: mcxrs13@nottingham.ac.uk

Ian Staples is Development Manager for Medical Appraisal with NHS Education for Scotland, Edinburgh, Scotland, UK
  Email: ian.staples@nes.scot.nhs.uk

Wim Verstappen MD PhD is a general medical practitioner and coordinator of GP vocational training and senior researcher for IQ healthcare (Scientific Institute for Research on Quality of Healthcare) at Radboud University Nijmegen Medical Centre, the Netherlands
  Email: w.verstappen@elg.umcn.nl

Katharine Wallis MBChB MBHL Dip Obst, FRNZCGP is a general medical practitioner and a researcher at the University of Otago, New Zealand
  Email: katharine.wallis@otago.ac.nz

Michel Wensing PhD is Professor of Implementation Science at Radboud University Nijmegen Medical Centre, the Netherlands.
  Email: m.wensing@iq.umcn.nl

Christopher Williams is a fifth-year medical student in the Faculty of Medicine at the University of Glasgow, Glasgow, Scotland, UK
  Email: chris_williams118@hotmail.com

Nigel Williams MSc FRCGP is a general medical practitioner and Associate Medical Director for Primary Care in NHS Lothian, Edinburgh, Scotland, UK
    Email: nigel.williams@nhslothian.scot.nhs.uk

Steven Wilson PgDip MSc MCMI is Senior Programme Manager with Healthcare Improvement Scotland, Glasgow, Scotland, UK
    Email: steven.wilson@nhs.net

Malcolm Wright OBE is Chief Executive of NHS Education for Scotland, Edinburgh, Scotland, UK
    Email: malcolm.wright@nes.scot.nhs.uk

Dedication

This book is dedicated to Professor T Stuart Murray, Emeritus Professor of General Practice at the University of Glasgow and former Director of Postgraduate GP Education in the west of Scotland and National GP Director in Scotland. Under Stuart's visionary leadership and strong belief in scholarship and professional development, the Department of Postgraduate GP Education was quickly imbued with a culture of innovation and creativity and gained an international reputation in the field of medical education and research & development. During much of this time, Dr Murray Lough was Assistant Director of Postgraduate GP Education to Stuart and he, too, deserves equal plaudits for his mentorship, leadership and inspirational approach to research and development. Both of us owe a great debt of gratitude to Murray and Stuart on personal and professional levels.

Paul Bowie
Carl de Wet
March 2014

Acknowledgements

We also offer sincere thanks to Professor Moya Kelly, Director of Postgraduate GP Education in the west of Scotland, who has continued where Stuart left off by providing the necessary leadership, as well as a creative platform, for scholarly developments in support of patient safety and quality improvement to flourish in the department. Other NES leaders and colleagues, particularly Dr John McKay, Professor Philip Cachia, Dr David Bruce, Dr Niall Cameron, Dr Kenneth Lee, Dr David Cunningham, Marion Macleod, Susan Kennedy, Professor Rose Marie Parr, Anne Watson, Dr Ailsa Power, Dr Elaine McNaughton, Dr Gordon McLeay, Dr Ronald MacVicar, Dr Diane Kelly and Dr Fiona Gailey, have all been extremely supportive of the safety and improvement development work reported in this book, providing ongoing advice, constructive feedback, encouragement or opportunities to apply for funding.

We are grateful also to colleagues such as Jill Gillies, Dr Neil Houston, Steven Wilson and Dr Brian Robson from our 'sister' organisation, Healthcare Improvement Scotland (www.healthcareimprovementscotland.org), as well as colleagues in wider NHS Scotland and further afield, such as Dr Paul Ryan, Dr Grant McHattie, Dr Jean Robson, Andy Crawford, Dr Gregor Smith, Professor Mike Pringle, Professor Susan Dovey and members of the west of Scotland GP Audit Development Group, who have all acted as 'critical friends' over the years, with many being instrumental in enabling us to test and implement our developments within the service to gather much-needed feedback. In the same vein our academic colleague, Professor Kate O'Donnell of the University of Glasgow, is providing expert research advice and support in the complex study of patient harm in general medical practice.

Most of the work described in this book would not have been possible without the initial advice, guidance and support of the following GP educator colleagues from NES, many of whom personally participated in small pilot studies and often recruited their own practices to help us test and refine our early ideas: Drs Alison Garvie, Colin Hodgson, Rhona McMillan, Duncan McNab, Janice Oliver, Linsey Semple and David Sutherland. A steady stream of GPs on fixed-term fellowships have also played their role and we thank them all for their contributions: Drs Annabel Shepherd, Lindsey Pope, Mark Russell, David Blane, Esther Curnock, Karyn Devlin, Francesca Gray, Marie Jamieson, Kate Lewin, Catriona Nesbit, Claire Reid, Sarah Capewell and Kirsty Stewart.

We acknowledge also the important role played by external funding bodies, most notably the UK Health Foundation (www.health.org.uk/) and the European Union-funded LINNEAUS Euro-PC collaboration (www.linneaus-pc.eu/) led by Professor Aneez Esmail and project managed by Annette Barber of the University of Manchester. Involvement with these groundbreaking initiatives has enabled us to participate in and learn from national and international development networks of healthcare leaders, academics and researchers who all have a keen interest in advancing knowledge of safety and improvement in primary care.

We also salute and sincerely thank the dedicated and hard-working efforts of our GP department staff colleagues, past and present, without whom we would be floundering much more so than usual on a daily basis: Jane Gordon, June Morrison, Karen Miller, Isabel Robertson, Emily Watt, Hazel Baillie, Liz Cook, Julie Ogilvie, Cath Kelly, Irene Lynch, Kelly O'Donnell, Nicola Fraser, Gillian Jamieson, Danielle Finlay, Jill Havlin and Kirsten McDonald. Special thanks is also due to education and research colleagues, Lynn Railston, Ian Colthart and Drs Julie Ferguson, Suzanne Bunniss, Nick Bradley, Hannah Hesselgreaves, Helen Allbutt, Judy Wakeling and Clare Tochel who have contributed to, supported or championed much of our development work. We are particularly indebted and thankful to the NES lead for communications, Christine Patch, for her very welcome contribution to the development and promotion of this book.

Finally, it would be utterly remiss of us not to acknowledge and thank profusely the many, many general practitioners, practice managers, practice nurses, administrative support staff, patients, pharmacists, GP clinical directors, GP appraisers, GP trainers and GP trainees across Scotland who have made, and continue to make, vital contributions to the design, development, testing and implementation of the tools, techniques and concepts outlined in this book – the sole purpose of which is to help them to improve the quality and safety of healthcare they provide to their patients.

Paul Bowie and Carl de Wet
March 2014

Introduction

I was delighted to be invited to write a short introduction to this excellent book on safety and improvement in primary care. Its key messages and guidance will clearly be of great benefit to many clinical practitioners, healthcare managers and leaders, educators, safety improvement advisers and decision-makers working to enhance the quality and safety of patient care in the National Health Service in Scotland, and much further afield.

As NHS Scotland's national body for education, training and lifelong learning, we have a pivotal role to play in ensuring that the Service has the right staff in the right place at the right time. This means that they will have had appropriate evidence-based education and training that enables them to provide safe, effective and person-centred care for the people of Scotland.

This book will make a major contribution to our continual efforts to improve quality and safety standards in the primary healthcare field. It fits perfectly with our organisational mission to innovate, develop and implement creative educational solutions that support excellence in healthcare. Whilst largely focused on the work of NHS Scotland, Paul Bowie and Carl de Wet's approach of blending practical examples supported by contemporary theory and empirical evidence ensures that their first book together has international significance and will, I am sure, rapidly become an essential text for all those with an interest in improving the safety of patients in the primary care setting, wherever they are based in the world.

Malcolm Wright OBE
Chief Executive
NHS Education for Scotland
March 2014

Part I

Understanding Systems

CHAPTER 1

'The heart of the matter': a parent's perspective

Margaret Murphy

More than anything, this is what distinguishes the great from the medio-cre. They didn't fail less. They rescued more.[1]

This chapter is about what I like to call 'the heart of the matter' – the patient's experience of healthcare and how that experience can drive improvement in clinical practice. I would like to tell you about the patient journey of my own 21-year-old son Kevin through the Irish healthcare system in the closing years of the millennium as a means of first identifying and then discussing some of the challenges in providing safe care. Challenges that, if not appropriately met at primary care level, can have devastating consequences for patient, family and clinician. I would like to share some of my own reflections about Kevin's experiences before concluding with a 'wish list' of recommendations to help improve the quality and safety of care in the future.

KEVIN'S JOURNEY

I offer you the ultimate official data in relation to Kevin – his death certificate – which lists: 'multi-organ failure, hypercalcaemia, parathyroid tumour'. Nothing or no one had prepared us for this – we had no warning, we never considered his life to be in danger and no one had intimated that this was the case. We had questions and we needed answers. How can a 21-year-old boy be admitted to hospital on a Thursday and die on the Sunday? What went wrong?

During 1997 Kevin presented on a number of occasions with persistent back pain to his general practitioner (GP). He was referred to an orthopaedic consultant in the autumn when he didn't improve. Blood tests were requested at the clinic and revealed abnormally high levels of plasma calcium, at 3.51 mmol/L (normal range 2.05–2.60 mmol/L). There were also other abnormal measures – for example, a plasma creatinine level indicative of a more than 50% loss of overall renal function. All of the abnormal results were underlined in the laboratory report. However, when writing to the GP the consultant underplayed the high calcium levels and ignored the plasma creatinine level. That letter is not on the GP's file and the consultant's intention to see Kevin again early in the new year was therefore also never conveyed. Kevin was also unaware that he would have a follow-up appointment.

It is significant that throughout Kevin's care only one set of clinical eyes saw those particular test results – at no point in his care was the hard copy forwarded and neither did it travel with Kevin as part of a patient-held record – no one else, patient or clinician, had an opportunity to revisit them or question them again.

After repeated consultations in general practice, Kevin was on each occasion returned to us as seemingly healthy and without explanation for his sometimes unacceptable and erratic behaviour. Only later did we learn that this behaviour was due to the chemical imbalance caused by his undiagnosed medical condition and the fact that while his bones were being starved and softening, the viscosity of his blood was being altered and putting a huge strain on his heart.

Kevin's medical record contains an entry made by the GP's secretary:

> Telephone call from patient's mother. She is extremely worried about her son. She wishes you to know that she thinks he may be depressed also. Failed his first year exams, Repeating and not doing well either, finding it hard to study. He is now remaining in bed a lot. She has arranged an appointment with Dr X (a psychiatrist) tomorrow and would like to have results of bloods, bone scan, etc for the consultation. She wonders if he really has a back problem. What can I tell the mother? She wishes to speak to you. Results in file.

The GP's response: 'Fax results to Dr X.' There was no direct contact with the mother or the patient.

Kevin spent the summer of 1999 in the United States. On his return he again consulted his GP, complaining of lethargy, occasional vomiting and continuing bone pain. Blood and urine samples were taken and the test results were telephoned to the surgery the next day. The practice nurse wrote the results on a Post-it note and drew attention to the high calcium level, now 5.73 mmol/L.

The GP seemingly ignored the high calcium levels, and in his referral to the hospital included only those elements of the blood test results that supported his own diagnosis of leptospirosis – although he did send the Post-it note with the letter. It was at this point that Kevin's contact with primary care came to an end. Our next interaction with his primary care physician was to inform him of Kevin's death.

When compiling the file in the hospital on admission on the Thursday, the Post-it note containing those vital calcium results was stuck to the back of the letter and was not seen until 6 weeks *after* Kevin's death. The standard blood tests in that particular hospital did not include calcium. So, throughout Kevin's time there, they remained unaware of his dangerously high calcium levels. Instead, a diagnosis of nephritis was made.

Despite his continuing decline, no alarm was raised. He became dehydrated and described worsening muscle pain and neurological problems. His medical record quotes him as saying: 'I have crazy thoughts coming into my head.' The same notes also show advancing renal failure. At this time, no medical personnel seemed to appreciate how ill Kevin had become as his condition continued to deteriorate rapidly. Finally, he was transferred to Cork University Hospital (CUH).

I can recall speaking with a consultant in the hospital corridor on the afternoon before Kevin was transferred to CUH. I asked: 'Are you concerned at all about the delay in his transfer, because I have this desperate sense of urgency (hand on my chest)?' Kevin's brother interjected and inquired: 'What will they do differently in CUH?' The consultant replied: 'They'll do nothing different. Perhaps they'll take a biopsy on Monday or Tuesday.' Kevin was dead on Sunday.

It was at CUH where we first heard concerns about his high calcium levels, then 6.1 mmol/L! Unfortunately, Kevin was managed at registrar level. Senior personnel and more aggressive treatments were not available at the weekend. We cannot say if that would have resulted in a better outcome, but it would be nice for me, his mother, to know that he was given every chance.

During Sunday, Kevin was lucid but very sleepy, giving a thumbs-up sign to his father when he left his bedside. At 3.30 p.m. the young intern checked on Kevin in the intensive care unit, and before the intern had reached the door on his way out of the unit, Kevin suffered a heart attack while his sister and I sat at his bedside. Attempts at resuscitation failed. Kevin had died right before my eyes.

I asked about organ donation, as Kevin carried a donor card. The doctor shook his head, 'no'. Kevin had been allowed to deteriorate to the point where his organs were of no use to any other human being. That was very difficult to hear. It was almost like Kevin dying twice. The doctor then asked if we would like him to enquire about Kevin's eyes. So Kevin's corneas were donated and we later learned that two people, a 42-year-old woman, and a 60-year-old man, now have sight because of Kevin.

And that is Kevin's journey. A journey that could have been considerably shortened, and successfully shortened, had appropriate interventions occurred during earlier contacts in primary care. Adverse events happen to real people. Kevin was more than a statistic, he was more than a medical condition. He was a real person, a young man, full of life. But, above all, he was my beautiful boy – handsome, strong and carefree.

A DAVID AND GOLIATH EXPERIENCE

And *after* his death? What was the outcome of our (his family's) interactions with the healthcare system? There were initial honest and humane reactions from individuals for which I will always be grateful – especially the nurse. But in a short space of time this was replaced by a process of damage limitation.

What we encountered was closing ranks, lame excuses, muddying of the waters and protestations of loyalty to colleagues. One doctor described his dilemma as an issue with 'loyalty to colleagues'. Another suggested, when referring to the Post-it note, that even if it had been seen by his consultant colleague, it would not have meant anything to him. He said this was because it was not written as they would write it in 'scientific notation' – for example, 'Cal' might not mean 'calcium' and 'Sod' might not mean 'sodium'. It was at that point that I lost faith.

Our confidence and any hope of ascertaining the truth through honest dialogue was shattered and that is why we undertook litigation. It also became clear that the legal system favours the defendant in these cases, especially in the areas of finance and resources. For ordinary people, like ourselves, it is a David and Goliath experience. Until the eleventh hour every effort was made by the defendants to settle without admission of liability – a wearing-down strategy that lacks compassion and consideration for heartbroken people.

Disappointed and frustrated, we retraced Kevin's medical history over the previous 3 years. The story slowly and painfully unfolded. Failings and short-comings were many in number and serious in nature. They were indicative of system breakdown and were compounded by misdiagnosis, inappropriate treatment and management, together with issues of miscommunication and errors in data handling.

Almost 5 years later, a judge of the High Court declared: 'It is very clear to me that Kevin Murphy should not have died.' Two GPs, a private consultant, a hospital consultant and a hospital all admitted liability, expressed their regret at Kevin's death and sympathised with the family. Sadly, this was not done in person, but through legal representatives.

When adjudicating on the quality of Kevin's care in the autumn of 1997, medical experts later stated:

> The combination of bone pain, hypercalcaemia and renal failure in a young patient points either to a diagnosis of primary hyperparathyroidism or metastatic malignancy and these ominous results should have been investigated as a matter of urgency

and

> All the evidence indicates that the patient was suffering from a solitary parathyroid adenoma at that time and removal would have been curative with a normal life expectancy.

It becomes all the more poignant when research tells us that the procedure to remove what was discovered at autopsy to have been a *benign* tumour has a 96% success rate, with only a 1% complication rate. Our family experience bears this out. Three months after Kevin's death, his father successfully underwent this surgery. Wonderful odds in Kevin's favour! Kevin could have had surgery to remove his overactive parathyroid gland. He would have been cured and would still have been alive today.

But we now know that every point of contact failed him. The necessary referral to an endocrinologist did not happen, the diagnosis of primary hyper-parathyroidism was not made and his hypercalcaemia was allowed to progress for a further year and 10 months until his plasma calcium level was higher than any ever recorded in that university hospital and was described as 'inconsistent with life'.

As patients we do understand that the practice of medicine is a complex and risk-laden endeavour. I accept unreservedly that no one intended any harm to Kevin. I recall a chance meeting with the senior house officer (SHO), 6 weeks after Kevin's death. He said: 'Kevin was very unlucky.' That was all he brought away from the tragedy. What a waste of an opportunity for learning and self-growth for that young man. The organisation took the easy way out and left him with a superficial perception of what had happened.

We have a special memory of that young SHO on the afternoon of Kevin's death. Kevin's friends started to arrive at the hospital – they were confused, bewildered and in a state of shock, many of them sitting on the hospital corridor floor with their backs to the wall, heads in hands. That SHO passed by, stopped, took off his white coat (the barrier), rolled it up, placed it on the ground and, saying nothing, he just sat with them – a most wonderful spontaneous demonstration of solidarity. He showed himself to be a decent, empathic and insightful young man. He deserved better than a superficial explanation.

I also accept that it is a great burden for healthcare professionals when tragedy occurs. To this day I am concerned for the registrar, who clearly found the outcome so difficult. At a chance encounter I identified myself as Kevin's mother; he looked shocked, blurted the words 'I didn't think he'd die' and fled the scene. Clearly no one had taken care of him either.

Monetary compensation was never an issue for us as a family. The truth is that the sum of money does not exist that would equate to Kevin and neither could we imagine any circumstance in which we would derive benefit or pleasure from that money. Consequently, we donated the settlement figure to two charities.

EVERY POINT OF CONTACT FAILED KEVIN

When we reflect on Kevin's journey the potential to achieve a proper diagnosis and treatment was sabotaged by a combination of filtering of the results and inaction. There were errors at primary care level right through to a tertiary training hospital. In fact, every point of contact failed him before and after his death.

At the primary care level
- Inability to recognise the seriousness of Kevin's condition
- Appropriate and timely interventions were not taken
- Selective and incomplete transmission of laboratory test results

- Non-receipt of vital information
- Absence of integrated pathways
- Link between his uncharacteristic behaviour and test results was not made; the mnemonic 'moans, bones and groans' describes the textbook presentation of primary hyperparathyroidism
- There was absolutely no tracking of his deteriorating test results – for example, there was no longitudinal approach
- Serious absence of direct communication with the patient or family; I would argue that you ignore at your peril the concerns of a mother . . .
- There was no system to flag the abnormally high calcium readings in a way that triggered an automatic referral

At secondary and tertiary care levels
- His transfer from secondary to tertiary care was delayed, losing 2 crucial days
- The impact of transferring him to CUH over the weekend meant treatment was provided at a registrar rather than consultant level
- Team dynamics: how come somebody in his team, whether junior or senior, did not speak up on Kevin's behalf?
- An absence of complete records – for example, the hospital did not have the benefit of access to his original blood tests from 1997 or the more recent 'off the Richter scale' calcium levels
- Lack of effective communication between primary and secondary care professionals was a significant contributory factor to his needless death

At the levels of analysis and learning
I am convinced that proper disclosure and dialogue with us as a family would have been far more beneficial to all parties and would have avoided almost 5 years of trauma and uncertainty brought about by the litigation process and the inappropriate responses that forced us down that route.

The healthcare culture
It is necessary to at least briefly comment on systems and culture. Error is often attributed to system failures. However, in some cases there is also an individual component and we have to take responsibility for that. It is also very certain that something called a system did not walk through the front doors of our institutions and say 'from now on I'm running the show around here'.

Systems are designed by people, they are maintained by people and they can certainly be changed by people. People are the culture; people are the system. In my opinion an effective safety culture is one where the system, the organisation and individual clinicians take pride in but can also demonstrate:
- their level of adherence to procedures, protocols, best practice
- their commitment to their professional oaths and to the ethical guides of each profession
- that they practise inclusively, which is reflected in their engagement and partnership with patients and carers

- their transparent and open handling of critical incidents coupled with supporting patient, family and staff – a combination of acknowledging error, achieving learning, preventing recurrence, allowing staff to recover and be more effective in the future; in essence, advancing patient safety.

A PATIENT AND FAMILY WISH LIST

The patient is the single constant throughout the full journey, with a variety of professionals that dip in and out of the care continuum. It is also good to remember that the patient is the individual with the greatest vested interest in the outcome of the journey. This makes patients a wonderful repository of useful information and gives them a valuable perspective to offer because they see through a different lens from healthcare professionals. I therefore consider it a great pity that this valuable resource is not utilised to a greater degree. So, what have I learned from all of this? Yes, I have my own wish list, a patient and family wish list.

Wish list for clinicians

- Be aware of and follow existing guidelines and be prepared to challenge one another when deviating from them
- Listen to and respect patients and families
- Know your personal limitations; respond to your patient's needs by making appropriate and timely referrals
- Keep impeccable records and refer to them constantly
- Resist the temptation to over-rely on past experience; while experience can serve one well, it also has the potential to result in 'tunnel vision'
- Communicate effectively with one another and with patients

Wish list for organisations

- Acknowledge errors
- When adverse events occur, investigate them using appropriate methods and include patients and families in the process
- Disseminate good practice and be constantly vigilant for opportunities to further improve
- Disseminate learning by implementing a fully compliant and just reporting and learning system
- Practise dialogue and collaboration – for example, meaningful engagement with patients and families
- Create a partnership between healthcare professionals and patients
- When things go wrong, be honest and open and seize the opportunity to give some meaning to tragedy
- Identify those times in the patient journey that are associated with increased risk – for example, transition from one care setting to another
- Greater consideration of team dynamics; how do you facilitate intervention by concerned team members other than 'the boss'?

- Provision of necessary support for patients, families and clinicians following adverse events
- Above all, do not allow yourself be seduced by the notion that a similar incident could not possibly happen in your organisation

Open disclosure *has* to be part of the culture of each organisation if learning and improvement are to be achieved. Disclosure is not about blame. It is not about accepting blame or about apportioning blame. It is about integrity and being truly professional. We cannot change the past but we can use the past to inform the present and in the present we can influence the future. Isn't it so much better if we do that together in partnership? Cases like ours need to be heard in a non-adversarial environment, where the focus is not on blame but, rather, on honestly arriving at the truth, acknowledging what happened and identifying ways to prevent a recurrence – in short, learning from the tragedy.

CONCLUSION

My personal experience of collaboration and partnership now spans the international, national and local arenas. It would never have come about were it not for the vision of those in healthcare who believe in patient involvement and engagement. These are the true leaders and innovators – they invite participation and offer opportunities for engagement.

The story does have motivational impact for students and professionals. I was particularly moved to receive an email from one student following my presentation to her class: 'Since then I say to myself I will always speak up and will always be honest.' Could I, as Kevin's mother, ask anything more of a young professional embarking on his or her career? What is critical is that we preserve the very precious relationship of trust between doctor and patient. While there is no acceptable level of error, error will occur and it is at that time we are challenged to behave with integrity and seize the opportunity to give some meaning to tragedy.

I am asking each of you to resolve to always be in rescue mode, that you practise truly patient-centred care – in that you do what is best for your patient. In doing so, I can guarantee that all of the other asks that will be made of you will be fulfilled, because if your focus is your patient and the best outcome for that patient then best practice will be achieved and you will be the kind of doctor you want to be, as well as the kind of doctor your patients want as their physician.

Finally, I want say: I was present at Kevin's birth. I know every detail of that birth. I was also present when he died. As his mother, I needed and deserved to know everything relating to how that came about. Over and above that, it is essential that I be assured that lessons will be learned, that those lessons will be disseminated – all in the hope of preventing a recurrence.

REFERENCE

1. Gawande A. Failure and rescue. *New Yorker*. 2012 June 4. Available at: www.newyorker. com/online/blogs/newsdesk/2012/06/atul-gawande-failure-and-rescue.html (accessed 24 December 2013).

CHAPTER 2

Improvement strategies and challenges

Sander Gaal, Wim Verstappen & Michel Wensing

INTRODUCTION

One of the most consistent findings in health services research is the gap between best practice (as determined by scientific evidence) on the one hand, and actual clinical care on the other. Studies in countries such as the United States, the Netherlands and the United Kingdom (UK) suggest that at least one in three patients does not receive care according to current scientific evidence, while one in five patients receives healthcare that is not needed and which is potentially harmful.[1] While patient safety incidents with serious adverse outcomes are rare in primary care, the incidence of avoidable risks is substantially higher. The challenge for general practice is to improve patient safety but to avoid defensive medicine and unnecessarily heavy administrative procedures. In this chapter we outline practical guidance on how to improve healthcare practice, with a particular focus on making patient care safer.

IMPLEMENTATION CHALLENGES

Most experts in healthcare improvement, when reflecting on (possible) failures of implementing strategies for change, emphasise the crucial importance of first acquiring a good understanding of the problem – the target group, its setting and the obstacles to change – in order to develop effective interventions.[2] This is similar to clinical practice, where a diagnosis usually precedes a treatment choice. Regarding patient safety in primary care, this means understanding and clearly mapping out the specific problems and areas for potential improvements. The first challenge to improvement is that this is a process that is still in an early phase.[3]

The second challenge to improve patient safety in primary care, but also in other healthcare settings, is that it constitutes a very broad field of items and different definitions. Defining 'patient safety' is not easy.[4-6] The literature provides many different definitions (more than 25 in total),[7] varying from the quite extensive, such as:

> A failure to perform an intended action which was correct given the circumstances. It can only occur if there was or should have been an appropriate intention to act on the basis of a perceived or remembered state of events and if the action finally taken was not that which was or should have been intended

to the much simpler:

> preventable incidents that result in a perceived harm.[8]

The World Health Organization defines *patient unsafety* as 'a process or act of omission, or commission that resulted in hazardous healthcare conditions and/or unintended harm to the patient'.[9] Regardless of which definition is chosen, an important question to ask is what does it mean in daily practice? When asked in interviews, general practitioners (GPs) named more than 300 items relating to patient safety. This ranged from the safety of the practice building through to polypharmacy and to the difficulties in the diagnostic process.[3] The most important items were keeping up medical knowledge, a poor doctor–patient relationship, managing elderly patients and polypharmacy.[10]

To improve patient safety, we must first identify the causes of patient safety incidents, before devising solutions and measuring the success of improvement efforts.[5,11] The literature shows that many different aspects of primary care can lead to patient safety incidents. A Canadian study on this subject classified incidents into six groups, depending on whether they relate to (1) administration, (2) communication, (3) diagnosis, (4) documentation, (5) medication or (6) procedures.[12] Another study of reported patient safety incidents classified potential risk factors[13] into recall and reminder systems,[14] knowledge and skills errors,[15] errors related to medical records,[16] communication between hospital and primary care[17] and management of medical emergencies.[18] However, there is still no unambiguous classification of the types and severity of patient safety incidents.[7,11] Most patient safety incidents also have more than one cause[19] and often result from a 'string' of mistakes (the so-called 'Swiss cheese model'). Implementation of patient safety improvements is only feasible when they connect with the views of primary care workers themselves. For instance, why do some clinicians adopt strict surveillance of patients with diabetes mellitus and conduct regular examination of feet and eyes and cardiovascular and renal risk assessments, while others do not? Is it because they have a better understanding of guidelines, more support staff, a group of patients who are more motivated to self-care and/or greater financial incentives to adopt these practices? The answers to these questions will be crucial to help develop targeted and effective patient safety implementation strategies. Unfortunately, there is still a dearth of evidence about the factors relevant to effective implementation of evidence-based medicine,[1] and this is also true in the case of patient safety improvement. The rest of this chapter will provide a brief description of how barriers and incentives to improvement can be identified, categorised and used to tailor interventions to facilitate desired change in practice.

DESIGNING IMPROVEMENT INITIATIVES

Current knowledge of barriers to and incentives for change is derived from observational studies and theoretical reflections, rather than well-designed prospective studies. Many of the proposed theories overlap and the majority have not been validated as having the ability to facilitate, describe or predict change in clinical practice. Nevertheless, they are useful for identifying potential barriers and promoters of change. For example, a study to understand the failed implementation of a hand hygiene improvement initiative identified various barriers including lack of awareness, knowledge, reinforcement, control, social norms, leadership and facilities.[1] Furthermore, the study showed that *different* theories could indeed contribute to explaining the failure to adopt best practice.

Engaging healthcare professionals

Individual healthcare professionals need to be informed, motivated and perhaps trained to incorporate the latest evidence regarding patient safety into their daily work. For instance, Cabana *et al.*[20] used a 'professional perception model'. Based on a review of 76 studies on barriers to clinical guideline adherence, they identified salient factors as lack of awareness, lack of familiarity, lack of agreement, lack of self-efficacy (i.e. the belief in one's ability to perform a behaviour), low expectancy of favourable outcomes, inertia/lack of motivation and perceived external barriers beyond the control of individuals. Empirical data showed that lack of awareness and motivation, as well as perceived external factors, were particularly important barriers to adopting guidelines. Other models describe the stepwise change process that individuals need to undergo to alter their behaviour. 'Stages of change' theories[21-23] have mostly been used to distinguish between patients with different degrees of motivation to adopt better lifestyles, but they are increasingly being used in research of implementation strategies.

Contextual factors

Healthcare professionals work in specific social, organisational and structural settings, with potentially many factors at different levels that may support or impede improvement efforts. A scientific model[22,24] makes the distinction between 'predisposing factors' (e.g. knowledge and attitudes in the target group), 'enabling factors' (e.g. capacity, resources, availability of services) and 'reinforcing factors' (e.g. opinions and behaviour of others). Systematic reviews of the effective implementation of evidence and guidelines[25,26] found that initiatives that considered and accounted for factors at all three levels (predisposing, enabling and reinforcing) were the most successful. Similarly, failure to implement evidence into practice usually involves factors at different levels of the healthcare system, including characteristics of professionals and patients; team functioning; influence of colleagues; organisation of care processes; available time, staff and resources; policymaking; and leadership.[27]

Tailoring strategies to bring about improvement

Information about potential barriers and incentives to improvement can be obtained from various sources, including interviews, surveys, focus groups, consensus-building methods, direct observation, retrospective record review, clinical audit and analysis of documentation. It is widely accepted that this information can and should be used to adapt implementation strategies to the context of the specific organisation or team. However, there is limited evidence that tailoring interventions makes them more effective. In fact, some efforts at tailoring interventions have been unsuccessful. For instance, a study of UK GPs used face-to-face interviews, guided by psychological theory, to identify barriers to implementing guidelines on the management of depression,[28] but this tailored intervention did not improve professional performance any more than simply distributing the guidelines. A further example is a Norwegian general practice study of guidelines for sore throat and urinary tract infections that used multiple methods to identify barriers to change: direct observation, telephone interviews, a postal survey and data extracted from medical records.[29] A multifaceted intervention was developed, tailored to the identified problems, which included a short summary of the guidelines, patient education materials, computer-based decision support, extra fees for telephone consultations and interactive courses for professionals. Despite this intensive intervention, no change in the main outcomes was found. An evaluation of the project suggested that lack of time and resources contributed significantly to this failure.

PRACTICAL SUGGESTIONS

Improving patient safety in primary care through effective improvement programmes seems a logical step. However, improving patient safety is a difficult and time-consuming process (as is any implementation process) and will need much effort from GPs and other practice employees to succeed. Because patient safety incidents usually have multiple causes, it may also be difficult to find a specific starting point when considering the practicalities of improving patient safety in front-line practice. Different practices may also identify different priorities after considering which aspects of patient safety they should attempt to improve first. For example, in one practice it may be ease of patient access while in another practice it may be their patient recall system.

As there is no single 'silver bullet' to improve patient safety, programmes should instead focus on specific aspects identified as important in each practice. However, safety improvement efforts can be undertaken by selecting from a range of standardised methods and approaches such as ensuring safe practice facilities, incident reporting and review (significant event analysis), measuring safety culture, conducting structured case note reviews (trigger review method) and clinical audit. A small number of these methods are briefly discussed here.

Incident reporting and analysis

Incident reporting is the most frequently researched improvement method in the field of patient safety. It has been and still is promoted as one of the more effective methods to improve safety of care.[30,31] In fact, in some countries it is mandatory, with national systems for incident reporting. Some of the studies in secondary care settings have been on a large scale (e.g. comprising 30 000 reported incidents).[32] In one primary care study in Australia, 805 incidents were reported. Of these, 27% had potential for severe harm and 76% were judged to have been preventable. The majority of the incidents were related to medication, clinical management and diagnosis.[33] Reported incidents were more likely to concern healthcare process than deficiencies in the knowledge and skills of healthcare professionals.[34] Incident reporting is typically promoted as a team-based activity, reflective learning is encouraged and there is evidence that the method can improve patient safety.[31]

SAFETY CULTURE

There is some evidence that the safety culture of an organisation or team is a relevant factor in their healthcare performance, but the exact nature of this relationship has proven difficult to articulate.[35] In an organisation or team with a negative safety culture, healthcare workers would be less inclined to report incidents and valuable learning opportunities would, therefore, be missed.[36] Different instruments have been developed to measure the culture of general practices. The MaPSaF (Manchester Patient Safety Framework)[37] and SafeQuest[38] instruments are examples of validated instruments taking a qualitative and quantitative approach, respectively, to assessing perceptions of practice culture and helping to facilitate team-based discussions and learning on related issues. The association (if any) between a positive safety culture in general practice and improved clinical outcomes has yet to be determined. However, there is some evidence that a positive culture improved outcomes in the care of patients with diabetes mellitus.[39]

Potential targets for safety interventions

A number of factors are potential targets for patient safety interventions.
- A high workload and job stress has been associated with reduced performance in general practice, although no causal relation was found with patient safety.[40]
- An investigation of practices with higher than average mortality rates found the rates could be explained by their large number of nursing home residents.[41]
- Medication-related errors have been identified as a major threat to patient safety.

Orientation

1 **Promote awareness of innovation**
   • Level of interest in reading and continuous education
2 **Stimulate interest and involvement**
   • Degree of contact with colleagues
   • Experience of need for innovation

Insight

3 **Create understanding**
   • Available knowledge and skills
   • Ability to remember information
4 **Develop insight into own routines**
   • Attitude (open-minded or defensive)
   • Willingness to acknowledge gaps in performance

Acceptance

5 **Develop positive attitude to change**
   • Ability to perceive advantages of change
   • Opinion of scientific merit of change
   • Opinion of credibility of innovation source
   • Degree of involvement in development process
6 **Create positive intentions/decision to change**
   • Perception of self-efficacy; degree of confidence in our skills
   • Perception of potential problems of putting change in practice

Change

7 **Try out change in practice**
   • Perception of practical barriers (time, staff, money)
   • Opportunity to try change on small scale
8 **Confirm value of change**
   • Whether first experiences positive or negative
   • Degree of cooperation experienced and reaction of patients and colleagues
   • Side effects (e.g. higher or lower costs)

Maintenance

9 **Integrate new practice into routines**
   • Willingness and ability to redesign processes
10 **Embed new practice in organisation**
   • Whether procedures in place for constant reminding
   • Availability of supportive resources
   • Degree of support from management

FIGURE 2.1 Potential barriers and incentives in relation to a proposed 10-step model for inducing change in professional behaviour[47]

● Computer systems with safety 'prompts' are a potential intervention, although it is known that GPs often do not read these warnings.[42]
● Discharge counselling: When 30-minute discharge medication counselling was performed in the hospital, medication accuracy in the home setting improved, resulting in significantly fewer GP consultations and fewer hospital readmissions.[43]
● Polypharmacy is one of the reasons for the high rate of medication-related patient safety incidents that disproportionately affects the elderly.[44]

An international panel of primary care physicians and researchers agreed that many different strategies to improve patient safety were important: specifically, building a positive safety culture, clinician education and patient safety guidelines.[45]

Patients have an important role in improving their own safety by becoming actively involved in their healthcare. It has been shown that when patients are given access to their own medical records, they may identify incidents.[46] However, there is a lack of empirical data to inform the extent to which patients could or should take on this role.[47] In an interview study with patients, poor communication with clinicians was identified as a more important cause of medical errors than diagnostic and treatment errors.[48]

CONCLUSION

Although there is an increasing awareness of the importance of understanding factors that facilitate or hinder the improvement of safety in general practice, it remains unclear which factors are critical to ensure the success of improvement initiatives in specific clinical settings and contexts. Better use and testing of existing theories in prospective trials may help to clarify this. Improving safety is likely to be different in every general practice, and improvement programmes should take this into account during development and implementation.

REFERENCES

1. Grol R, Grimshaw J. From best evidence to best practice: effective implementation of change in patients' care. *Lancet.* 2003; **362**(9391): 1225–30.
2. Grol R. Personal paper. Beliefs and evidence in changing clinical practice. *BMJ.* 1997; **315**(7105): 418–21.
3. Gaal S, van Laarhoven E, Wolters R, *et al.* Patient safety in primary care has many aspects: an interview study in primary care doctors and nurses. *J Eval Clin Pract.* 2010; **16**(3): 639–43.
4. Elder NC, Pallerla H, Regan S. What do family physicians consider an error? A comparison of definitions and physician perception. *BMC Fam Pract.* 2006; **7**: 73.
5. Jacobson L, Elwyn G, Robling M, *et al.* Error and safety in primary care: no clear boundaries. *Fam Pract.* 2003; **20**(3): 237–41.
6. Grober ED, Bohnen JM. Defining medical error. *Can J Surg.* 2005; **48**(1): 39–44.
7. Sandars J, Esmail A. The frequency and nature of medical error in primary care: understanding the diversity across studies. *Fam Pract.* 2003; **20**(3): 231–6.
8. Kuzel AJ, Woolf SH, Gilchrist VJ, *et al.* Patient reports of preventable problems and harms in primary health care. *Ann Fam Med.* 2004; **2**(4): 333–40.
9. World Health Organization World Alliance for Patient Safety. *The Conceptual Framework of an International Patient Safety Event Classification.* Copenhagen: WHO; 2006.
10. Gaal S, Verstappen W, Wensing M. Patient safety in primary care: a survey of general practitioners in the Netherlands. *BMC Health Serv Res.* 2010; **10**: 21.
11. Dovey SM, Meyers DS, Phillips RL Jr, *et al.* A preliminary taxonomy of medical errors in family practice. *Qual Saf Health Care.* 2002; **11**(3): 233–8.

12. Jacobs S, O'Beirne M, Derfiingher LP, *et al*. Errors and adverse events in family medicine: developing and validating a Canadian taxonomy of errors. *Can Fam Physician*. 2007; **53**(2): 271–6, 270.

13. Makeham MA, Kidd MR, Saltman DC, *et al*. The Threats to Australian Patient Safety (TAPS) study: incidence of reported errors in general practice. *Med J Aust*. 2006; **185**(2): 95–8.

14. Makeham MA, Saltman DC, Kidd MR. Lessons from the TAPS study: recall and reminder systems. *Aust Fam Physician*. 2008; **37**(11): 923–4.

15. Makeham MA, Mira M, Kidd MR. Lessons from the TAPS study: knowledge and skills errors. *Aust Fam Physician*. 2008; **37**(3): 145–6.

16. Makeham MA, Bridges-Webb C, Kidd MR. Lessons from the TAPS study: errors relating to medical records. *Aust Fam Physician*. 2008; **37**(4): 243–4.

17. Makeham MA, Mira M, Kidd MR. Lessons from the TAPS study: communication failures between hospitals and general practices. *Aust Fam Physician*. 2008; **37**(9): 735–6.

18. Makeham MA, Saltman DC, Kidd MR. Lessons from the TAPS study: management of medical emergencies. *Aust Fam Physician*. 2008; **37**(7): 548–50.

19. Woolf SH, Kuzel AJ, Dovey SM, *et al*. A string of mistakes: the importance of cascade analysis in describing, counting, and preventing medical errors. *Ann Fam Med*. 2004; **2**(4): 317–26.

20. Cabana MD, Rand CS, Powe NR, *et al*. Why don't physicians follow clinical practice guidelines? A framework for improvement. *JAMA*. 1999; **282**(15): 1458–65.

21. Grol R. Implementing guidelines in general practice care. *Qual Health Care*. 1992; **1**(3): 184–91.

22. Davis D, Evans M, Jadad A, *et al*. The case for knowledge translation: shortening the journey from evidence to effect. *BMJ*. 2003; **327**(7405): 33–5.

23. Prochaska JO, Velicer WF. The transtheoretical model of health behavior change. *Am J Health Promot*. 1997; **12**(1): 38–48.

24. Green LW, Eriksen MP, Schor EL. Preventive practices by physicians: behavioral determinants and potential interventions. *Am J Prev Med*. 1988; **4**(4 Suppl.): S101–7.

25. Davis DA, Thomson MA, Oxman AD, *et al*. Changing physician performance. A systematic review of the effect of continuing medical education strategies. *JAMA*. 1995; **274**(9): 700–5.

26. Solomon DH, Hashimoto H, Daltroy L, *et al*. Techniques to improve physicians' use of diagnostic tests: a new conceptual framework. *JAMA*. 1998; **280**(23): 2020–7.

27. Solberg LI. Guideline implementation: what the literature doesn't tell us. *Jt Comm J Qual Improv*. 2000; **26**(9): 525–37.

28. Baker R, Reddish S, Robertson N, *et al*. Randomised controlled trial of tailored strategies to implement guidelines for the management of patients with depression in general practice. *Br J Gen Pract*. 2001; **51**(470): 737–41.

29. Flottorp S, Havelsrud K, Oxman AD. Process evaluation of a cluster randomized trial of tailored interventions to implement guidelines in primary care: why is it so hard to change practice? *Fam Pract*. 2003; **20**(3): 333–9.

30. Rosser W, Dovey S, Bordman R, *et al*. Medical errors in primary care: results of an international study of family practice. *Can Fam Physician*. 2005; **51**: 386–7.

31. McKay J, Bradley N, Lough M, *et al*. A review of significant events analysed in general practice: implications for the quality and safety of patient care. *BMC Fam Pract*. 2009; **10**: 61.

32. Shaw R, Drever F, Hughes H, *et al*. Adverse events and near miss reporting in the NHS. *Qual Saf Health Care*. 2005; **14**(4): 279–83.

33. Bhasale AL, Miller GC, Reid SE, *et al*. Analysing potential harm in Australian general practice: an incident-monitoring study. *Med J Aust*. 1998; **169**(2): 73–6.

34. Makeham MA, Stromer S, Bridges-Webb C, *et al*. Patient safety events reported in general practice: a taxonomy. *Qual Saf Health Care*. 2008; **17**(1): 53–7.

35. Scott T, Mannion R, Marshall M, *et al*. Does organisational culture influence health care performance? A review of the evidence. *J Health Serv Res Policy*. 2003; **8**(2): 105–17.

36. Leape LL. Reporting of adverse events. *N Engl J Med*. 2002; **347**(20): 1633–8.

37. Parker D, Kirk S, Claridge T. *The Manchester Patient Safety Assessment Tool*. Manchester: National Primary Care Research and Development Centre, University of Manchester; 2002.

38. de Wet C, Johnson P, Mash R, *et al*. Measuring perceptions of safety climate in primary care: a cross-sectional study. *J Eval Clin Pract*. 2012; **18**(1): 135–42.

39. Bosch M, Dijkstra R, Wensing M, *et al*. Organizational culture, team climate and diabetes care in small office-based practices. *BMC Health Serv Res*. 2008; **8**: 180.

40. Van den Hombergh P, Kunzi B, Elwyn G, *et al*. High workload and job stress are associated with lower practice performance in general practice: an observational study in 239 general practices in the Netherlands. *BMC Health Serv Res*. 2009; **9**: 118.

41. Billett J, Kendall N, Old P. An investigation into GPs with high patient mortality rates: a retrospective study. *J Public Health (Oxf)*. 2005; **27**(3): 270–5.

42. Isaac T, Weissman JS, Davis RB, *et al*. Overrides of medication alerts in ambulatory care. *Arch Intern Med*. 2009; **169**(3): 305–11.

43. Al-Rashed SA, Wright DJ, Roebuck N, *et al*. The value of inpatient pharmaceutical counselling to elderly patients prior to discharge. *Br J Clin Pharmacol*. 2002; **54**(6): 657–64.

44. Leendertse AJ, Egberts AC, Stoker LJ, *et al*. Frequency of and risk factors for preventable medication-related hospital admissions in the Netherlands. *Arch Intern Med*. 2008; **168**(17): 1890–6.

45. Gaal S, Verstappen W, Wensing M. What do primary care physicians and researchers consider the most important patient safety improvement strategies? *BMC Health Serv Res*. 2011; **11**: 102.

46. Pyper C, Amery J, Watson M, *et al*. Patients' experiences when accessing their on-line electronic patient records in primary care. *Br J Gen Pract*. 2004; **54**(498): 38–43.

47. Davis RE, Jacklin R, Sevdalis N, *et al*. Patient involvement in patient safety: what factors influence patient participation and engagement? *Health Expect*. 2007; **10**(3): 259–67.

48. Grol R, Wensing M. What drives change? Barriers to and incentives for achieving evidence-based practice. *Med J Aust*. 2004; **180**(6 Suppl.): S57–60.

CHAPTER 3

Safety culture

Paul Bowie & Carl de Wet

When leaders begin to change their responses to mistakes and failure, asking what happened instead of who made the error, the culture within healthcare institutions will begin to change.[1]

INTRODUCTION

The evidence for patients suffering preventable harm in well-funded, technologically advanced healthcare settings staffed by highly educated clinical workforces is incontestable.[2] However, improving the safety of patient care is a complex, multifaceted challenge that will require a significant change in thinking, and improvements in human–system interactions and organisational safety culture throughout most modern healthcare systems.[3,4] As a consequence, making patient care safer is of international concern[5] and is gradually becoming a key priority of national governments.[6,7]

In primary care a number of established strategies are already in use to mitigate risk, improve clinical effectiveness and enhance patient safety; for example, the Quality and Outcomes Framework, continuing professional development, professional appraisal and significant event analysis. As this book highlights, newer interventions such as the trigger review method, safety climate assessment, clinical care bundle application and Never Event lists are beginning to be implemented, or are in early development and testing, as a means of improving the reliability and safety of patient care.

The safety focus in primary care was previously very much centred on the skills and competence of the individual clinician – with the patient largely peripheral in this clinical risk model. In contrast, there is now the beginnings of a slow but gradual move towards a safety culture agenda that has a greater emphasis on systems thinking and design, stronger team working and more effective clinician–patient communication – all supported by a framework of accountability and regulation (*see* Table 3.1). Few would argue with this new direction.

TABLE 3.1 Clinical risk management versus patient safety[8]

Clinical risk management (past)		Patent safety (present)
Competence	→	Performance
Individual oriented	→	Team and systems centred
Voluntary code	→	Regulatory framework
Clinician centred	→	Patient centred

However, although these efforts are a step in the right direction, primary healthcare is still often unsafe.[2] If patient safety is to be improved further and avoidable harm reduced, a more explicit emphasis on upskilling the primary care workforce to better understand system design, human performance and organisational factors is also needed. In this respect, much can be learned from other healthcare systems and high-risk industries worldwide in improving safety behaviours, job task design, the organisation of work, and creating the right system conditions to ensure that safety is truly valued as a front-line priority.[2,4,8] Recognising and acting upon the prevailing safety culture within a healthcare team and organisation is a fundamental starting point in what is, undoubtedly, a highly important public health concern in primary care settings worldwide.[2]

At the core of 'safety culture' as a concept is the assumption that by exploring and assessing this topic at the work group level then a care team can begin to understand the contexts and conditions in which an undesirable safety-related situation can materialise in the clinical or administrative workplace, without being mitigated or acted upon before a serious incident occurs.[9] Take general practice systems for handling laboratory results as a prime example. There are known variations in the quality and safety of primary care results handling systems internationally.[10] Different professional and staff assumptions, attitudes and perspectives (perhaps often conflicting) exist around how the systems work, who performs which specific tasks, the complexity of those tasks, how safe and reliable the system actually is and how much effort and resource should go into involving staff in making it work more reliably. Additionally, different team members will be aware of recent errors or existing system problems, risks and incidents that others do not (but should) know about. The related people–system interactions (including inadequate systems and other external influences) will also be contributors to the added levels of ongoing daily frustration, anxiety, stress, and irritation in the workplace, which will all impact on staff (human) capabilities and performance, and ultimately patient safety. Poor system design is a major contributory factor in most significant events related to the handling of laboratory results in primary care.[10,11] In essence the evaluation of care team perceptions of the prevailing safety culture can shine a light on these types of issues by providing all staff with a valuable opportunity to begin to explore how things *really* work in the general practice.

WHAT IS MEANT BY 'SAFETY CULTURE'?

Adequately defining a potentially intangible concept such as safety culture is clearly problematic. This is evident in the academic debate, ambiguity, uncertainty and confusion over the often interchangeable nature of two commonly used key terms: 'safety culture' and 'safety climate'. Although both terms are inextricably linked and interchangeably used for convenience, they are different theoretical concepts.[9,12]

Safety culture can be defined as 'the sub-facet of organisational culture that is thought to affect members' attitudes and behaviour in relation to an organisation's ongoing health and safety performance'.[9] The concept is organic in that the culture evolves over time and is influenced by many factors, including the working environment, health and safety policy and practice, the workforce and management as well as leadership characteristics.[13] Organisational culture can be defined simplistically and perhaps ambiguously 'as the way we do things around here'.[14] It can be argued in high-risk, complex organisations (such as the aviation, nuclear power and healthcare industries) that, because 'safety' is of such critical importance to routine organisational goals, then this is essentially the dominating cultural construct within the organisation.[9]

Safety climate, on the other hand, refers to the measurable 'surface' components of safety culture – 'the individual and group values, attitudes, perceptions and patterns of behaviour that determine how seriously safety management is taken in the workplace'.[15] Assessing the safety climate perceptions of the workforce, usually using cross-sectional questionnaire surveys, can provide a 'snapshot' of the prevailing culture at a given moment in time and is a widely used approach among many diverse high-risk industries, including healthcare and nuclear power.[15,16]

A recent review takes a pragmatic view by concluding that safety culture can be 'viewed as an enduring characteristic of an organisation' whereas safety climate can be thought of in terms of a 'temporary state of an organisation that is changeable'.[17] It criticises current attempts at defining both concepts for failing to include, directly or indirectly, any reference to the science of human factors, the twin goals of which are to improve the performance, health and well-being at the individual and organisational level.

IMPORTANCE OF SAFETY CULTURE

There is strong agreement that safety culture is a highly important concept because it is such a decisive factor in many organisational performance and safety failures.[18,19] Safety culture is important because organisations with a positive safety culture are more likely to learn openly and effectively from failure and adapt their working practices appropriately.[9] The converse is true for a weak safety culture, which has been implicated as a causal factor in many catastrophic organisational incidents – for example, the Piper Alpha oil platform explosion, the space shuttle *Challenger* disaster and the Zeebrugge ferry incident.[13] Comparable National Health Services incidents where a poorly developed safety culture was cited as a contributory factor[18,20] would include the failings highlighted in Stafford Hospital (high mortality rates from emergency admissions), Bristol Royal Infirmary (high infant surgical mortality rates) in England and the Vale of Leven hospital (deaths associated with *Clostridium difficile*) in Scotland.

Media-highlighted failings in patient safety, as illustrated through these examples, are typically related (often erroneously) to the performance of individuals rather than to groups or organisations. What the aforementioned major incidents have shown us is the influence of high-level organisational factors on safety performance and related failures, rather than much of the previous (simplistic) focus in decades past, which was often on improving local system or technical designs or eradicating front-line human error issues.[18,21] It is really only in the past decade that we have begun to look seriously at how we can assess safety culture in healthcare settings to identify related issues of critical importance (such as the strength and effectiveness of team working, communication, leadership, and commitment to safety improvement and so on) and consider their implications in relation to practice systems, performance and safer care.

When considering how to improve the safety culture within an organisation, the generalised accident scenario by Wagenaar *et al.*[22] outlines four important characteristics that underpin most safety incidents and which are useful in helping to evaluate and learn from past incidents in order to better design current and future systems, deal more effectively with risks, and minimise or eradicate the chances of accidents happening or recurring within these systems. First, the circumstances surrounding the incident generally occur over a period of time (minutes, days, weeks or years). Second, during this time period it is possible that individuals may prevent the accident or minimise its impact. Third, the accident occurs within the confines of a 'system' (i.e. any work-based safety incident will take place within a sociotechnical system). Fourth, that latent failures and risks may lie dormant and undetected within the system ready to line up, like the holes in Reason's Swiss cheese model metaphor,[18] and create the conditions for the incident to occur.

In Cooper's[9] summary of safety culture research, a number of organisational systems, behaviours and psychological attributes were identified as having a distinguishing impact on organisations with low accident rates compared with those with higher rates. Examples with direct relevance to primary care include:

- strong senior management and leadership commitment and involvement in safety
- a mature, stable workforce
- good personnel selection and retention, job placement and promotion procedures
- good induction and follow-up safety training
- ongoing safety schemes reinforcing the importance of safety, including near miss reporting
- accepting that promotion of a safety culture is a long-term strategy that requires sustained effort and interest

- thoroughly investigating all accidents and near misses
- regular auditing of safety systems to provide feedback on performance and ideas for improvement
- capturing attitudes towards accident causation, job-induced stress and poor working conditions
- regularly assessing safety climate and improving safety behaviours.

Acting, where appropriate, on regular information from these activities combined with knowledge of what can go wrong can lead to the creation of an 'informed' safety culture. This is also the 'best way to stay cautious' about safety performance while taking a systematic approach to potentially predicting and preventing accidents.[1]

TRANSLATING SAFETY CULTURE FOR PRIMARY CARE

The prevailing safety culture influences clinicians and staff to choose behaviours that enhance – rather than compromise – safety practices and thinking. This poses an important question: can a primary care organisation implement a safety culture capable of both predicting and avoiding patient safety incidents? It is fair to say at this very early stage in the safety culture journey that the answer is highly likely to be negative, but this need not prevent practices from taking on the challenge.

The first step involves a very basic requirement to actually discuss the concept of a 'practice safety culture'. This implies that something as intangible, perhaps ethereal, can be adequately defined, understood, measured, acted upon and improved by healthcare leaders, clinicians, managers and staff in the way that policymakers assume. Perhaps more important, even if safety culture can be adequately measured, can we attribute these metrics with explicitly linked clinical and organisational outcomes such as reductions in healthcare errors and avoidable patient harm, or improvements in the safety attitudes, knowledge and behaviours of the primary care workforce? Again, the answer at this stage is unknown, but largely because the necessary depth of research and evaluation has yet to take place.

For general practices, therefore, the big challenge is to think more critically and smartly about how they perceive and approach issues of patient safety and improvement, and perhaps draw some inspiration from the principles, ideas and multiple methods outlined in the forthcoming chapters in this book. It is important to recognise that the leadership commitment to patient safety within a practice is strongly linked to the maturity level of the prevailing safety culture. The practice leadership ultimately creates the necessary workplace culture to ensure that patient safety and care improvement are valued as everybody's business.[23] Establishing a 'just' culture that enables the whole team to support and advance patient safety is, therefore, only possible with strong leaders (see Table 3.2). It is for the practice leadership – general practitioners, management and senior nursing staff – to facilitate and build a culture of trust that encourages effective team working, collective learning from significant events and strong communication across the clinical disciplines and administrative staff. They have both the responsibility and the authority to ensure that there is a continued focus on improving the safety of patient care – in essence, to establishing safety as a cultural 'value' as well as a practice 'priority'.

TABLE 3.2 Leadership influence on types of safety culture[2,7]

Element of safety culture	Characteristics
Open culture	Clinicians and staff feel comfortable discussing patient safety incidents and raising safety issues with both colleagues and senior staff
Just culture	Clinicians, staff, patients and carers are treated fairly, with empathy and consideration when they have been involved in a patient safety incident or have raised a safety issue
Reporting culture	Clinicians and staff have confidence in the local incident reporting system and use it to notify healthcare managers of incidents that are occurring, including near misses
	Barriers to incident reporting have been identified and removed:
	• clinicians and staff are not blamed and punished when they report incidents
	• they receive constructive feedback after submitting an incident report
	• the reporting process itself is easy
Learning culture	The practice:
	• is committed to learning safety lessons
	• communicates them to colleagues
	• remembers them over time
Informed culture	The practice has learned from past experience and has the ability to identify and mitigate future incidents, because it learns from events that have already happened (e.g. incident reports and investigations)

CULTURAL CHANGE: POTENTIAL 'QUICK WINS'

So how does a practice team go about considering and improving its safety culture? The first realisation should be that this is an evolving journey, often fraught with multiple challenges and obstacles – it can take time for attitudes to shift, behaviours to alter, systems-thinking to take hold and cultural changes to embed. However, there is the possibility for practices to introduce some 'quick wins' by keeping basic things simple, for example:

- ensure that messages are taken safely through the use of a formal message system
- ensure that patients' records are accessed by date of birth and then full name
- place sharps boxes in consulting rooms on a shelf out of the reach of children
- offer patients who do not attend for their warfarin checks a safer alternative

- make sure GPs' bags and on-call or emergency bags contain a sharps box
- routinely search your practice information system for events that should rarely, if ever, happen (e.g. patients being co-prescribed warfarin and aspirin or those who are co-prescribed two different non-steroidal anti-inflammatory drugs).

How confident would most practice teams feel that patient care delivery in these areas is completely safe and reliable? Given what we know about significant events and preventable harm in primary care,[2] it is possible but probably unlikely that the supreme confidence of a single practice is matched by the front-line reality in each of these areas. Therefore, practices may consider taking one or more of these issues to a formal or informal meeting as a first stepping stone to engaging the team more explicitly with the patient safety agenda.

Increasingly in hospital-based care we are seeing a cultural change in the way National Health Service leaders, clinicians and managers perceive the issue of patient safety. One manifestation of this is the introduction of 'patient safety' as a standing agenda item at board and other committee-level meetings. This conveys the very real message to patients, staff and the wider public that safety is taken seriously and that accountability for this issue goes straight to the top of the organisation. It may be the case that a practice team has placed significant event analysis as a standing item on the agenda at regular business or practice team meetings. Although this is commendable, the patient safety issue is of course much broader than just significant event analysis and therefore deserves greater recognition and respect. In the next 12 months – and with patient safety firmly established as a standing agenda item – the practice could consider some of the following tasks as one way of slowly developing the prevailing safety culture:

- create a manual or intranet-based log to capture significant events or important near misses
- gain the commitment of all clinicians to formally report at least one patient safety incident in the next 12 months
- begin to assess practice safety culture using a suitable instrument, repeating every 18–24 months
- appoint a 'patient safety champion' to galvanise and lead the team – for example, a practice nurse or doctor with a passion and enthusiasm for the topic
- try out the primary care trigger review method on the electronic records of 25 high-risk patients to identify safety-related learning needs
- interview a few regular patients or set up small focus groups (e.g. those taking warfarin) to enable you to begin exploring and capturing their experiences of the healthcare you provide and identify small changes for improving safety.

CONCLUSION

The concept of safety culture is relatively new to healthcare and more research, development and evaluation work is required to provide a better understanding of what a positive safety culture entails and how this can be further validated, particularly in primary care settings. Importantly, safety culture may be too complex as a construct to determine its measureable relationship with key organisational outcomes,[24-26] which in general practice terms could refer to, for example, rates of safety incidents from high-risk prescribing. In that case, no matter how much the prevailing safety culture matures within the context of a clinical setting where dealing with high levels of complexity and uncertainty is a constant, general practice may always be in state of 'chronic unease'.[1,13] This is arguably the default position in many high-risk industries, despite the strong priority, leadership backing and resources often given to organisational safety. However, this level of support is still highly variable in healthcare, with the recent focus on the substandard patient care highlighted in the mid-Staffordshire scandal in the United Kingdom unfortunately illustrating that the concept and influence of safety culture are still poorly understood.[19]

REFERENCES

1. Reason J. Achieving a safe culture: theory and practice. *Work Stress.* 1998; **12**(3): 293–306.
2. Health Foundation. *Evidence Scan: levels of harm.* London: Health Foundation; 2011. Available at: www.health.org.uk/public/cms/75/76/313/2593/Levels%20of%20harm. pdf?realName=PYiXMz.pdf (accessed 30 October 2012).
3. Marshall M, Parker D, Esmail A, *et al.* Culture of safety. *Qual Saf Health Care.* 2003; **12**(4): 318.
4. Department of Health. *Doing Less Harm: improving the safety and quality of care through reporting, analysing and learning from adverse incidents involving NHS patients – key requirements for healthcare providers.* London: HMSO; 2001.
5. World Health Organization. *Patient Safety Research: better knowledge for better care.* Geneva: WHO; 2009.
6. Scottish Government. *Delivering Quality in Primary Care National Action Plan: implementing the Healthcare Quality Strategy for NHS Scotland.* Edinburgh: Scottish Government; 2010.
7. Department of Health. *An Organisation with a Memory.* London: HMSO; 2000.
8. Hickey J. Risk management, patient safety and a medical protection organisation. In: Haynes K, Thomas M, editors. *Clinical Risk Management in Primary Care.* Oxford: Radcliffe Publishing; 2005. pp. 3–22.
9. Cooper MD. Towards a model of safety culture. *Safety Sci.* 2000; **36**(2): 111–36.
10. Elder NC, Graham D, Brandt E, *et al.* The testing process in family medicine: problems, solutions and barriers as seen by physicians and their staffs. A study of the American Academy of Family Physicians' National Research Network. *J Patient Safety.* 2006; **2**: 25–32.
11. McKay J, Bradley N, Lough M, *et al.* A review of significant events analysed in general

practice: implications for the quality and safety of patient care. *BMC Fam Pract.* 2009; **10**: 61.

12. Cooper D. Treating safety as a value. *Prof Saf.* 2001 Feb: 17–21.
13. Reason J. *The Human Contribution: unsafe acts, accidents and heroic recoveries.* Farnham: Ashgate; 2008.
14. Deal TE, Kennedy AA. *Corporate Cultures: the rites and rituals of corporate life.* Harmondsworth: Penguin Books; 1982.
15. Flin R, Burns C, Mearns K, *et al.* Measuring safety climate in health care. *Qual Saf Health Care.* 2006; **15**(2): 109–15.
16. de Wet C, Spence W, Mash R, *et al.* The development and psychometric evaluation of a safety climate measure for primary care. *Qual Saf Health Care.* 2010; **19**(6): 578–84.
17. Guldenmund FW. The nature of safety culture: a review of theory and research. *Saf Sci.* 2000; **34**: 215–57.
18. Reason J. Human error: models and management. *BMJ.* 2000; **320**(7237): 768–70.
19. Francis R. *Report of the Mid Staffordshire NHS Foundation Trust Public Inquiry.* London: The Stationery Office; 2013.
20. National Patient Safety Agency. *Seven Steps to Patient Safety for Primary Care.* London: NPSA; 2005.
21. Gadd S, Collins AM. *Safety Culture: a review of the literature.* Report No. HSL/2002/25. Sheffield, UK: Health & Safety Laboratory; 2002.
22. Wagenaar WA, Hudson PTW, Reason JT. Cognitive failures and accidents. *Appl Cogn Psychol.* 1990; **4**: 273–94.
23. Apekey TA, McSorley G, Tilling M, *et al.* Room for improvement? Leadership, innovation culture and uptake of quality improvement methods in general practice. *J Eval Clin Pract.* 2011; **17**(2): 311–18.
24. Flin R. Measuring safety culture in healthcare: a case for accurate diagnosis. *Saf Sci.* 2007; **45**: 653–67.
25. Hopkins A. Studying organisational cultures and their effects on safety. *Saf Sci.* 2006; **44**: 875–89.
26. Guldenmund FW. The use of questionnaires in safety culture research and evaluation. *Saf Sci.* 2007; **45**: 723–43.

CHAPTER 4

The wisdom hierarchy

Susan Dovey & Katharine Wallis

BACKGROUND

'Patient safety' is a term that has now become part of the vernacular language of medicine worldwide. It wasn't always this way. Before the Institute of Medicine's *To Err is Human*[1] report in 1999 it was a familiar phrase to certain sections of the health enterprise (mainly anaesthetics and surgery), but not one that was often spoken throughout most of the rest of the health system, including general practice.

It is a medical term, but one that has considerable lay currency, having been rapidly picked up by the media since late 1999. It is a term with inherent threat to the self-perceptions of healthcare providers, as it implies that, contrary to the fundamental purpose of their role in the health system, patients are not always safe in their care and that there are lapses in personal professionalism. This interpretation is softened by discussions about patient safety being a characteristic of health systems, rather than of the professional practice of individual doctors and nurses, but for some the implied criticism of their care may remain a real deterrent to getting serious about addressing patients' safety and improving their daily practice of medicine.

This book is about improving the safety of patients in general practice by building a culture that supports ideas that are directly opposed to the ideas of required perfection imparted by the medical culture that most general practitioners have learned and lived with for most of their lives. This chapter reviews why there is a need to talk about safety culture, and why a focus on patient safety in primary care is important. Ackoff's[2] theoretical 'wisdom hierarchy' framework is described and its relevance to safety culture is explored before the current state of readiness for transformative change in general practice safety culture is considered.

WHY IS THERE A NEED TO TALK ABOUT SAFETY CULTURE?

Most patient harm is caused by highly trained, competent, well-intentioned doctors who are working in systems that set them up to fail.[3] Appealing to internal motivation and individual virtue is insufficient to ensure patient safety because most harm stems from doctors who are already trying to do the right thing. Doctor integrity and competence, while important, are insufficient to guarantee quality and avoid harm. An individual 'trying harder next time' is not likely to improve outcomes even if, as shown in the LINNEAUS (Learning in an International Network About Errors and Understanding Safety) Collaboration's first study, it is the solution most general practitioners first propose.[4] As most preventable errors are caused by flaws in the system rather than flaws in the individual, the dominant strategy of blaming individuals for error and harm and recommending further education and more intensive training is unlikely to be effective.[5] Many safety experts therefore recommend a systems approach to patient safety.[5-8]

Pivotal to a systems approach is the development of a culture of openness and learning, or a culture of safety, in healthcare settings.[5] Safety culture concerns the shared assumptions that underlie how people perceive and act upon safety issues,[9,10] and has been defined as 'shared values, attitudes, perceptions, competencies and patterns of behaviour'.[11] In an organisation with a strong safety culture, the focus is on sharing information about medical error and injury, rather than seeking to identify and allocate blame when things go wrong, and learning from past problems to improve patient safety.[12-14]

According to Professor James Reason,[15] safety culture is made up of a *reporting* culture, where easy reporting of errors and near misses is possible; a *just* culture, where staff are encouraged and rewarded for reporting rather than punished (but where there is also a clear line for unacceptable behaviour); a *flexible* culture, which is minimally hierarchical; and a *learning* culture, where there is a willingness to learn from mistakes and to make reforms. Aspects of a positive safety culture include communication based on mutual trust and openness, shared perceptions of the importance of safety, confidence in the efficacy of preventive safety measures, organisational learning, committed leadership and executive responsibility, and a 'no-blame' approach to incident reporting and analysis.

WHY SHOULD THERE BE A FOCUS ON PRIMARY CARE?

Despite the majority of patient contacts taking place in primary care, most patient safety initiatives to date have focused on counting errors and tallying the cost of harm in hospitals.[16,17] Although there has been effort in recent years to redress the imbalance the problem of patient safety in primary care is yet to be well defined. Both the extent of primary care use and the impact of harm in primary care make addressing patient safety in primary care important. Given its scale, even if the error rate in primary care were only low, the burden of harm is potentially great; even if only one in 550 prescriptions were in error, considering the number of prescriptions written in primary care each year the burden of harm from incorrect prescriptions could be high. Addressing the problem of patient safety in primary care is made more urgent by increasing care shifts from hospital to community settings.

The systems approach to safety attempts to redefine medical uncertainty as quantifiable clinical risk, and then seeks to measure and reduce risk or error. However, the notion of risk is contestable. Despite medical advances, much uncertainty in primary care remains irreducible; it is not feasible to investigate everyone presenting with flu-like symptoms to exclude meningitis, for example. In primary care, clinicians make decisions and take responsibility in uncertainty, and the emphasis is less on reducing risk and more on coping in uncertainty. In this context, instead of trying to identify and reduce error through a systems approach, improving accessibility and communication between doctors and patients and between providers might better protect patient safety; instead of seeking to identify and reduce prescribing error, it may be better to reduce harm-prone practices such as prescribing, overall. The greatest threat to patient safety in primary care may not be improperly delivered care or error, so much as the care itself. The treatment itself may be the problem, rather than the (incorrect) delivery of the treatment. Doctors might be striving to work perfectly in a system that is heading off course.

Illich[18] was one of the early writers on the harm caused by medicine – iatrogenesis – in the 1970s. He described three types of iatrogenesis: (1) clinical iatrogenesis, which includes harm to individuals such as adverse drug events and hospital-acquired infections and harm to society such as drug resistance; (2) social iatrogenesis, which is about the medicalisation of life, where every deviation becomes a medical problem, rendering people anxious and dependent on healthcare; and (3) cultural iatrogenesis, which is about the war against suffering that undermines patients' ability to face their reality and accept pain and inevitable decline.[18] The current patient safety debate is largely confined to what Illich called clinical iatrogenesis – specifically, the harm to individuals – but in primary care, social and cultural iatrogenesis may be the greater problem. Some groups of individuals may be at greater risk of clinical, social and cultural iatrogenesis – such as women, because they take more drugs,[19] have more cosmetic surgery,[20] participate more in cancer screening and experience more over-diagnosis.[21]

ACKOFF'S 'WISDOM HIERARCHY' FRAMEWORK

Russell Ackoff was an American systems theorist who 30 years ago drew attention to the uselessness of data without the application of further effort beyond data collection.[22] He articulated a five-level process by which data becomes information, information becomes knowledge, knowledge becomes understanding, and understanding becomes wisdom – the ultimate goal. Wisdom about building a culture for patient safety in general practice is about knowing how to tolerate variability, uncertainty and risk, while also judiciously accommodating new knowledge (from information and data), understanding when to intervene and when not, and actually undertaking only those actions understood to be necessary. This framework will now be used to consider the currently available tools in primary care to protect patient safety, and the culture changes (values, attitudes, perceptions, competencies and patterns of behaviour) that might make these tools more effective.[11] Table 4.1 summarises key changes in culture that might leverage gains in patient safety from each layer in Ackoff's hierarchy.

TABLE 4.1 Summary of key changes to promote a patient safety culture in primary care practices

Levels in the wisdom hierarchy	Target of potential change to improve safety culture	Element of culture most likely to change
1 Data	• A practice's patient records • Aggregated datasets of patients' clinical records • Data from research projects • Sentinel event data	Values, attitudes, perceptions
2, 3 Information and knowledge	• A practice's patient records • Relevant research, published in a wide array of journals	Values, attitudes, perceptions, competencies
4, 5 Understanding and wisdom	• 'Translated' research in some form • Trigger tools	Values, attitudes, perceptions, competencies, changed patterns of behaviour

Level 1: data

Data are the critical building blocks of wisdom. In simpler times, data were precious because each data item (datum) had to be created and recorded and recording resources (pen, paper, writing skills) were much scarcer than they are today. The digital age has enabled the creation of more data than a human mind can process, which is perhaps fortunate, since much of it is not accessible to most people.

The most valuable and most accessible source of data about patient safety for general practice is each practice's set of clinical records. If these records are created and stored electronically, a searchable resource exists that can provide information for a practice about their own patients who consult with doctors, nurses and others in the practice; why they consult; where they consult; and what advice, investigations, treatments and health effects result from these consultations.

These data are used every day to tell stories of patients' experiences, to signal indications for screening and timed interventions, and to improve general practice care far beyond what it would be in the absence of records, or where records are distributed across many agencies, or where records remain on paper and unsearchable. Comprehensive electronic health records are a key to maintaining and improving patient safety in general practice – a culture is needed that recognises and values them as the first level of patient safety protection.

General practice research networks aggregate patient records data from a number of separate clinics. These networks have been defined as the 'laboratories' for general practice.[23] They now exist in a variety of configurations in most countries and there are one or two international networks. Historically most research networks have collected small slices of the data held in the records base of their contributing practices. There are one or two exceptions. In the United Kingdom (UK), the Clinical Practice Research Database (CPRD, formerly the General Practice Research Database (GPRD)) is arguably the world's largest computerised database of anonymised longitudinal medical records from primary care, currently holding data about the healthcare of about 5 million patients. Until funding dried up, a similar database used to exist in New Zealand – the Royal New Zealand College of General Practice Computer Research Group.[24] All patient data from the contributing general practices are held in these databases and they can be (and are) used as either the sole source of research data or linked to other health databases such as cancer, birth and death registries, and hospital and medicines dispensing data. Importantly, the purpose of these collections of data from multiple practices is not simply to aggregate data but to draw information from the data that is often explicitly intended to improve general practice care for patients. Data from one-off research projects is another data resource, albeit unpredictable in its accessibility and usefulness for individual general practices and the people working in them.

Finally, in most countries institutional and public data exist on sentinel events, patient complaints and litigation. The raw data files are seldom accessible but the institutions and organisations that manage these data generally produce reports summarising the types of patient safety events represented in their data and sometimes providing tips for healthcare providers about how to make their clinical practices safer.[25–27] These data are overwhelmingly generated by secondary and tertiary level healthcare institutions and have very limited relevance for general practice. The UK has made specific efforts to include general practice in its publicly funded safety databases, but despite these efforts only a tiny proportion of all sentinel event reports come from general practice.

Therefore, data to help general practices build a safety and improvement culture abound, but most sources of data are probably not very useful. The outstanding exception is the data held closest to home – in general practices. If culture can change towards viewing these data as more than individual records of patient encounters or data for other organisations to use to hold us to account, there may be lessons to learn from them to help change the way clinicians think and act, and there will be a stronger investment in building safety and improving our practices.

Levels 2 and 3: information and knowledge

Information is the messages created from the analysis of data. So, with respect to the data resources already described, *information* is the sense made from patient records, the analysis of data from aggregated general practice databases and research projects, and the written reports prepared from sentinel events, patient complaints and injury databases. *Information* influences the creation of meaningful patterns, but it doesn't recognise them: *knowledge* is the process of taking information and deriving meaning from it. Both information and knowledge are created by research. They are massively more useful than *data* alone, but still quite a distance from *understanding* and *wisdom*.

There are some key examples of how general practice data have been used to create information and knowledge beyond the walls of individual practices. The GPRD is frequently used for patient safety research that has been published and is passively accessible for people to read. The following are some examples of things we know from the GPRD analyses published in 2011 alone.

- Although selective serotonin reuptake inhibitor medicines are associated with increased risk of bleeding in many sites, they are not associated with haemorrhagic stroke.[28]
- Opiate analgesics and oral corticosteroids are associated with an increased risk of perforated diverticular disease, but calcium channel blocker and aspirin use is not.[29]
- People with more than one chronic condition have higher consultation rates in general practice than other people and more problems with continuity of care.[30]
- Symptoms similar to Parkinson's disease can follow influenza, but influenza is not associated with a higher risk of developing idiopathic Parkinson's disease.[31]

These messages are only a fraction of the information and knowledge generated by the CPRD. During the 2002–11 decade, 683 papers reporting research based on these general practice data were published. However, in most years less than 5% of CPRD research papers were published in the primary care journals that are most likely to be read by general practitioners, and in occasional years *none* of the CPRD analyses of UK general practice data was reported in the primary care literature.

Since 2011, Thomson Reuters Web of Science has grouped together 14 scientific journals in its 'primary care' category. Together, these journals published 1041 citable articles in 2010 alone. Each year, at least this amount of new information and knowledge specific to primary care is created and made widely available through easily accessible media. Extrapolating from the CPRD's record, most relevant primary care research will be published in a much wider array of journals than would typically be read by general practitioners and other primary care providers. Therefore, there is a lot of existing information and knowledge. Obviously, there are also gaps in this literature, where no answers have yet been found to primary care practices and tools that have implications for patient safety.

General practice as a research discipline is still in a relatively early stage of development and hindered by low levels of professional engagement, limited training opportunities for developing expertise in primary care research[32] and an inhospitable funding environment.[33] A primary care provider responsibility to create knowledge from primary care data through research is not yet recognised as a professional imperative and there needs to be a cultural shift before this happens – perhaps concern for patient safety will be the catalyst for this culture change. Research must be a key component of a safety culture.

Levels 4 and 5: understanding and wisdom

Much of the information and knowledge generated from medical research contains messages for protecting the safety of patients in primary care clinics. If one were to read *only* the reports cited here, primary care patients may become safer by continuing to receive appropriate antidepressant medication even if they became at increased risk of stroke;[28] having opioids and corticosteroids withheld if they had diverticular disease;[29] their general practitioner becoming sensitive to risks of care continuity problems arising for patients with more than one chronic disease;[30] and avoiding investigations designed to diagnose Parkinson's disease if the symptoms became apparent just after an episode of influenza.[31] The trouble is that most general practitioners probably will not have the chance to make these changes towards safer care because the likelihood that they will have read these research reports is very small.

There is a gap between what is known from research that analyses data and what is understood and changed into safer clinical practice, simply because most research does not reach people who can understand it best and change that understanding into wise actions. For specialty medicine, Hoffman *et al.*[34] estimate that 167 journals need to be read in a narrow specialty area (otolaryngology) to ensure all new trials are known about, and in a wider area (neurology), 896 journals would need to be read. General practice is of course broader in scope than any other medical specialty and it is impossible to access and understand all the research relevant to primary care. This is all known. Moreover, it is also known that very little impact follows most interventions designed to remedy the problem of relevant research not reaching those who could use it. In the past, mechanisms such as clinical practice guidelines have been the backbone of the process of 'translating' research into clinical practice, but it is now know that multifaceted interventional programmes are needed before evidence-based guidelines have a chance of being implemented.[35,36] A culture that prioritises alternative means of conveying research results to frontline primary care providers (other than by publications in scientific journals) will therefore help to promote patient safety.

New Zealand developed an efficient programme for bringing research 'brief messages' to the attention of primary care providers, using a *marketing* strategy. The Best Practice Advocacy Centre New Zealand (bpac[nz]) is a public university and private primary care provider collaboration established to *market* 'best' clinical practice in primary care.[37] Survey data show that almost 100% of recipients rank bpac[nz] information highly in terms of trustworthiness, quality and usefulness.[38] This, in turn, means bpac[nz] recommendations are widely adopted.[39] Theoretically, if care is changed in the direction suggested by research, it should be better and safer than care previously provided. However, no research has yet specifically tested this theory of the effect of bpac[nz] interventions.

Wikipedia defines *wisdom* as 'a deep understanding and realisation of people, things, events or situations, resulting in the ability to apply perceptions, judgements and actions in keeping with this understanding.'[40] In essence, wisdom is about judging (understanding) followed by deliberate *action* to promote well-being. Wisdom is ultimately what is needed if healthcare is to be as safe for patients as it can be.

THE NEXT STEPS

If patients are to become safer in primary care, the culture of the care environment needs to change to recognise existing and emerging opportunities for more and less safe care, and patients and providers need to be oriented towards changing the safer option. This may start by simply resolving to create clearer medical records. It is necessary to have such data before primary care providers are in a position to provide safe care for patients. It is necessary to become informed by these data and to know what they say. Research is the process by which data is given meaning. This research may be as informal as a clinician reading a patient's health record before making a decision about his or her clinical care, to as formal as a large, multi-centred, multinational randomised controlled trial. For formal research to have a greater impact on a primary care safety culture, it needs to become more accessible than it is at present. A change is needed in the academic culture that values publication in the scientific literature above other research dissemination methods. Accessibility of research is a problem across the whole of healthcare, but is particularly problematic for primary care because of the very wide scope of healthcare problems brought to primary care doctors and nurses. There is a new focus on research translation that has already seen some efforts to bring research to where it is needed, but so far these initiatives are only marginally effective and most of healthcare is delivered without the wisdom that access to research might allow.

REFERENCES

 1. Kohn L, Corrigan J, Donaldson M, editors. *To Err is Human: building a safer health system*. Washington, DC: National Academy Press; 1999.
 2. Ackoff R. From data to wisdom. *Informatie*. 1990; **32**(5): 486–90.
 3. Gawande A. *The Checklist Manifesto: how to get things right*. New York, NY: Metropolitan Books; 2010.
 4. Tilyard M, Dovey S, Hall K. Avoiding and fixing medical errors in general practice:

prevention strategies reported in the LINNEAUS Collaboration's Primary Care International Study of Medical Errors. *NZ Med J.* 2005; **118**(1208): U1264.

5. Reason J. Human error: models and management. *BMJ.* 2000; **320**(7237): 768–70.

6. Leape LL. Error in medicine. *JAMA.* 1994; **272**(23): 1851–7.

7. Studdert DM, Brennan TA. No-fault compensation for medical injuries: the prospect for error prevention. *JAMA.* 2001; **286**(2): 217–23.

8. Leape LL, Berwick DM, Bates DW. What practices will most improve safety? Evidence-based medicine meets patient safety. *JAMA.* 2002; **288**(4): 501–7.

9. Parker D, Kirk S, Claridge T. *The Manchester Patient Safety Assessment Tool.* Manchester: National Primary Care Research and Development Centre, University of Manchester; 2002.

10. Haukelid K. Theories of (safety) culture revisited: an anthropological approach. *Saf Sci.* 2008; **46**(3): 413–26.

11. Flin R. Measuring safety culture in healthcare: a case for accurate diagnosis. *Saf Sci.* 2007; **45**(6): 653–67.

12. Wachter RM, Pronovost PJ. Balancing 'no blame' with accountability in patient safety. *N Engl J Med.* 2009; **361**(14): 1401–6.

13. Scott A, Mannion R, Davies H, *et al.* Implementing culture change in health care: theory and practice. *Int J Qual Health Care.* 2003; **15**(2): 111–18.

14. Kirk S, Parker D, Claridge T, *et al.* Patient safety culture in primary care: developing a theoretical framework for practical use. *Qual Saf Health Care.* 2007; **16**(4): 313–20.

15. Reason J. *Managing the Risks of Organizational Accidents.* Aldershot: Ashgate; 1997.

16. Gandhi TK, Lee TH. Patient safety beyond the hospital. *N Engl J Med.* 2010; **363**(11): 1001–3.

17. Joyce P, Boaden R, Esmail A. Managing risk: a taxonomy of error in health policy. *Health Care Anal.* 2005; **13**(4): 337–46.

18. Illich I. Medical nemesis. *Lancet.* 1974; **1**(7863): 918–21.

19. Gu Q, Dillon C, Burt V. *Prescription Drug Use Continues to Increase: US prescription drug data 2007–2008.* Atlanta, GA: Centers for Disease Control and Prevention; 2010.

20. Spence D. The gender agenda. *BMJ.* 2011; **343**: d7753.

21. Jørgensen KJ, Gøtzsche PC. Overdiagnosis in publicly organised mammography screening programmes: systematic review of incidence trends. *BMJ.* 2009; **339**: b2587.

22. Eliot T. *The Rock: a pageant play written for performance at Sadler's Wells Theatre.* London: Faber & Faber; 1934.

23. Green L, Dovey S. Practice based primary care research networks: they work and are ready for full development and support. *BMJ.* 2001; **322**(7286): 567–8.

24. Dovey S, Tilyard M. The computer research network of the Royal New Zealand College of General Practitioners: an approach to general practice research in New Zealand. *Br J Gen Pract.* 1996; **46**(413): 749–52.

25. Health Quality and Safety Commission. *Making Our Hospitals Safer: serious and sentinel events 2009/2010.* Wellington, New Zealand: Health Quality and Safety Commission; 2010.

26. National Patient Safety Agency: National Reporting and Learning Centre. *Organisation Patient Safety Incident Reports.* London: NHS England; 2011. Available at: www.nrls.npsa.nhs.uk/patient-safety-data/organisation-patient-safety-incident-reports/directory/ (accessed 12 December 2011).

27. Department of Health. *Building Foundations to Support Patient Safety: sentinel event*

program annual report 2009/10. Melbourne: Quality, Safety and Patient Experience Branch, Victorian Government Department of Health; 2010.

28. Douglas I, Smeeth L, Irvine D. The use of antidepressants and the risk of haemorrhagic stroke: a nested case control study. *Br J Clin Pharmacol.* 2011; **71**(1): 116–20.

29. Humes D, Fleming K, Spiller R, *et al.* Concurrent drug use and the risk of perforated colonic diverticular disease: a population-based case-control study. *Gut.* 2011; **60**(2): 219–24.

30. Salisbury C, Johnson L, Purdy S, *et al.* Epidemiology and impact of multimorbidity in primary care: a retrospective cohort study. *Br J Gen Pract.* 2011; **61**(582): e12–21.

31. Toovey S, Jick S, Meier C. Parkinson's disease or Parkinson symptoms following seasonal influenza. *Influenza Other Respir Viruses.* 2011; **5**(5): 328–33.

32. Bolon S, Phillips R. Building the research culture of family medicine with Fellowship training. *Fam Med.* 2010; **42**(7): 481–7.

33. Lucan S, Barg F, Bazemore A, *et al.* Family medicine, the NIH, and the medical-research roadmap: perspectives from inside NIH. *Fam Med.* 2009; **41**(3): 188–96.

34. Hoffman T, Eruti C, Thorning S, *et al.* The scatter of research: cross sectional comparison of randomised trials and systematic reviews across specialties. *BMJ.* 2012; **344**: e3223.

35. Cabana M, Rand C, Powe N, *et al.* Why don't physicians follow clinical practice guidelines? *JAMA.* 1999; **282**(15): 1458–65.

36. Black M, Schorr C, Levy M. Knowledge translation and the multifaceted intervention in the intensive care unit. *Crit Care Med.* 2012; **40**(4): 1324–8.

37. Gauld R, Dovey S, Tilyard M, *et al.* How physicians can drive comparative-effectiveness research: lessons from New Zealand. *Am J Med.* 2011; **124**(2): 93–4.

38. Dovey SM, Fraser TJ, Tilyard MW, *et al.* 'Really simple, summary, bang! That's what I need.' Clinical information needs of New Zealand general practitioners and the resources they use to meet them. *N Z Fam Physician.* 2006; **33**(1): 18–24.

39. Tomlin A, Dovey S, Gauld R, *et al.* Better use of primary care laboratory services following interventions to 'market' clinical guidelines in New Zealand: a controlled before-and-after study. *BMJ Qual Saf.* 2011; **20**(3): 282–90.

40. Wikipedia. *Wisdom.* Available at: http://en.wikipedia.org/wiki/Wisdom (accessed 9 November 2013).

CHAPTER 5

Measuring harm

Carl de Wet, Catherine O'Donnell,
Paul Johnson & Paul Bowie

INTRODUCTION

It is now widely accepted that approximately one in ten patients admitted to hospital may suffer harm as a result of their interaction with healthcare.[1] In general practice, knowledge about care safety continues to increase, but the incidence of harm has not yet been reliably quantified.[2] There are at least two important reasons why harm *should* be measured in the general practice setting and why harm rates should be calculated. The first reason is that knowledge of the scale of a problem helps to guide decisions about the amount of resources required to invest in or reallocate to the potential problem and can inform the design and implementation of improvement initiatives. The second reason is that safety improvement interventions need to be evaluated through serial measurements to determine whether they are leading to safer care or otherwise adapt them to ensure they do.

Before measuring (and improving) the safety of general practice, a number of important challenges have to be acknowledged.

- There is currently no single method that can detect and measure *all* harm.
- The reliability of the majority of the available metrics is poor or unknown.
- Measurement is typically very time and resource intensive.
- The quality of the results (harm rate estimates) is determined by many inter-related factors, not least the attitudes, training and experience of the staff applying it.

This chapter aims to address these challenges and also to propose that clinical record review (CRR) is the most suitable metric to measure harm in general practice. A simple formula is described – developed from previous research – that can help to ensure harm rate estimates are sufficiently precise and adequately powered, thereby ensuring their clinical usefulness. Finally, the feasibility of CRR as a method to measure harm rates at the regional and national level of a healthcare system is considered.

CLINICAL RECORD REVIEW

The findings of landmark studies utilising the review of clinical records have shaped our understanding of the scale of the safety problem in secondary care settings worldwide; this evidence was the primer for the development and implementation of national policies to make patient care safer.[3,4] CRR is a well-established approach to detecting and quantifying suboptimal care issues.[5,6] It allows estimation of harm rates for specific patient populations at given points in time and, if repeated, allows comparisons to detect significant changes across time. Other methods such as incident reporting systems, analysing complaints or mortality data are methodologically deficient in comparison, because they rely on self-report data or they focus on a small subset of the patient population.[7-10]

One of the strengths of the CRR method is its flexibility – there is no single 'correct' adaptation. In recent years the Institute for Healthcare Improvement has popularised the 'global trigger tool' as a means for front-line clinicians to estimate harm rates using this rapid, focused and structured approach to record review.[9] Their rationale for the trigger tool method is 'the ability to quantify [harm] accurately with relatively small samples [of medical records] and to follow changes [in harm rates] longitudinally over time'.[10] Specific trigger tools are now routinely used in many acute hospital settings worldwide[11-14] and have been piloted in other settings, including primary care,[15-18] to test their feasibility in measuring rates of harm.

However, the reliability (and therefore potential usefulness) of the harm rates detected with CRR are dependent on the method's many constituent parameters (factors). Examples of these are as follows:

- *the quality of the clinical records* – in particular the completeness and reliability of data recording across a practice population
- *individual reviewer factors* – inter-rater reliability, quality and extent of previous training and experience, if the reviewer is internal or external to the practice (or organisation) and if one or more individuals review each record
- *specific characteristics of the review process* – number of months or patient encounters reviewed in each record, how many records are reviewed and how often reviews are conducted
- *the 'frailty' of the patient population whose records are reviewed* – inter-patient and inter-practice variation, which are reflections of the likelihood of patients experiencing harm.

A selection of CRR parameters and their effects on the precision and power of the detected harm rate estimates are shown in Table 5.1. Examples of potential factor values are included for interest only and may vary even more in real life.

STATISTICAL PRECISION AND POWER

The parameter values (*see* Table 5.1) can potentially be combined in thousands of different ways, each resulting in a slightly modified but unique CRR scenario. Any of these CRR scenarios can be used (if we temporarily suspend feasibility considerations) to measure harm and estimate harm rates, but they will all produce uniquely different results. Many of the results will *not* be sufficiently reliable or have adequate precision to make them clinically useful. Unfortunately, researchers and policymakers often overlook this crucial point, appearing to accept *any* reported harm rate or reduction in harm at face value. Therefore, while the CRR method and its various adaptations are potentially of great use, it is essential to resolve this methodological and statistical challenge.

TABLE 5.1 Clinical record review (CRR) parameters and their effect on the precision and power of harm rate estimates

CRR parameter	Example of value range	Affects precision	Affects power
Number of practices conducting CRRs	1–1000	✓	✓
Number of unique patient records reviewed by each practice at a given point in time	20–200	✓	✓
The real harm rate in the sampled patient population, expressed as incidents per 100 patients per year	2, 5, 10, 20	✓	✓
The reduction in the real harm rate over a period of time	20%, 50%		✓
Inter-patient variation in harm susceptibility (MRR)*	1.2–3	✓	✓
Inter-practice variation in harm susceptibility (MRR)*	1.2–2	✓	✓
Period of time reviewed in each record (calendar months)	3–12	✓	✓
Period of time over which changes in harm rates are examined (months)	3–48		✓
Number of reviews during a 12-month period	2–4		✓
Reviews at different time points are conducted on the same or different samples of patient records	Same		✓

* MRR = median rate ratio. This expresses the relative difference in underlying harm susceptibility between an average pair of patients or practices; for example, an inter-practice MRR of 2 implies that a typical pair of practices will differ by a factor of 2 in the rate at which patient safety incidents occur.

To do so, it is important to first distinguish between two important but different ways in which measurement and rates can be used. A clinical analogy may help to illustrate this best. Imagine a patient presents to her general practitioner (GP) with an acute exacerbation of asthma. As part of the initial assessment the GP measures the patient's peak expiratory flow rate (PEFR, or peak flow). The measure is dependent on the patient's clinical condition, her understanding of the method and technique, the type of peak flow meter used and the number of times the test is repeated (usually three times). The estimated rate at that specific point in time informs the GP's management plan, which includes scheduling a follow-up appointment. A week later the patient returns, and the GP again measures her PEFR and compares the result with the previous to determine whether there is an improvement (or not).

Harm rate estimates can be used for the same two purposes. First, to quantify the incidence of harm in defined patient populations at given points in time. The findings are typically expressed as a rate such as 'number of harm incidents per 100 patients per year'. For example, a study of patients with diabetes mellitus found an estimated harm rate of 5 per 100 patients per year. Second, harm rates at different points in time can be compared and the observed increases or reductions can be described – usually as a percentage. For example, during a 5-year national patient safety programme, the estimated rates of harm reduced by 15%. The terms 'precision' and 'power' apply to the two different ways in which harm rates can be used (and *to* the clinical analogy) and are defined here.

Precision

The precision of a harm rate estimate is its repeatability or reproducibility – in other words, the degree to which repeated measurements (in unchanged conditions) will produce the same results. The term 'accuracy' implies how close an estimated harm rate is to the true harm rate and is often used colloquially as synonymous with precision. A high level of precision is desirable for any estimate but usually requires substantial resources (e.g. more time, multiple reviewers and larger numbers of patient records). It is therefore important to consider what level of precision will be acceptable and whether that can be achieved with the available resources before selecting a CRR design.

In this chapter we pragmatically define a harm rate estimate as having 'acceptable precision' if its estimation error is less than ±25% (low estimation error implying high precision). We use 'estimation error' as a proxy for precision because it is easier to quantify and interpret and we define it as the distance from the 95% confidence limits to the harm rate estimate (expressed as a percentage). For example, a harm rate of 10 incidents per 100 patients per year with a 95% confidence interval of 8–12 could also be expressed as 10 ± 2. Expressing ±2 as a percentage of 10 gives an estimation error of ±20%.

Power

'Power' gauges the probability that specific CRR scenarios are able to detect real changes in harm rates over a given period of time. In statistical terms, ≥80% power is considered adequate by convention. For example, a given CRR design has 92% power to detect a 15% reduction in harm during a 12-month period. The (perhaps oversimplified) interpretation is that the probability of detecting the reduction is 92% while the chance of failing to detect it is 8%.

A recent general practice study examined the potential precision and power of individual harm rate estimates for a wide range of CRR scenarios.[19] The selected method was Monte Carlo simulation, which allows computerised modelling of many multiple, complex 'real-life' scenarios in non-deterministic systems – that is, those that are characterised by substantial inherent uncertainty – making it the ideal choice for the general practice setting.

The key study finding was that the precision and power of the harm rate estimates of any given CRR scenario are mainly determined by the number of

detected harm incidents. The number of detected harm incidents is, in turn, determined by the underlying 'real' harm rate and the total amount of time spent reviewing the records of all the selected patient records – or, in other words, the review 'effort'. The review 'effort' is the combined product of the:
- period of time reviewed in each record
- number of records reviewed per practice
- number of practices reviewing records
- number of times each record is reviewed.

The relationship between the number of detected harm incidents and CRR parameters can be simplified and expressed as a statistical formula (*see* Figure 5.1).

$$\frac{eHR(prec)}{eHR(pow)} \longrightarrow nHI = rHR \times Ltr \times nPrac \times nRec \times nTimes$$

Precision or power of harm rate estimate	Number of detected harm incidents	Real harm rate	Length of time reviewed in each record	Number of practices reviewing records	Number of records reviewed in each practice	Number of times each record is reviewed
←	=	x	x	x	x	x

FIGURE 5.1 A formula to express the relationship between the variable parameters of a given clinical record review scenario and the number of detected harm incidents, which is associated with the degree of precision and power of the estimated harm rates

The close link between the number of harm incidents and precision and power has the following 'real-life' implications (insofar as reality is encompassed by the range of scenarios simulated in de Wet *et al.*[19]).
- Any CRR scenario (e.g. any combination of parameter values) that results in the detection of at least 100 harm incidents will yield a harm rate estimate with acceptable precision (as defined in this chapter).
- Any CRR scenario that results in the detection of at least 500 harm incidents will have adequate power ($\geq 80\%$) to allow a 'real' reduction of $\geq 20\%$ over a specified period of time (12 months in this study) to be found. To detect a larger reduction in harm will require relatively less 'effort' – for example, a reduction in harm of $\geq 50\%$ requires the detection of a minimum of 100 harm incidents.
- A single general practice cannot generate harm estimates with acceptable precision or adequate power with any feasible combination of parameter values.

FEASIBLE APPLICATION OF THE CLINICAL RECORD REVIEW METHOD
Healthcare researchers, clinicians, policymakers and others can combine different parameter values to create unique CRR scenarios to fit their aims and resources. By applying the formula in Figure 5.1, they can judge whether their

selected CRR scenarios are likely to yield harm rate estimates with adequate precision and acceptable power. As a general rule of thumb, a CRR aiming to determine the incidence of harm at a given point in time in general practice will require approximately 2000 records (assuming a high baseline harm rate) to be reviewed; this increases to 20 000 records if the harm rate is low. However, if the aim is to detect changes in general practice harm rates with adequate power over time, as many as 120 000 records may have to be reviewed, depending on the prevalence of the harm in the patient population of interest.

These estimates may seem large, but they represent 'best case' scenarios and are likely to still underestimate the amount of records that may have to be reviewed. One reason for this is that the calculations are based on 'harm', rather than *preventable* patient safety incidents (PSIs). While a substantial proportion of PSIs may not be preventable because they originated in different settings, or are recognised as side effects of appropriate treatment or are dependent on patient factors, current estimates suggest between 10% and 50% are preventable.[7,16,20,21,22] Therefore, when reductions in harm are being measured, the 'non-preventable' proportion of PSIs has to be removed, or at the very least considered. Otherwise, the observed reduction will appear 'smaller' (as a percentage) and the power of the CRR method will decrease.

Consider the following study as an example to further illustrate this point: Takata et al.[14] detected 107 adverse drug events, of which 24 (22%) were judged preventable, when they reviewed 960 paediatric records in 12 US hospitals. Say they then aimed to reduce the number of *preventable* incidents by an ambitious 50% (e.g. a reduction from 24 to 12 incidents) over a given period of time, this reduction would 'only' be 11.2% of the overall harm rate.

Despite these challenges, there is still considerable political and policy interest in a measure to reliably quantify and then track rates of harm in primary care records over time. The ideal attributes of such a measure are that it should be relevant, valid, reliable, discriminative, credible, timely, feasible, accessible and actionable.[22] The CRR method has these attributes but may be limited by feasibility concerns (e.g. number of practices reviewing records and number of records reviewed per practice).

While a single general practice cannot feasibly measure its rate of harm with acceptable precision or adequate power, there are many potential CRR iterations that can yield harm rate estimates with adequate precision and acceptable power, especially if implemented at regional or national level. There are approximately 1000 general medical practices in Scotland.[23] Applying the formula suggests that if 300 or more practices each reviewed 25 records twice during a 12-month period of time, the harm rate estimates will have acceptable precision and adequate power to detect a 50% reduction in the baseline harm rate. Even smaller reductions in harm could be detected if every practice in Scotland participated. This is now a real possibility because of the trigger review method (a form of CRR) being contractually incentivised in 2013, as well as it being a key component of the recently launched Scottish Patient Safety Programme in Primary Care.[24]

The relationship between measurement and improvement, and the challenge of 'getting one to follow the other' has previously been described.[22] We still do not know which interventions can successfully improve patient safety in general practice. What little evidence there is suggests successful interventions will likely require a multi-method approach, rigorous evaluation and small, local clinician-led pilots.[25] Future research is therefore now being undertaken to examine the utility of the trigger review method as a learning and improvement tool, 'working on the nuts and bolts of how we turn measurement for improvement into tangible change in practice'.[22]

REFERENCES

1. Health Foundation. *Evidence Scan: levels of harm*. London: Health Foundation; 2011. Available at: www.health.org.uk/public/cms/75/76/313/2593/Levels%20of%20harm.pdf?realName=PYiXMz.pdf (accessed 30 October 2012).
2. Bates DW. Mountains in the clouds: patient safety research. *Qual Saf Health Care*. 2008; **17**(3): 156–7.
3. Vincent C, Neale G, Woloshynowych M. Adverse events in British hospitals: preliminary retrospective record review. *BMJ*. 2001; **322**(7285): 517–19.
4. Brennan TA, Leape LL, Laird NM, *et al.* Incidence of adverse events and negligence in hospitalized patients: results of the Harvard Medical Practice Study I. 1991. *Qual Saf Health Care*. 2004; **13**(2): 145–51, discussion 151–2.
5. Resar RK, Rozich JD, Classen D. Methodology and rationale for the measurement of harm with trigger tools. *Qual Saf Health Care*. 2003; **12**(Suppl. 2): ii39–45.
6. Sharek PJ, Parry G, Goldmann D, *et al.* Performance characteristics of a methodology to quantify adverse events over time in hospitalized patients. *Health Serv Res*. 2011; **46**(2): 654–78.
7. Field TS, Gurwitz JH, Harrold LR, *et al.* Strategies for detecting adverse drug events among older persons in the ambulatory setting. *J Am Med Inform Assoc*. 2004; **11**(6): 492–8.
8. Wetzels R, Wolters R, van Weel C, *et al.* Mix of methods is needed to identify adverse events in general practice: a prospective observational study. *BMC Fam Pract*. 2008; 9: 35.
9. Christiaans-Dingelhoff I, Smits M, Zwaan L, *et al.* To what extent are adverse events found in patient records reported by patients and healthcare professionals via complaints, claims and incident reports? *BMC Health Serv Res*. 2011; **11**: 49.
10. Classen DC, Lloyd RC, Provost L, *et al.* Development and evaluation of the Institute for Healthcare Improvement global trigger tool. *J Patient Saf*. 2008; **4**(3): 169–77.
11. Griffin FA, Classen DC. Detection of adverse events in surgical patients using the trigger tool approach. *Qual Saf Health Care*. 2008; **17**(4): 253–8.
12. Matlow A, Flintoft V, Orrbine E, *et al.* The development of the Canadian paediatric trigger tool for identifying potential adverse events. *Healthc Q*. 2005; **8**(Spec No): 90–3.
13. Sharek PJ, Horbar JD, Mason W, *et al.* Adverse events in the neonatal intensive care unit: development, testing, and findings of an NICU-focused trigger tool to identify harm in North American NICUs. *Pediatrics*. 2006; **118**(4): 1332–40.

14. Takata GS, Mason W, Taketomo C, *et al.* Development, testing, and findings of a pediatric-focused trigger tool to identify medication-related harm in US children's hospitals. *Pediatrics.* 2008; **121**(4): e927–35.
15. de Wet C, Bowie P. The preliminary development and testing of a global trigger tool to detect error and patient harm in primary-care records. *Postgrad Med J.* 2009; **85**(1002): 176–80.
16. Singh R, McLean-Plunckett EA, Kee R, *et al.* Experience with a trigger tool for identifying adverse drug events among older adults in ambulatory primary care. *Qual Saf Health Care.* 2009; **18**(3): 199–204.
17. Gaal S, Verstappen W, Wolters R, *et al.* Prevalence and consequences of patient safety incidents in general practice in the Netherlands: a retrospective medical record review study. *Implement Sci.* 2011; **6**: 37.
18. Bowie P, Halley L, Gillies J, *et al.* Searching primary care records for predefined triggers may expose latent risks and adverse events. *Clin Risk.* 2012; **18**(1): 13–18.
19. de Wet C, Johnson P, O'Donnell C, *et al.* Can we quantify harm in general practice records? An assessment of precision and power using computer simulation. *BMC Med Res Methodol.* 2013; **13**: 39.
20. Barber ND, Alldred DP, Raynor DK, *et al.* Care homes' use of medicines study: prevalence, causes and potential harm of medication errors in care homes for older people. *Qual Saf Health Care.* 2009; **18**(5): 341–6.
21. Morris CJ, Rodgers S, Hammersley VS, *et al.* Indicators for preventable drug related morbidity: application in primary care. *Qual Saf Health Care.* 2004; **13**(3): 181–5.
22. Scott I, Phelps G. Measurement for improvement: getting one to follow the other. *Intern Med J.* 2009; **39**(6): 347–51.
23. Information Services Division Scotland. *Practices and their Populations.* Edinburgh: NHS National Services Scotland; 2012; Available at: www.isdscotland.org/Health-Topics/General-Practice/Practices-and-Their-Populations/ (accessed 28 September 2012).
24. NHS Scotland. *Welcome to the Scottish Patient Safety Programme.* Edinburgh: NHS Scotland; 2013; Available at: www.scottishpatientsafetyprogramme.scot.nhs.uk/programme (accessed 5 April 2013).
25. Siriwardena AN. Quality improvement projects for appraisal and revalidation of general practitioners. *Qual Prim Care.* 2011; **19**(4): 205–9.

CHAPTER 6

Systems thinking

Michelle Beattie & Clare Carolan

A systems view of the world is part of the essential literacy of our age.[1]

INTRODUCTION

The complexity of primary healthcare is set to increase,[2] driven by factors such as advances in technology, polypharmacy, public expectations, ever-changing political influence and the current restrained financial climate. The drive to deliver safe, effective, person-centred care has brought quality improvement (QI) to the forefront of healthcare, which recognises that improving current and future healthcare services will require significant change within the healthcare system. This chapter will examine the theory of systems thinking within the context of primary care and the utility of adopting a 'systems thinking' approach to implementing QI initiatives.

Much of the theory embedded within safety and QI initiatives derives from systems thinking. Systems thinking has its origins in general systems theories[3,4] and acknowledges the complexity, influence and interrelationships of the systems in which we live and work; thus, explaining how each part of the system affects the whole and vice versa. There is recognition that changes required to improve future health services will not be achieved by simply working 'harder' or employing more staff, but rather will require changes within the system. For example, to ensure that patients in primary care obtain a consultation within 48 hours of their request for an appointment, one cannot simply assume that asking general practitioners (GPs) to work harder will resolve the issue. For one, there is unlikely to be the 'buy-in' to implement such a solution and even if GPs were to work harder by working longer hours, or seeing patients quicker, this would both be unsustainable and potentially compromise the quality of care. Furthermore, employing more GPs is limited by resource and financial constraints. Solutions need to be system focused. For example, enhancing patient education on self-care and when and how to use other healthcare service providers such as local pharmacists or optometrists; prioritising appointments based on the needs of the patient; and offering alternatives to face-to-face appointments (i.e. telephone consultations).

There is no single definition of systems thinking, so therefore terms such as complex adaptive systems, complexity theory and complex evolving systems are often used interchangeably. Although some would argue there are clear distinctions between aspects of these terms, there appears to be a shared view that change requires more than a simple cause and effect relationship and that the evolving interrelationships among component parts of the system need to be considered.[5] As such, implementing improvement in practice is not a linear process. It is not a simplistic reductionist process of doing X and the outcome equals Y; rather, an acknowledgement of the complexity of interactions of the healthcare system is needed. It is also recognised that even when there is empirical evidence to implement a change in practice, the process of change management may frequently be impeded by other variables and relationships within the healthcare systems.

THEORY OF PROFOUND KNOWLEDGE

Deming[6] offers a theoretical framework to consider the complexity of such systems. Edward Deming, an American statistician and renowned quality management systems guru, devised a theoretical model coined the 'theory of profound knowledge'.[6] This model is based on the principle that each organisation is composed of a complex system of interrelated processes and people. The model has four interlinked parts:

1. *Appreciation of the system* – understanding the overall processes involving suppliers, producers and recipients (or customers, or patients) of goods and services; it is the structure of the entire organisation rather than simply the employees alone that holds the key to improving the quality of output
2. *Knowledge of variation* – the range and causes of variation in quality, and use of statistical sampling in measurements (systems vary in performance, exhibiting two kinds of variation: 'normal' or common cause variation, i.e. the background noise, and 'special cause' variation, i.e. caused by something specific)
3. *Theory of knowledge* – the concepts explaining knowledge and how it is built up in improvement
4. *Psychology* – the concepts of human nature in relation to change.

Successfully implementing and sustaining change within any organisation will only occur when all four parts of the system have been considered. For example, a general practice would like to change their diabetes mellitus protocol to incorporate the HbA_{1c} blood test for screening and diagnosing diabetes as an alternative to using either random blood sugar or fasting plasma glucose blood tests. Before actually making such a change, they would need to understand the effect of such a proposal within the current system. Is the test available locally? How long would the proposed test take? What are the cost implications? Will the costs be incurred by the laboratory or primary care facility? Knowledge of variation would also need to be considered, such as the average number of diagnoses made in a specified time frame, and the rate of false positives or negatives. The theory of knowledge would require an exploration with other colleagues within the practice about their thoughts and perceptions of the proposed change. For example, is there evidence to support this change? Will this improve patient care? What will the new system actually improve? The psychology of any proposed change usually differs among the individuals involved – who will be the early adopters and who will be those who will resist the change? How can the negative effects of change be mitigated? The example is summarised in Box 6.1.

BOX 6.1 An example of Deming's framework to understand a practice as a system

The practice needs to gain a shared understanding through communication of the following.

- *The actual practice system*: identify the resources and the organisational structure; consider the current service provision (e.g. number and type of patients seen, tests undertaken).
- *Variation within the system*: fluctuations in staffing or patient demand (common variations, e.g. Monday mornings; special variations, e.g. during a flu pandemic).
- *The evidence base for the current system*.
- *The mindset of their colleagues!*

UNDERSTANDING MACRO-, MICRO- AND MESOSYSTEMS

Systems thinking also incorporates consideration of the multiple systems within a system; these are sometimes referred to as macro-, micro- and mesosystems, with the term mesosystem describing the relationships and connections between microsystems.[7] For example, a macrosystem could be a National Health Service board; a microsystem could be a GP practice; and a mesosystem, a community nursing team. Each macrosystem will have multiple meso- and micro-subsystems, which are interdependent and interrelated to one another, or to the larger macrosystem. Any improvement in one aspect of a macrosystem, or micro- or meso-subsystems, will influence and affect other aspects of the macrosystem and subsystems. Consideration needs to be given to the potential impact on other components of the system to enable buy-in and to limit negative effects on other systems and subsystems. Conversely, the culture of a larger macrosystem will likely influence other subsystems.

Appreciating 'systems thinking', including the influence of the culture within macrosystems, is of significant importance when examining adverse events in healthcare. Historically, adverse events in healthcare have been managed in a punitive manner, where the blame apportioned for errors and the proposed solutions have merely focused at the level of the individual involved. This punitive approach very likely prevented the openness and transparency of error reporting, thereby reducing the opportunity for learning. Moreover, it is apparent that the operational mechanisms within systems have a significant influence on the behaviour of individuals within the system. This perspective has altered the management of adverse events to focus on aspects of the system for improvement, rather than the individual, to reduce the likelihood of a similar adverse event reoccurring. Clinical areas now use root cause analysis or significant event analysis tools (*see* Box 6.2) to facilitate the learning and subsequent system improvements required following an adverse event.

BOX 6.2 Using system's thinking in significant event analysis*

When undertaking significant event analysis, use the following four questions:
1. What happened?
2. Why did it happen?
3. What was learned?
4. What was changed?

Use a systems thinking approach when answering questions 2 and 4.

(*See Chapter 31 for more on significant event analysis)

For example, a community nurse takes a blood sample from the wrong patient. Previously, the nurse would likely be reprimanded and required to conduct a training course on venepuncture. Adopting a systems approach would identify both the human and the system factors that contributed to the error. For example, what was the mechanism for requesting the blood test? Was the nurse carrying a particularly high caseload that day? Was the nurse suitably experienced and supported? Is the system for patient identification in the community robust, and what is the mechanism for labelling and checking samples? Furthermore, how errors are communicated to the patient after the event can be examined by using a systems approach. By examining the mechanism of the error at the systems level rather than simply at the individual level, improvements to the system can be implemented with the aim to reduce the likelihood of the error reoccurring in the future. Simply retraining the nurse would not reduce the likelihood of the error reoccurring in another part of the system, while improving the system for patient identification in the community might. In addition to the culture of the macrosystem, the influence of laws, ethics and current governmental policies of the societal exosystem within which the healthcare system exists must also be acknowledged.

COMPLEXITY AND QUALITY IMPROVEMENT IN HEALTHCARE

Much of systems theory is derived from complexity theory. Complexity theory acknowledges the enormity of change, the need to work in constant chaos and that the constituent parts of healthcare are all related at some level.[8] QI requires a systems mindset, where aspects of a service need to be considered in the wider context of available health and social care services. Barriers to QI in general practice are multifaceted and include social, organisational and cultural factors,[9] and therefore understanding and overcoming barriers to QI in primary care requires a systems approach.

Clinicians generally focus on improvement and safety from the perspective of improving their own practice.[10] This is likely more so in primary care where GPs and other primary healthcare professionals often work independently with a significant degree of autonomy. While it is recognised that individuals can and should focus on improvement, an individual perspective may limit the view and subsequent relevance for the wider systems involved. Clinicians were generally taught that improvement results from hard work and knowledge acquisition,[11] which is at odds with underpinning philosophy of systems theory. Systems theory acknowledges that improvements will come not from working harder, but working differently. Being able to view improvement through a systems perspective will require a shift in what are often deeply held ideologies and assumptions.

Yet, primary care clinicians are well placed to implement and benefit from a systems approach to quality and safety. Changes in GP contracts have shifted an emphasis from quantity to quality, with a particular focus on rewarding quality aspects of long-term conditions.[12] For some QI initiatives it can be difficult to see a direct relationship between improving processes and systems and actual better outcomes for patients. However, some aspects of primary care offer distinct advantages in such processes. Adopting change within a relatively static and known population may be easier than other settings. Primary care practitioners are also more likely to witness the direct impact of quality and safety initiatives and improved outcomes for patients. Such positive feedback may enhance further uptake of QI initiatives. Continuity of care in general practice also allows GPs to follow patients through their patient journey including transitions of care between hospital and home. This allows primary care to identify areas for improvement in service provision, and identify areas of duplication or even waste within the system.

The World Health Organization's 'Ten Steps to Systems Thinking'[13] provides a framework for designing (steps 1–4) and evaluating (steps 5–10) improvement initiatives (or system changes) in general practice using a systems thinking approach. Table 6.1 outlines the 10 steps and provides a practical example of how they can be applied, using the following scenario.

> *Clinical scenario: the Welcome Practice has had a recent significant increase in unwanted teenage pregnancies. The nearest family planning clinic and genitourinary medicine clinic are more than 40 miles away.*

TABLE 6.1 The 'Ten Steps to Systems Thinking' framework for designing and evaluating an improvement initiative[13]

The 10 steps	Example of application in practice
Step 1: Convene stakeholders Identify and convene stakeholders	The practice manager arranged a meeting in protected learning time and invited all staff (clinical and non-clinical) as well as the community midwife and public health nurse to attend.
Step 2: Collectively brainstorm What are the system dynamics and possible system-wide effects of the proposed intervention?	At the meeting, staff considered the following questions: • Are the contraceptive needs of young teenagers in the area being met? • Is there an unmet need for sexual health services in young people in the area? • Is the practice teenage friendly? • The main issue they identify is that no one locally has been trained to provide long-acting reversible contraception (LARC).
Step 3: Conceptualise effects Develop a conceptual pathway by mapping how the intervention(s) may affect patients and the health system through its subsystems	*Agreed interventions* • Set up new nurse-led teenage-dedicated clinics once a week. • A GP and practice nurse volunteer will be trained to insert subcutaneous LARC. *Mapping* • Improved LARC use will decrease unwanted pregnancies and reduce pressure on maternity services. • Improved sexual health advice and sexually transmitted infection (STI) screening will reduce infertility rates in the long term. • Providing LARC will increase contraceptive choices for all female patients. • Providing LARC could increase practice income, which could be reinvested in staff and services.
Step 4: Adapt and redesign Adapt and/or redesign the proposed intervention to optimise synergies, while proactively avoiding or minimising potential unwanted consequences	• Uptake of new services can be promoted through clinic timing (after-school hours) and a 'drop-in' clinic. • Nursing time comes at an opportunity cost. Initially the new clinic will be from 4.15 p.m. to 5 p.m once a week only. • Increasing STI screening will increase laboratory workload. • Other health problems may opportunistically be detected, including substance abuse, mental health problems and child protection issues. This may increase referrals to other services. • Confidentiality issues: raise awareness through posters. Results handling protocol to be expanded to include email and text notification, rather than a home telephone. • Required staff training: What are the cost and time implications, including continuing professional development of these skills? • GP undertaking new role: how will workload be shared?

Design (row label spanning Steps 3 and 4)

(*continued*)

The 10 steps	Example of application in practice
Step 5: Determine indicators Select indicators that are important to track in the redesigned intervention across the affected subsystems	The Welcome Practice identifies the following indicators: • number of patients who attends new clinic • number of LARCs inserted • teenage pregnancy rates • number of STI screens • number of brief interventions for alcohol abuse • number of referrals to alcohol and drug action teams
Step 6: Choose methods Select evaluation methods that would best track the indicators	The practice will obtain baseline data for the indicators (*see* previous step). They will audit these indicators on a monthly basis.
Step 7: Select design Select the evaluation design that best fits the methods and nature of the intervention.	The Welcome Practice team decides clinical audit will fit the design best.
Step 8: Develop plan and timeline Develop and agree an evaluation plan with a timeline as a team	The practice manager will arrange a further meeting in 3 months' time. During this time she will lead on the implementation of the interventions.
Step 9: Set a budget Set a budget for the project costing the intervention and the evaluation	The team identifies the following expenses: • cost of staff training • funding extra hour of staff's time to provide the new clinic • miscellaneous – advertising, educational and health promotion materials, condoms, additional STI screen, administrative costs.
Step 10: Source funding Allocate funding to support the evaluation before the intervention begins	Initial practice investments likely to be recouped from additional income generated through the Quality and Outcomes Framework and a local enhanced service agreement for LARCs.

(Left margin label spanning the table: Evaluation)

SUMMARY

The majority of decision-making in primary healthcare occurs in the context of complex social interactions, which is often not addressed by the available evidence base.[14] Systems thinking provides a conceptual framework that accounts for the wider influences affecting change and improvement that are not influenced by traditional forms of evidence, and it furnishes healthcare providers with a powerful tool by which to implement safe and cost-effective quality improvements in healthcare.

REFERENCES

1. Laszlo E. *The Systems View of the World: a holistic vision for our time.* Advances in Systems Theory, Complexity and the Human Sciences. Cresskill, NJ: Hampton Press; 1991.
2. Katerndahl D, Wood D, Jaen C. A method for estimating relative complexity of ambulatory care. *Ann Fam Med.* 2010; **8**(4): 341–7.
3. Von Bertalanffy L. The theory of open systems in physic and biology. *Science.* 1950; **111**(2872): 23–9.
4. Parsons T. *The Social System.* Glencoe, IL: The Free Press; 1951.
5. Health Foundation. *Research Scan: complex adaptive systems.* London: Health Foundation; 2010.
6. Deming WE. *Out of the Crisis.* Cambridge: Cambridge University Press; 1986.
7. Brofenbrenner U. *The Ecology of Human Development.* Cambridge, MA: Harvard University Press; 1979.
8. Porter-O'Grady T, Malloch K. *Quantum Leadership: advancing innovation, transforming health care.* 3rd ed. Sudbury, MA: Jones & Bartlett Learning; 2011.
9. Grol R. Implementing guidelines in general practice care. *Qual Health Care.* 1992; **1**(3): 184–91.
10. National Leadership and Innovation Agency for Healthcare. *Engaging Clinicians in a Quality Agenda.* Llanharan: NLIAH; 2008. Available at: www.wales.nhs.uk/sitesplus/documents/829/EngagingCliniciansinaqualityagendaApril08.pdf (accessed 12 November 2013).
11. Wensing M, Grol R. Single and combined strategies for implementing changes in primary care: a literature review. *Int J Qual Health Care.* 1994; **6**(2): 115–32.
12. Steel N, Maisey S, Clark A, *et al.* Quality of clinical primary care and targeted incentive payments: an observational study. *Br J Gen Pract.* 2012; **57**(539): 449–54.
13. Alliance for Health Policy and Systems Research. *Systems Thinking for Health Systems Strengthening.* Geneva: World Health Organization; 2009.
14. Martin CM, Sturmberg JP. General practice: chaos, complexity and innovation. *Med J Aust.* 2005; **183**(2): 106–9.

CHAPTER 7

Task analysis

Eleanor Forrest & Paul Bowie

INTRODUCTION

Ergonomics and human factors practitioners promote the development of 'user-centred' systems in the workplace that are intuitive, efficient and pleasurable to use, enabling people to achieve their work-related goals while taking account of natural human limitations and capabilities.[1] Obtaining a clear understanding of what staff actually need to achieve is critical to the design of such work systems. This can be accomplished by asking some key questions.

- What work tasks are performed? (*See* Box 7.1)
- What is the nature of those tasks?
- How can risks be eliminated and performance improved?
- How can staff well-being in the workplace and patient satisfaction with the service be enhanced?

BOX 7.1 Examples of risk-prone work tasks and systems in general practice

- Vaccinating patients
- Booking appointments
- Diagnosing specific illness
- Handling laboratory results
- Prescribing drugs
- Referring patients
- Monitoring high-risk medications
- Communicating with patients
- Communicating with colleagues (internally and externally)
- Using electronic clinical records
- Triaging patients
- Dispensing drugs
- Repeat prescribing

Task analysis methods can be used to help answer these questions by providing a rigorous, structured description of user activity and by outlining a framework for the investigation of existing work practices to facilitate the design or redesign of complex systems. The methods are highly adaptable and flexible and provide a step-by-step description of the specific work task under analysis. Task analysis methods are widely used across a range of industry sectors including aviation, air traffic control, energy, military defence and increasingly in healthcare. Their use and application should lead to the 'more efficient and effective integration of the human element into system design and operations'.[2] Given the extent of human–system interactions in primary care and what we know from significant events related to system failures and (un)reliability, using task analysis methods to create or modify work systems has the potential to improve patient safety by designing more efficient and safer methods of working, and also enhancing staff well-being and job satisfaction.

BENEFITS OF TASK ANALYSIS

Task analysis provides a wide range of practical methods for collecting data on specific work tasks, which can help to:
- identify potential hazards or opportunities for human error in the system
- improve the design of work tasks and activities
- determine what changes need to be made to prevent hazards from recurring
- understand tasks as a step in incident investigation.

Omitting necessary steps when performing a specific task is the single most common type of human error.[3] The inherent properties of some work task steps (such as related complexities, risks, reliance on short-term memory or the potential for distractions) are more likely to result in errors (e.g. handling test results or clinically managing complicated illness) than other tasks (e.g. answering the telephone or photocopying). These properties can be identified and prioritised in advance using information from task analysis methods to enable us to devise and implement appropriate strategies to minimise risks.

Task analysis methods can be used whenever a practice needs to understand exactly what a specific work task involves in terms of the expected knowledge, skills and behavioural requirements of different staff members. They can be applied during the design stage of a new practice system, or the modification of an existing system, or as part of an audit of an existing system.[4] This type of analysis should provide the foundation for all ergonomics and human factors interventions and analysis techniques (e.g. human error analysis and training needs analysis).

WHAT IS TASK ANALYSIS?

Task analysis has been defined as 'the study of what an operator (or team of operators) is required to do (their actions and cognitive processes) in order to achieve system goals'.[5] It helps the analyst to understand and represent human and system performance in a particular task or scenario[6] by breaking it down into the actions, decisions and cognitive processes that are necessary to complete it (e.g. arranging patient appointments).

It is not one specific technique but a range of methods for collecting and recording information about tasks in a systematic way.[7] The aim is to obtain detailed descriptions of what people do, represent those descriptions graphically or by documenting them, predict difficulties, and evaluate systems against the functional requirements of the practice.[8] Studying the work task in detail helps to identify areas that are, or have the potential to be, inefficient, unsafe or unsatisfactory. It can be used to understand the context within which tasks are performed to help us to:

- identify, predict and analyse the types of failures that are likely to occur at each step of a task or sub-task level, and the potential consequences of these errors
- assess the adequacy of risk control measures at each step
- identify ways to mitigate against failures at each step.

The Clinical Human Factors Group has described task analysis as a means to provide a 'window on the system',[9] as it assists with the identification of the points in a process where patient safety risks are prevalent. It can help staff to capture the physical (e.g. staff musculoskeletal problems due to poor workstation design), cognitive (e.g. over-reliance on memory or decision-making difficulty), psychosocial (e.g. staff stress, motivation or dissatisfaction) and sociocultural (e.g. an overbearing practice hierarchy) problems and challenges in a particular system. The practice can use this information to identify (and design for) health and safety issues, workload peaks, safety-critical tasks, interactions among care providers and how allocation of roles and responsibilities is best distributed.

HOW TO PERFORM TASK ANALYSIS

The method involves breaking down clinical, or non-clinical, processes into their constituent subtasks, collecting task data, analysing the data so that tasks are understood and then producing a documented representation of the analysed tasks. Rather than describing all the available task analysis methods, this chapter provides an overview of those most commonly used. There are many specialist publications that provide a comprehensive and detailed description of the various approaches,[5,10] which range from observational methods to sophisticated software programs.

It should be noted that task analysis is only one technique for identifying the human element of tasks. In practice, as task analysis can be applied to a diverse range of topic areas, analysts frequently 'tailor the technique(s) to fit the purpose of the evaluation'.[5] The following sections describe some of the key methods used to collect information about the task, describe and represent the data collected and how to suggest ways to make the task more efficient and safe to effectively support the task goals. It is important to note that the information and outputs from each part of the task analysis process feed into the next activity. The information obtained as part of the task analysis should provide the foundation to all human factors analyses.

The key steps when conducting a task analysis are to:
- identify the task to be analysed
- decompose the task
- describe and represent the data collected
- conduct further human factors analysis.

Identify the task to be analysed

Deciding on which task to be analysed is typically based on a number of factors including priority, criticality and/or frequency of task. The practice should ensure that the most appropriate task is analysed to make the best use of time and resources. An example of a task is the test ordering and results handling system used in primary care (*see* Figure 7.2 of the case study at the end of this chapter). It is made up of a number of subtasks or activities (e.g. order test or results reviewed).

Decompose the task

The high-level goal that the users are trying to accomplish needs to be identified. The aim of the high-level task decomposition is to break the tasks down into their constituent subtasks and operations (typically four to eight discrete subtasks that cover the entire task of interest). It is important to decide the correct level of detail required to ensure consistency across the analysis. Taking the analysis to a lower level may result in decomposing subtasks further into task flows, decision processes and screen layouts.

There is no right or wrong level of analysis, and the level the analysis is taken to will depend on what level data is required by any follow-on analyses. In order to break down a task, it is necessary to ask the question 'How is this task done?' and to repeat this question until satisfied that a sufficient level of detail has been obtained.

The task decomposition should always be conducted from the perspective of the end users, although who they are will depend on the tasks being investigated (e.g. nurse, doctor, pharmacist, patient, receptionist). It is important to get users involved in the task analysis process and through consultation and engagement to identify how the task actually occurs in practice. All users who are involved in the task should be consulted and as many engaged in the process as the project time and budget allows. To gather data about the task to enable the task decomposition it is often necessary to collect a number of different types of data about the task, including:
- information about users (e.g. different types of clinical or non-clinical staff involved in the system)
- description of the environment (where tasks are performed)

- major goals (what will result in a successful end state)
- user preferences and needs
- tasks and subtasks (physical, cognitive and emotional)
- conditions under which tasks are performed (e.g. environmental conditions)
- results or outcomes of tasks (e.g. successful completion criteria)
- requirements to perform task (e.g. information, communication with others, equipment)
- design (System, Training, Interface, Workplace and Job).

The output of the task decomposition needs to be validated and approved, where possible, with experts in the task. When a system is not yet in operation the tasks analysis should be reviewed with users who have relevant experience of similar or comparable systems. This can be done using a variety of qualitative data collection including:

- observation methods (e.g. walk-through or talk-through)
- questioning methods (e.g. interviews, questionnaires)
- workshop methods (e.g. walk-through, focus groups).[5]

By using these methods the reality of how tasks are actually performed is often revealed to differ from the actual task-related policies and procedures in place. The task analysis may highlight 'work-arounds' or procedure deviance developed by staff due to deficiencies in equipment, environment, staffing and so on.

Describe and represent the data collected

The output of the task decomposition is best represented as a diagram showing the sequence of activities by ordering them from left to right. It is useful to accompany the diagram with a written account of the task. Sometimes task flow diagrams are produced, which show the specific details of current processes and can include details of interactions between the user and the current system, or other individuals, and any problems related to them. They can be used to highlight areas where task processes are poorly understood, or are carried out differently by different staff, or are inconsistent with the higher-level task structure. To ensure the outputs accurately represent the task, it is important to present the resulting analysis to someone else who has not been involved in the decomposition but who knows the task well enough to check for accuracy and consistency.

Organising the results of the data collection into clear statements and/or diagrams describing the task requirements and goals enables the task to be analysed systematically. The resulting task diagram provides a broad overview of the task and helps to highlight areas for further investigation. Types of possible task diagram that can be produced are:

- task outlines – good for illustrating sequential tasks
- flow charts and task steps – useful for understanding a process and identifying bottlenecks
- hierarchies and network diagrams – helpful for depicting relationships

- workflow diagrams – good for demonstrating a sequence of work-related operations of an individual, group or organisation.

Providing clear representation of the collected task data serves three purposes.
1. The resulting data can be used to present the findings to the wider team so the task analysis can be validated and approved by the users.
2. Written and/or graphical representation can help to clarify the complexities of the task.
3. The way in which the task is represented will assist in developing solutions to improve the effectiveness, safety and efficiency of the task.[11]

Many different approaches are available and there is no one ideal method. The method chosen should be based on the purpose of the output (e.g. error identification or training needs analysis), design phase and/or expertise of the analyst.

One of the most well-known and commonly used methods is hierarchical task analysis, which produces a nested hierarchy of goals, operations and plans. It arose out of the need to understand the components of complex real world tasks in safety-critical industries. Another approach is procedural task analysis. It breaks down each of the individual steps and decisions that are required to achieve it and allows identification of the information, devices and clinical or non-clinical staff involved in each task. This method is useful for identifying points within a task that are challenging, are time-consuming, result in errors or are in other ways inefficient or hazardous (e.g. results handling).

Other task analysis methods include:
- tabular task analysis
- GOMS (Goals, Operators, Methods and Selection rules)
- cognitive task analysis.[5]

The task analysis methods described in this chapter focus on providing a *physical* description of the tasks and activities taking place within a system. A number of other methods exist that can be used to explore the *cognitive* processes used by people in the system. These cognitive task analysis methods can be used to explore, describe and represent cognitive elements such as decision-making and judgements. A number of different approaches are available (e.g. cognitive work analysis, applied cognitive task analysis, cognitive walk-through). The outputs of these types of analyses can be used to guide interface design, evaluation of training procedures and the evaluation of team performance in complex systems.[8] Cognitive task analyses can be very time-consuming and rely on the users to recall events or incidents in the past and be able to explain their cognitive processes when performing tasks.

Conduct further human factors analysis

The outputs produced by task analysis methods are useful as they provide a step-by-step description of the activity under analysis and are often required by further human factors analysis activities such as usability evaluation, human error identification or performance evaluation. Whatever method is used to describe and represent the tasks, the resulting output can be analysed in a number of different ways. Stammers and Shepherd[11] describe how task analysis produces the following kinds of information that can be used for follow-on analysis:

- identification of tasks and subtask components
- grouping of components
- importance, priority and critically of subtasks
- frequency of subtasks
- sequence of subtasks
- decisions that must be made
- trigger conditions for subtasks
- goals for task or subtask
- performance criteria for each subtask
- information required by each subtask
- information generated by each subtask
- knowledge of the system employed in making decisions – understanding the users must have of the system and its functions in order to fulfil their role
- identification of potential errors and hazards.

PRACTICAL CONSIDERATIONS
How long should each analysis take?
Most task analysis methods are easy to learn and apply and can be conducted by non-human factors specialists, although it can be time-consuming and labour intensive to gather and analyse the data. The length of time spent conducting a task analysis will vary widely depending on the expertise of the analyst, the nature and complexity of the task, and the level of detail generated in the task decomposition.

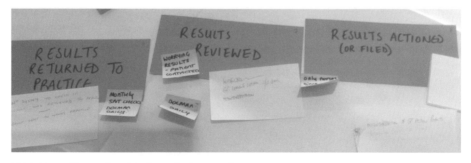

FIGURE 7.1 Example of task analysis raw data output

What resources should be involved?
It is unlikely that practices and most healthcare organisations will choose to train up specialists to conduct task analysis – so are more likely to conduct

them largely on their own. They should, therefore, make use of groups and workshops to ensure that end users (e.g. staff or patients) are involved in the process. No additional specific additional resources are needed. Specialist computer programs exist to facilitate task analysis – however, Post-it notes, pens and paper can often suffice (*see* Figure 7.1).

SUMMARY

Task analysis methods include a wide variety of techniques that can be applied by front-line staff in a primary care setting to consider the human element of their systems. The advantages of these types of improvement methods are as follows.

- Task analysis is highly adaptable, useful and flexible and it provides a step-by-step description of the task under analysis, which is often the first time this has been undertaken.
- Most methods are easy to learn and apply and can be conducted by non-human factors specialists.
- Using task analysis methods allows the practice to gain a deeper understanding of the task, system or scenario under analysis.
- The outputs (especially the graphical representation) are useful for communicating findings with the wider team.
- The outputs are important for inputting into further human factors analysis methods (e.g. human error identification, training needs analysis).

CASE STUDY: SAFE TEST ORDERING AND RESULTS HANDLING

This case study illustrates the impact that can be achieved in a primary case setting by using task analysis methods.

Background and aims

The systems-based management of laboratory test ordering and results handling is a significant source of error in primary care. Evidence-based guidance is required to assist care teams with minimising the risk associated with the test ordering and results handling system to improve patient safety. The study sought to build consensus on 'good practice' guidance statements to inform the implementation of safe systems for ordering laboratory tests and managing results.

Method

An initial workshop was conducted to identify the tasks for analysis. Seven subsequent workshops were run with a range of clinical and non-clinical staff (e.g. practice nurses, reception staff, general practitioners) to gain an understanding of the test ordering and results handling process. The process was then broken down into a number of high-level subtasks based on the conceptual model of the testing process developed by Hickner *et al.*,[12] who divided the process into three key phases:

1. Pre-Analytic Phase – structured around ordering and implementing test
2. Analytic Phase – lab analysis (out of scope)
3. Post-Analytic Phase – tracking *and* returning the test, responding to and documenting the results, notifying patient of results, following up with needed action.

The data were then described and represented in a resulting task flow diagram (*see* Figure 7.2), which identified the key steps in the process and the main transitions where communication of information is critical.

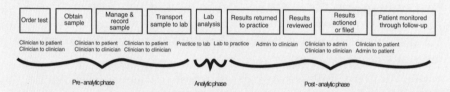

FIGURE 7.2 Task analysis for test ordering and results handling

To gain approval of the task decomposition and task flow diagram, six primary care practice visits were conducted. The output from the task analysis was used to structure the visits to:

- confirm that a complete set of pre- and post-analytic steps had been identified from the workshops for the test ordering and results handling process
- identify examples of where potential errors could occur at each step in the generic process
- identify examples of good practice activities currently used in practices to reduce the likelihood of these errors occurring.

A range of human factors data collection methods was used during the practice visits. The task analysis diagram developed as an output from the workshops was used as a checklist pro forma to conduct a 'walk-through/talk-through'[5] analysis of the process steps. Each step was considered separately, along with transitions between each step, and each person who interacted with that step was identified and then encouraged to 'think aloud'[13] as they worked through performing activities. The analysis took place for each person who had a role at that step in his or her normal workspace (i.e. general practitioner at his desk, administrative staff at the reception desk or in the back office and healthcare assistant in treatment room). As well as clarifying and approving the task analysis output, further analysis was conducted by encouraging each clinical and/or non-clinical member of staff to identify opportunities for error during his or her steps and to describe how the practice had barriers in place to reduce the likelihood of those errors occurring. In addition to documenting these errors and good practice activities, observations (e.g. where blood samples were stored) were made and photographs were taken where appropriate.

Key findings

The research highlighted that no one single issue or task step is responsible for errors in the process and no one type of 'good practice' activity would solve the problems that can occur. It was recommended that a system-wide approach be implemented with multiple checks put in place.

Project outputs

Each step in the generic process was analysed and reported in the following ways.
- *Issue*: each issue was assigned a high-level category of communication, system or process issues.
- *Description*: a description of the issue or potential error or human failure.
- *Identified good practice*: examples of good practice were identified and generated as 'good practice statements' for each task step. The resulting outputs are being generated as guidance documents for primary care practices.[14]

Summary

This case study illustrates how a number of convergent methods were systematically applied to obtain task analysis data. The outputs of the tasks analysis were subsequently used for further error analysis and for the development of good practice statements and guidance.

FURTHER READING

The following documents offer more guidance on task analysis methods:
- www.ahrq.gov/downloads/pub/advances/vol2/karsh.pdf
- www.who.int/hrh/tools/job_analysis.pdf

REFERENCES

1. Preece J, Rogers Y, Sharp H. *Interaction Design: beyond human-computer interaction.* New York, NY: John Wiley & Sons; 2002.
2. Energy Institute. *Human Factors Briefing Note Number 11: task analysis.* London: Energy Institute: 2011. Available at: www.energypublishing.org/publication/ei-technical-publications/process-safety/management-systems/human-factors-briefing-note-no.-11-task-analysis (accessed 12 November 2013).
3. Reason J. Combating omission errors through task analysis and good reminders. *Qual Saf Health Care.* 2000; **11**(1): 40–4.
4. Embrey D. *Task Analysis Techniques.* Human Reliability Associates; 2000. Available

at: www.cwsvt.com/Conference/Functional%20Assessment/Task%20Analysis%20Techniques.pdf (accessed 18 October 2013).

5. Kirwan B, Ainsworth L. *A Guide to Task Analysis*. London: Taylor & Francis; 1999.

6. Stanton N, Salmon P, Walker G, *et al*. *Human Factors Methods: a practical guide for engineering and design*. Aldershot: Ashgate; 2005.

7. Rail Safety and Standards Board. *Understanding Human Factors: a guide for the railway industry*. London: RSSB; 2008.

8. Jordan P. *An Introduction to Usability*. London: Taylor & Francis; 1998.

9. Clinical Human Factors Group. *Implementing Human Factors in Healthcare: 'taking further steps'*. 'How To' Guide: Volume 2. CHFG; 2013. Available at: www.chfg.org/wp-content/uploads/2013/05/Implementing-human-factors-in-healthcare-How-to-guide-volume-2-FINAL-2013_05_16.pdf (accessed 29 October 2013).

10. Shepherd A. *Hierarchical Task Analysis*. New York, NY: Harper & Row; 2001.

11. Shepherd A, Stammers RB. Task analysis. In: Wilson JR, Corlett N, editors. *Evaluation of Human Work*. 3rd ed. Boca Raton, FL: CRC Press; 2005. pp. 129–57.

12. Hickner J, Fernald D, Harris D, *et al*. Issues and initiatives in the testing process in primary care physician offices. *J Qual Patient Saf*. 2005; **31**(2): 81–9.

13. Jordan P. *Designing Pleasurable Products: an introduction to the new human factors*. London: Taylor & Francis; 2000.

14. Bowie P, Forrest E, Price J, *et al*. Expert consensus on safe laboratory test ordering and results management systems in European primary care. *Eur J Gen Pract*. In press.

CHAPTER 8

Process mapping

Brian James

INTRODUCTION

The world does not change itself in the social milieu – people change the world, sometimes on purpose. If quality improvement (QI) methods are considered as ways of getting better at purposeful change, 'process mapping'[1] would be the equivalent of a QI Swiss army knife. Process mapping is a versatile and simple technique that can be used at many different stages in a QI project, or when redesigning a system or introducing a new care service. For the purposes of this chapter, it will be considered as anything that organises or maps system processes in or between workplaces.

The approach can help map a whole patient journey or the steps in a work process with the help of people who represent all of the different roles involved. In doing this, opportunities for improvement can be visualised and it can pinpoint areas of inefficiency in a process by identifying duplication, variation and unnecessary steps – it also helps the care team to develop good ideas and focus on where to start to make improvements that will have the greatest impact in improving care quality for patients. A range of practical benefits using this approach is reported in the evidence base, which outlines potential clinical benefit across a variety of specialties, multidisciplinary teams and healthcare systems.[2-4]

To understand how process mapping might best be used, it is useful to first consider a conceptual model of QI methods (*see* Figure 8.1).[5]

QI in healthcare can be defined as the planned interaction between 'technical/rational approaches to change' on the one hand, with 'social psychological (behavioural) approaches to change' on the other, in order to achieve improved patient and care outcomes. While much QI literature specifically identifies the importance of combining these two approaches to achieve sustainable improvement, there is little consideration of *how* they should best interact.[6-8] The nature of the interactions between these two processes (whether positive or negative) is often the major determinant of an improvement initiative's success.

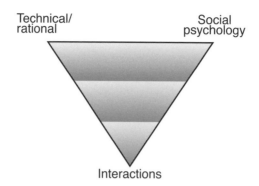

FIGURE 8.1 A conceptual model of quality improvement methods

In Figure 8.1 the inverted triangle can be likened to a spinning top, with the 'interactions' at the bottom providing the momentum and fulcrum that keeps the top (technical and social processes) spinning.[5] The model's key implication is that everyone, whether senior leadership or front-line staff, has a responsibility for ensuring the interactions between 'rational/technical' and 'social/psychological/behavioural' processes remain positive. Staff engagement is therefore a vital component of any successful improvement initiative.[9]

Social psychological approaches to change

Just a couple of concepts will be used to illustrate the importance of the right-hand side of the triangle. QI is a complex social intervention.[10] Without engagement at all levels it is unlikely to succeed, be sustained and spread. The most commonly cited reason for QI projects to fail is mismanagement of the human dimensions of change.[9] A key concept is that the external manifestation of improvement is change, but transition is a psychological process internal to each individual involved in the change that they go through in order to come to terms with the new situation.

Three consecutive stages of transition have been described:
1. the ending, where something needs to be let go
2. the neutral zone, where the old way has gone but the new way has not yet taken hold (a state of flux)
3. the beginning, when the new way feels like the norm.[11]

How might a leader translate insight of these stages into supportive action?

Individuals vary in their readiness for change. Rogers[12] divides people into five categories according to their willingness to adopt innovations:
1. Innovators
2. Early adopters
3. Early majority
4. Late majority
5. Laggards.

QI projects should therefore recruit the innovators, who in turn recruit the early adopters and so on until, finally, the laggards are also recruited. The term 'Laggards' may seem pejorative but it includes a heterogeneous group, including people with valid reasons to resist change. Taking their concerns seriously could therefore pay dividends. Resistance to change is in many cases a normal and necessary response. Rather than simply being wilful, resistance is a sign of a group's resilience, with individuals adhering to coherent group standards.[13]

QI depends greatly on accessing the collective knowledge, wisdom and experience of the people in clinical teams. They should therefore be considered active participants, rather than passive targets. Effective 'leadership for improvement' facilitates transitions by informing, involving, engaging, and empowering staff participation. Leadership utilises their knowledge, skills and energy in imaginative ways to deliver reliable improvement by integrating change (and associated data collection) into existing work tasks. Key concepts include 'shared mental models', 'pull rather than push' motivators, and 'coaching and facilitation'.[14] From the technical/rational side of the model, process mapping tools are ideal for empowering staff participation.

PROCESS MAPPING

Process mapping tools range from the very simple to the extremely complex, but their purpose is to expose, scrutinise and analyse system processes. This is done in order to achieve two main aims: (1) understand the problem and (2) understand the solution.

There are three general *questions* to consider when creating process maps.

1. *What is the scope of the process?* That is, where does it begin and where does it end? For example, do general practitioner appointments start with patients coming through the surgery door, the clinician's door or when they drive into the premises of the surgery?
2. *Do all the steps or stages have clear definitions?* In other words, would you recognise a step in practice and would someone else recognise it too? It is essential to establish *shared* definitions.
3. *Does the map represent what actually happens?* This will be more likely if participants/stakeholders from all different parts of the process are involved, engaged and utilised in change, in identifying problems, analysing and understanding the causes of errors (and potential errors) and identifying, agreeing and testing solutions.

Often, there is an incorrect assumption that the problem is known. For example: 'The problem is no one is completing the referral form', when the actual problem is that there are no referral forms available to complete. The available methods to help teams and organisations correctly identify and understand the problem(s) can broadly be grouped into two types – diverging and converging methods. Examples are shown in Box 8.1. The methods are typically applied in a group context and a 'neutral' group facilitator can be a real asset. A number of methods are briefly discussed here.

BOX 8.1 Examples of diverging and converging process mapping methods

Diverging methods	Converging methods
• Brainstorming	• Dot voting
• 'High level' and 'detailed level' process mapping	• Force field analysis
	• Fishbone (Ishikawa) diagrams
• Patient shadowing	• Measurement/data/baseline
• Patient stories	• Pareto analysis

'High level' and 'detailed level' process mapping

A 'high level' process map is made when a small group of people quickly map out the major steps of a process. This can then be followed by a 'detailed level' process map. Participants often comment that, until they had mapped out their processes, they did not realise that they did not understand them. An example of a simple annotated process map is shown in Figure 8.2.

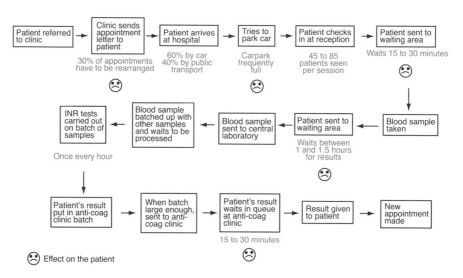

THE ANTICOAGULANT BLOOD TESTING PROCESS

FIGURE 8.2 An example of a simple process map[8]

Patient shadowing

Patient shadowing, or process activity mapping, is a method that provides a detailed snapshot of the patient journey and is best constructed by literally shadowing a patient. The steps in a detailed level map are numbered sequentially. Data are recorded in the table, such as the time taken for each step.

Having developed the map, questions can then be asked about the data. For example, 'How much time is spent between various activities?' Further analysis can be carried out – for example, using a Pareto chart to determine if there is 'waste' and if so, where it is occurring.

Dot voting

This is a useful method to include during a brainstorming session or when a process map or an affinity diagram has been created. With the dot voting method, every group member receives 10 'sticky' dots (the kind used on wall-charts). Everyone votes on the issues to prioritise. All 10 votes can be used for one thing, or they can be spread out.

Step 1: Identify the beginning and end of the process

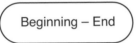

Step 2: Brainstorm potential solutions, activities or required steps and write them on Post-it notes

Solution/
Activity/Step

Step 3: Stick Post-its on a blank wall and insert decision points (yes/no)

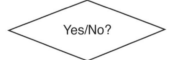

Step 4: Add where data are needed (and what they are)

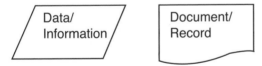

Step 5: Insert parallel steps/activities, feedback loops

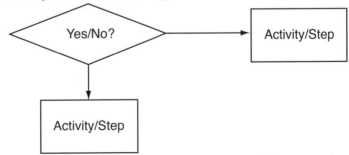

Step 6: The group organises and reorganises until they are satisfied with the proposed solutions before asking for stakeholder feedback

FIGURE 8.3 Practical steps to construct a flow chart of possible solutions

Force field analysis

Force field analysis is a method to analyse the causes of a problem. It is a particularly effective way to ensure clinical engagement if the person analysing the causes was involved in identifying the causes. Force field analysis allows the drivers and restraints to change to be compared and 'balanced'.[15]

Fishbone (Ishikawa) diagram

Fishbone diagrams (or Ishikawa diagrams) allow the graphical depiction of cause and effect. The head of the fish represents the problem, while the ribs represent all the possible causes in different categories.

Pareto chart

A Pareto chart can be used to identify the area with the greatest potential for improvement and for its visual impact. A Pareto chart is based on the 20/80 principle, where 20% of causes may be responsible for 80% of problems. Similarly, 20% effort could translate into 80% improvement.

Flow charts

By convention, flow charts are constructed from top to bottom. 'Yes' responses are placed on the vertical axis and 'no' responses on the horizontal axis. The practical steps involved in constructing a flow chart for helping groups to understand their potential solutions are shown in Figure 8.3.

TASK ANALYSIS VERSUS PROCESS MAPPING

In the interests of clarity and to avoid any potential confusion, there may appear to be superficial similarities between task analysis (*see* Chapter 7) and process mapping in that they both come from the same 'family' of mapping techniques. However, there are very clear differences. Task analysis is used to describe and represent the human and system performance of a particular workplace task. It is typically used for understanding the human–technology and human–human interactions and for breaking down very specific work tasks (actions and cognitive processes) into component steps or physical operations.

On the other hand, process mapping is used to generate a visual representation of work procedures in terms of the human and system elements (e.g. patient journey maps). It typically uses standardised symbols to graphically represent task sequences or processes in terms of component steps, sequential flow of the tasks, temporal aspects of the task, collaboration between different agents who perform each step and any technology or equipment used to perform the steps. It only takes into account error-free performance and does not represent the individual human cognitive (thinking) processes involved in work task and system performance.

SUMMARY

Process mapping techniques confer a number of potential benefits for primary care teams in improving the quality of care and services (particularly business efficiency) they provide to their patients.[6] These benefits can include:

- acting as a starting point for an improvement project specific for your own place of work
- creating a culture of ownership, responsibility and accountability for your team
- illustrating a patient pathway or process, understanding it from a patient's perspective
- acting as an aid or prompt to plan changes more effectively
- collecting ideas, often from staff who understand the system but who rarely contribute to change and improvement
- acting as an interactive means to engage staff in a meaningful improvement activity
- developing an end product (a process map) that is easy to understand and highly visual.

FURTHER READING

- Fishbone diagram and Five Why's method: www.nrls.npsa.nhs.uk/resources/?entryid45=75605
- Nominal Group technique: www.nrls.npsa.nhs.uk/resources/?entryid45=75604
- Timeline charting: www.nrls.npsa.nhs.uk/resources/?entryid45=75603
- Barrier Analysis Tool: www.nrls.npsa.nhs.uk/resources/?entryid45=75606
- Brainstorming: www.businessballs.com/brainstorming.htm and www.mindtools.com/brainstm.html

REFERENCES

1. Trebble TM, Hansi N, Hydes T, *et al.* Process mapping the patient journey: an introduction. *BMJ.* 2010; **341**: c4078.
2. NHS Modernisation Agency. *Process Mapping, Analysis and Redesign.* London: Department of Health; 2005.
3. Taylor AJ, Randall C. Process mapping: enhancing the implementation of the Liverpool care pathway. *Int J Palliat Nurs.* 2007; **13**(4): 163–7.
4. Ben-Tovim DI, Dougherty ML, O'Connell TJ, *et al.* Patient journeys: the process of clinical redesign. *Med J Aust.* 2008; **188**(Suppl. 6): S14–17.
5. James B, Beattie M, Shepherd A. *Quality and Safety in Practice: why theory matters* [Poster]. Enhancing Nursing Through Educational Research (ENTER): Inaugural Scottish Conference, University of Stirling, Scotland; 2012 November 28.
6. King DL, Ben-Tovim DI, Bassham J. Redesigning emergency department patient flows: application of Lean Thinking to health care. *Emerg Med Australas.* 2006; **18**(4): 391–7.
7. Deming W. *The New Economics.* 2nd ed. Cambridge, MA: MIT Press; 1994.

8. NHS Institute for Innovation and Improvement. *Quality and Service Improvement Tools. (2006–2011).* Coventry: NHS III. Available at: www.institute.nhs.uk/option,com_quality _and_service_improvement_tools/Itemid,5015.html (accessed 8 February 2013).

9. NHS Institute for Innovation and Improvement. *Managing the Human Dimensions of Change.* Coventry: NHS III; 2005.

10. Boaden R, Harvey G, Moxham C, *et al. Quality Improvement: theory and practice in healthcare.* Coventry: University of Warwick and NHS Institute for Innovation and Improvement; 2008.

11. Bridges W. *Managing Transitions: making the most of change.* Perseus Books Group, HarperCollins Publishers, New York, 1991.

12. Rogers E. *Diffusion of Innovations.* New York, NY: The Free Press; 1985.

13. Plsek P, Greenhalgh T. The challenge of complexity in health care. *BMJ.* 2001; **323**(7313): 625–8. Available at: www.ncbi.nlm.nih.gov/pmc/articles/PMC1121189/ pdf/625.pdf (accessed 10 November 2010).

14. Senge P. *The Fifth Discipline: the art and practice of the learning organisation.* 2nd ed. London: Random House Business Books; 2006.

15. Darnton A. *Reference Report: an overview of behaviour change models and their uses.* Government Social Research Service; 2008. Available at: www.civilservice.gov.uk/ wp-content/uploads/2011/09/Behaviour_change_reference_report_tcm6-9697.pdf (accessed 31 October 2013).

CHAPTER 9

Policies, protocols and procedures

Marion Foster & Paul Bowie

INTRODUCTION

Human memory and attention are imperfect, whether in the home or in the workplace. As a consequence, we all make mistakes. One way to mitigate errors or lapses in concentrations during everyday work tasks is through the use of policies, protocols and procedures (PPPs). The use of PPPs to improve the safety or reliability of work-based processes is standard practice in high-reliability industries, most notably in commercial aviation and petrochemical organisations. High reliability is an essential characteristic of any safe healthcare service. One way to ensure this is to standardise processes, where possible. Well-designed PPPs, therefore, have a critical importance as safeguards against potential healthcare risks[1] and breaching of statutory and contractual obligations.[2]

Unfortunately, there is still wide variation in the quality of care that is delivered in all healthcare settings.[3-8] Given what is known about human error theory and the often significant differences between general practice teams with regard to their culture, geographic, socio-economic contexts and available resources, variation may arguably be inevitable. However, when the variation is significant, so that fundamental and safety-critical tasks are inadequately performed (e.g. monitoring of patients prescribed disease-modifying anti-rheumatic drugs), the increased risk of harm to patients, and hence the practice, becomes unacceptable.

In recent years, major efforts have been made in most modern healthcare systems worldwide to improve the safety, effectiveness and reliability of patient care. In Scotland, these policy ambitions are clearly outlined in the national Quality Strategy and in the goals of the Scottish Patient Safety Programme.[9] Building a safety improvement culture in practices will be a key factor in reducing preventable harm and enhancing the effectiveness and efficiency of the care we provide to patients.[10,11] The National Patient Safety Agency recommends the integration of *risk management activity* within general practices as one way to achieve this: 'manage your risks and identify and assess things that could go wrong by developing systems and processes documented in the practice Policies, Protocols and Procedures'.[10]

This chapter discusses the important role of PPPs in supporting many aspects of everyday busy general practice. It is also a simple 'how-to' guide and offers practical recommendations for practice managers or anyone else tasked with the design, development and writing of PPPs.

DIFFERENTIATING BETWEEN POLICIES, PROTOCOL AND PROCEDURES

The following practical example illustrates the relation between the three terms: policy, protocol and procedure. A practice manager designed and wrote a new document: 'How to Register a New Patient'. This document explains how the practice deals with potential new patients and it is the *policy* of the practice. The *protocol* outlines the 'rules' that the practice will abide by during this process, and the *procedures* are the step-by-step instructions (the 'how-to' guide) explaining to staff exactly what they should do.

A simplified description, therefore, is that policies represent the 'external face' of the practice and procedures the 'internal face'. Practices tend to have fewer policies than procedures. Policies are normally freely available to staff, patients and the public, whereas procedures are normally only available to staff.

'Policy', 'protocol' and 'procedure' are terms that are often used interchangeably and which can be misunderstood. They are also sometimes confused with another commonly used term, 'guideline'. It is therefore important to be able to define each term and understand that they have different purposes (*see* Table 9.1).

- *Policies*: these are guiding principles that underpin service issues or topics of high importance and are practice specific. They are designed to ensure that high-level objectives of the team are delivered.
- *Protocols*: a protocol defines a set of procedures or steps to be followed for the accomplishment of a given task. In other words, to obtain a desired outcome, the protocol associated with the completion of a task (procedure) should be adhered to. Protocols are problem-oriented, measurable standards that determine a course of action to be taken. They comprise a *mandatory* set of decision-making rules, instructions or standards based on evidence-based guidelines or best practice specific to the organisation or general practice. Deviation from protocols can lead to confusion, misunderstanding and miscommunication – known contributory factors to many patient safety incidents.
- *Procedures*: these are about the required tasks to implement a policy. They are normally written as a series of steps and can usually be presented as a flow chart.
- *Guideline*: a guideline is a set of systematically developed standards or rules that assist in the decision about how to apply the policy or appropriate management of specific conditions. Guidelines are often used to underpin a policy.

TABLE 9.1 A comparison of the terms 'policy', 'protocol' and 'procedure'

	Policy	Protocol	Procedure
Meaning (definition)	Describes the team's commitment to key determinants of quality and safety	A mandatory set of standards based on best available evidence	Based on policies and procedures – it is the recipe to enact policies
	Guiding principles of the practice		Provides specific, step-by-step instructions: who does what, when and how
	The basis for procedures and protocols		
	Policies signpost what should be done, rather than how		
Nature and scope	Covers a broad range of activities and often intangible or less precise than protocols and procedures		Tangible, succinct, precise, exact and factual
Type of writing required	Standard sentence and paragraph format		Best expressed through special formats including playscripts, flow charts, lists and checklists

POTENTIAL BENEFITS OF POLICIES, PROTOCOLS AND PROCEDURES

All general practice teams should have effective clinical and administrative systems in place to ensure the delivery of safety and effective care. Clearly written and well-designed PPPs help to render these systems and tasks visible and can standardise and support them with a number of important potential benefits:

- improved efficiency of staff time and effort
- as a decision aid when important issues arise
- reduce conflict and the potential for misunderstanding within the team by depersonalising issues
- eliminate duplication (reinventing the wheel)
- provide the team, patients and stakeholders with clear information of everyone's rights, roles and responsibilities
- ensure stability and continuity of care during staff transitions
- decrease training time (e.g. for new staff or locums)
- clearly states the practice's future aims and intended direction
- simplify access to information
- act as a reminder to periodically review existing safety systems and services to ensure they are still fit for purpose.

However, the potential benefits of PPPs – as effective safeguards against potential harm while increasing workplace efficiency – are rarely fully realised. Analysis of incident reports and complaints[12-14] has shown the following.

- Compliance with PPPs is variable. Paradoxically, they seem to be followed less in those cases where they are arguably needed the most.
- Some practices do not have PPPs, while in others they are inadequate with evidence that the content was not always properly thought through.

- The very people they were developed for and who should apply them do not always understand them.
- The wider practice team is seldom involved in the development stage, which can cause them to feel disenchanted and thereby cause them to disengage with the PPPs.
- The written quality of some PPPs is poor, so that interpreting them becomes ambiguous, inconsistent or incoherent.
- PPPs are not always disseminated appropriately, so that team members may be unaware of their existence or where and how to access them.

In other words, there is evidence to suggest that many practices do not have 'fit for purpose' PPPs, and even when they do, these may not be 'living documents' that are used regularly by all relevant staff and updated and reviewed periodically. The implication is that there may be a need for practical guidance to help practice managers (and others) to design, develop and implement PPPs in an effective manner.

RECOMMENDATIONS FOR WRITING EFFECTIVE POLICIES, PROTOCOLS AND PROCEDURES[15–17]

PPPs are more likely to be used and be useful if they are clearly written. There are at least three rules of thumb that can help to achieve this goal: (1) keep the structure simple, (2) use everyday language that readers will understand easily and immediately and (3) be specific: mean what you say and say what you mean. A number of practical 'tips' to help produce clear and well-written PPPs are provided in Box 9.1.

Policy

- A policy addresses what the rule is, rather than how to implement it.
- The policy should deal with issues that are important (what staff need to know and want to know about).
- It should be consistent with the practice's overall vision.
- State who the policy is intended for and what the consequences are of non-compliance.
- There should be no duplication or contradiction of other policies.
- The content should be presented in an unambiguous, clear and concise manner, written in simple, everyday language.
- It should be implementable, compliant with legislation and draw on available evidence.
- Informed by relevant stakeholder input and feedback.
- It should be accessible.
- It should be reviewed and updated periodically.
- Try to use a standard template for all policies of the practice; as a minimum it should have the name of the practice, the date it was issued and the intended review date, the name of the person responsible for the policy and page numbers and total number of pages (e.g. page 2 of 14).

BOX 9.1 Practical 'tips' for clear and well-written policies, protocols and procedures

Keep the structure simple

- Use gender-neutral language – 'their' instead of 'he/she'
- Use short sentences (maximum of 15 words)
- Use short paragraphs (maximum of 100 words for policies; maximum 40 words for procedures)
- Use lists where possible – it makes the information easier to read and encourages short sentences
- List steps to follow in order to comply with a policy
- List responsibility for each step; use one action per step – steps that contain more than one action can confuse the reader
- Do not make assumptions about the reader's background knowledge
- Order the sequence
- Number points to facilitate referencing. Use 1, 2, 3, not one, two, three
- Use headings to help organise information
- Be consistent – repetition of terms increase the reader's retention

Use everyday language that readers will easily and immediately understand

- Use short words (one or two syllables)
- Use common words (e.g. 'use' instead of 'utilise')
- Use active rather than passive language
- Write as you would speak, editing out informal words or phrases
- Avoid the use of jargon, unnecessary technical expressions and fancy vocabulary
- Avoid the use of abbreviations or acronyms; if acronyms are necessary, use the full title/term first before using the acronym
- Avoid too much detail – additional information can be provided as links to the document

Be specific: mean what you say and say what you mean

- If action is mandatory, use the words 'must' or 'will'. If the action is recommended or if valid reasons to deviate from the requirement exist in particular circumstances, then use 'should'. If the action is permissive, use 'may'.
- Avoid using the word 'shall' unless there is a legislative requirement than prescribes its use. This word causes confusion between whether an action is mandatory or recommended.

Procedure

- Demonstrate the link between the proposed procedure and the practice policy.
- Describe the benefits to the staff members who have to follow the procedure.
- Engage the intended users during the development process – what are they already doing and how do they think this could be improved?
- Try to provide staff with options and explain possible instances where procedures may have to be flexible or may not be appropriate.
- Use the 'if . . . then' method and write with a single person in mind, describing the condition and action. For example, 'IF the fire alarm sounds [condition], THEN stop what you are doing and evacuate the premises [action].

UNWRITTEN POLICIES, PROTOCOLS AND PROCEDURES

There is a real danger of creating a policy or procedure for everything. When there are too many, it becomes difficult to manage them and staff begin to ignore them because of 'information overload'. So, paradoxically, too many PPPs can become a hazard and a barrier to safe and effective care processes.

TABLE 9.2 Examples of instances when a policy or procedure could be left unwritten or, conversely, should be written up

Leave unwritten if . . .	Write it up when . . .
it involves organisational culture and norms	unwritten rules that have been working well informally begin to break down
it cannot be enforced (if a member of staff realises that enforcement of a policy is lax, they think the same of all of the policies)	the practice grows, change increases and/or complexity arises
there will still be inconsistency	when the following happen: • accidents (involving injury or non-injury) • changes • complaints (internal and external) • confusion • cost overruns • external events or trends that have an impact (e.g. no-smoking policy) • frequent or recurrent questions • high waste factors • inconsistency • misunderstandings • changes in laws, regulations and contracts • sensitivity, volatility, stress or frustration • unique interpretations of unwritten policies or procedures

It is therefore acceptable, even desirable, to have unwritten policies and procedures, since it is impossible to write everything down. However, it is important to remain vigilant for signs that informal, unwritten rules are no longer sufficient or appropriate. Table 9.2 outlines some of the instances in which one would consider leaving a policy or procedure unwritten and, conversely, consider changing a policy from unwritten to written.

CONCLUSION

Implementation of PPPs is not always successful. They are 'technical solutions'[18] that are introduced into the complex, dynamic working environment of general medical practice. Pre-existing issues such as an overly controlling team hierarchy, poor team working, inadequate internal communication systems or an underdeveloped safety culture may have to be addressed first to create a suitable environment for their introduction.[19]

Some clinicians and managers may also resist or feel threatened by PPPs because they perceive them as impinging on their expertise, interfering with their decision-making or oversimplifying the working environment. This is particularly so when there is too much emphasis on protocols, which can lead to disengagement by staff and can draw their attention away from common practice problems – these need to have high value among those who are expected to use them and be simple so that they can be followed and understood. Otherwise steps will be skipped, particularly when staff are very busy or stressed, or staff will avoid using them altogether.[18,19]

Additionally, there is variation in perceptions of local safety climate within and between general practice teams. Similar variation exists in the strength of team working, the maturity of the learning environment and overall commitment to quality improvement in general practices.[20,21] Taking heed of these types of cultural issues is therefore equally important to supporting PPP development and implementation and essential if the whole team is to be engaged.

REFERENCES

1. Spath PL. *Error Reduction in Health Care: a systems approach to improving patient safety.* 2nd ed. San Francisco, CA: Jossey-Bass; 2011.
2. Primary and Community Care Directorate, The Scottish Government. *Clinical and Staff Governance for General Practice in Scotland.* Edinburgh: The Scottish Government; 2010. Available at: www.sehd.scot.nhs.uk/pca/PCA2010(M)18.pdf (accessed 9 September 2011).
3. Hines S, Joshi MS. Variation in quality of care within health systems. *Jt Comm J Qual Patient Saf.* 2008; **34**(6): 326–32.
4. Resar RK. Making noncatastrophic health care processes reliable: learning to walk before running in creating high-reliability organizations. *Health Serv Res.* 2006; **41** (4 Pt. 2): 1677–89.
5. Holmboe ES, Weng W, Arnold GK, *et al.* The comprehensive care project: measuring

physician performance in ambulatory practice. *Health Serv Res.* 2010; **45**(6 Pt. 2): 1912–33.

6. Tsimtsiou Z, Ashworth M, Jones R. Variations in anxiolytic and hypnotic prescribing by GPs: a cross-sectional analysis using data from the UK Quality and Outcomes Framework. *Br J Gen Pract.* 2009; **59**(563): e191–8.

7. Morrison J, Anderson MJ, Sutton M, *et al.* Factors influencing variation in prescribing of antidepressants by general practices in Scotland. *Br J Gen Pract.* 2009; **59**(559): e25–31.

8. Wang KY, Seed P, Schofield P, *et al.* Which practices are high antibiotic prescribers? A cross-sectional analysis. *Br J Gen Pract.* 2009; **59**(567): e315–20.

9. NHS Scotland. *Welcome to the Scottish Patient Safety Programme.* Edinburgh: NHS Scotland; 2013. Available at: www.scottishpatientsafetyprogramme.scot.nhs.uk/programme (accessed 5 April 2013).

10. National Patient Safety Agency. *Seven Steps to Patient Safety for Primary Care.* London: NPSA; 2009. Available at: www.nrls.npsa.nhs.uk/resources/?EntryId45=59804 (accessed 12 November 2013).

11. Kizer K. *Large System Change and a Culture of Safety: enhancing patient safety and reducing errors in health care.* Chicago, IL: National Patient Safety Foundation; 1999.

12. Kennedy I. *Learning from Bristol: the report of the public inquiry into children's heart surgery at the Bristol Royal Infirmary 1984–1995.* Command Paper CM5207. London: HMSO; 2001.

13. Kotter J. Leading change: why transformation efforts fail. *Harv Bus Rev.* 2007; **85**(1): 96–10.

14. Kohn L, Corrigan JM, Donaldson MS, editors. *To Err is Human: building a safer health system.* Washington, DC: National Academy Press; 2000.

15. Campbell. Nancy J. *Writing Effective Policies and Procedures.* New York, NY: AMACOM; 1998.

16. Dew J, Curtis MR. *Procedure Writing.* Available at: http://bama.ua.edu/~st497/pdf/procedurewriting.pdf (accessed 12 November 2013).

17. Edgerton E, Nicholson J. *The 'How To' of 'How To's': writing procedures like a pro* [Handout]. Dayton, OH: Woolpert; 2000. Presented at the STC 47th Annual Conference, Orlando, Florida; 2000 May 22. Available at: http://classes.engr.oregonstate.edu/mime/winter2011/ie366-001/Other_Resources/WE3M-Writing-Procedures.pdf (accessed 12 November 2013).

18. Bosk CL, Dixon-Woods M, Goeschel CA, *et al.* The art of medicine: reality check for checklists. *Lancet.* 2009; **374**(9688): 444–5.

19. de Wet C, Johnson P, Mash R, *et al.* Measuring perceptions of safety climate in primary care: a cross-sectional study. *J Eval Clin Pract.* 2012; **18**: 135–142.

20. Campbell SM, Hann M, Hacker J, *et al.* Identifying predictors of high quality care in English general practice: observational study. *BMJ.* 2001; **323**(7316): 784–7.

21. Apekey TA, McSorley G, Tilling M, *et al.* Room for improvement? Leadership, innovation culture and uptake of quality improvement methods in general practice. *J Eval Clin Pract.* 2011; **17**(2): 311–18.

CHAPTER 10

Patient and public involvement: part 1

Jill Murie & Julie Ferguson

Involving patients in their own healthcare has become a priority for healthcare policymakers and leaders, and is also strongly supported by leading professional and patient interest groups and organisations.[1-3] It is now widely accepted that, when patients are actively involved in safeguarding their own health, they receive an improved quality of care.[4,5] In the United Kingdom (UK) the vision of person-centred care is putting people and patients at the centre of the National Health Service (NHS) by delivering services as close to home as appropriate and ensuring safer, high-quality, reliable and effective primary healthcare. To achieve this vision requires, and will continue to require, working in partnership with patients, carers and the general public.

The policy priority of patient and public involvement (PPI) in healthcare planning, design, development and improvement is recognised by devoting two chapters to this important topic based largely on UK experiences. This chapter takes a 'macro' approach by providing a policy and evidence-based overview of PPI, while the second chapter describes the purpose and meaning of PPI at the 'micro' level perspective of the patient and healthcare professional. More specifically, this chapter begins with a summary of the history and current state of PPI in the NHS. Common PPI language and terminology is defined and a selection of related models and methods, including patient surveys, are described. Finally, some of the challenges to successful implementation of PPI in primary care are considered.

OVERVIEW OF PATIENT AND PUBLIC INVOLVEMENT

Involvement of the public in healthcare provision and planning at health authority, primary care and community levels has a long and sometimes turbulent history in the NHS. Over the past 60 years, patient-centred healthcare has risen to prominence internationally including in the UK. The concept of patient experience as a measure of quality and safety in healthcare is now firmly embedded within NHS policy[6] and the National Institute for Health and Care

Excellence guidelines.[7] The Royal College of General Practitioners has affirmed its commitment to involving patients and carers as equal partners in the provision of health and social care by supporting a 'Patient Partnership in Practice'.[8]

The names given to PPI-related initiatives have altered over time, as reflected in the many policy documents devoted to the subject, but the basic principles remain unchanged. In the mid 1990s, the emphasis was on a 'primary care-led NHS', in which users and carers had a greater voice. In 2013, the national Patients Association's stated aim is 'Listening to patients, Speaking up for change'.[9] The organisation is a healthcare charity, which campaigns for improvements to health and social care services across the UK. It captures stories about healthcare from thousands of patients, family members and carers every year via a helpline, surveys, focus groups, listening events and obtaining feedback from the organisation's 'Ambassador network'. In addition, the Patient Association Helpline provides signposting and information for patients and supports them as they navigate healthcare services. Similarly, the Scottish Patients Association, established in 1982, provides support and information to improve treatment options and facilitates effective communication between the public, health departments and local patient services.[10]

Single-interest groups such as Diabetes UK, Chest Heart and Stroke, the British Heart Foundation and the MS Society contribute to research and development, education and training and offer support and advice to patients and carers as well as health professionals. Strategic alliances between patient groups and clinicians and researchers have the potential to set priorities and research agendas[11] and all NHS research ethics committees now have lay representation. The Royal College of General Practitioners has an active national Public Participation Group, known as P3, which comprises general practitioners (GPs) and lay members. P3 advises the College on a range of medical issues from the patient's perspective and provides guidance to the public.[12]

The Care Quality Commission in England requires all general practices to have a patient participation scheme in order to comply with Care Quality Commission registration standards.[13] Practice patient participation groups have been a popular concept in primary care. Their parent organisation – the National Patient Participation Association, formed in 1978 – describes itself as a 'unique umbrella body supporting patient led groups in primary care'.[14] However, ensuring strong representation, avoiding tokenism and providing training are constant challenges to effective public participation, in addition to bias resulting from self-selection and self-interest in shaping local service provision.

Clinical commissioning groups in England are engaging with patients and the public to inform healthcare commissioning decisions and to identify their priorities and aspirations at the community level, while also taking an active role in improving and monitoring services. In the past, organisational approaches to involve people in commissioning seldom progressed beyond tokenism.[15] However, clinical commissioning groups are now expected to audit their level of PPI engagement activity and provide documentary evidence of how they involve those community organisations and patient representatives who are best placed to lead and contribute to constructive change and improvement in local healthcare services. The Department of Health will offer a choice of provider for 20.5 million tests annually by 2015, including endoscopy, audiology assessments and imaging such as computed tomography and DXA scans.[16] However, the consequences for patient choice[17] need to be questioned if commissioning decisions are not necessarily based on quality of care but on the need for fiscal balance instead.

PATIENT AND PUBLIC INVOLVEMENT TERMINOLOGY

The term 'patient-centred' as opposed to 'illness-centred' practice was used as early as 1955.[18] Since then, the language has evolved to the extent that, in 2013, jargon thrives amid a social and political arena in which expectation is raised by increasing 'consumerism' and 'choice' in wider society. As a result, it is now well recognised that there is a need for clarity and consistency in PPI terminology and related models and methods of evaluation (*see* Box 10.1).

PATIENT AND PUBLIC INVOLVEMENT METHODS AND MODELS

A range of different PPI models and methods is outlined in Box 10.2, while 'patient surveys', one of the more commonly used methods for capturing experiences and opinions of patients, are discussed here in more detail.

PATIENT SURVEYS

Patient surveys serve many purposes in the NHS. They can determine the health and social needs of a community[25] and contribute to health services research.[26] In primary care, patient surveys are now integral to incentive-based performance management of practices and the revalidation of individual GPs as regular systematic patient feedback is considered essential to improve quality of care and for public accountability within the NHS.

Assessing personal care

The quality of the consultation has been assessed using the Patient Enablement Instrument, which consists of six questions about the patient's ability to cope and the patient's change in his or her understanding of his or her problem after the consultation.[27] The CARE tool focuses on the patient's perceptions of empathy,[28] a 'holistic instrument on measuring patient-centredness of doctors'.[29] A General Medical Council (GMC) patient survey includes confidentiality and trustworthiness.[30]

Performance benchmarking

In addition to providing feedback on GPs' interpersonal and technical skills, the patient experience domain of the Quality and Outcomes Framework

BOX 10.1 Common patient and public involvement terms and their definitions

Subjects

Patient: person, service user, client, consumer, survivor, customer
Carer: parent, partner, spouse, family, formal or informal carer
Public: practice population, lay people, community, locality, voluntary group
Healthcare professional: doctor, nurse, service provider, clinician, manager

Interventions

Evidence-based practice: conscientious, explicit, and judicious use of current best evidence in making decisions about the care of individual patients[19]
Health education materials: a broad perspective to help patients understand their diagnosis, treatment and management in general terms and not personalised
Shared decision-making: interactive process between patients and clinicians who decide on healthcare together, maximising the potential of the consultation to translate evidence-based medicine into clinical decisions incorporating patients' values and preferences
Patient decision aid: a shared decision-making tool that involves patients in decisions by informing them of options and outcomes that help them clarify their personal values and choices
Patient-mediated intervention: aim at changing healthcare professionals' behaviour, either through provider–patient interactions or through information provided by or to the patients

Compliance, adherence and concordance

Compliance: 'The extent to which the patient's behaviour matches prescriber's recommendations'[20]
Adherence: 'The extent to which the patient's behaviour matches agreed recommendations from the prescriber'[21]
Concordance: an agreement reached after negotiation between a patient and a healthcare professional that respects the beliefs and wishes of the patient in determining whether, when and how medicines are to be taken[22]

Narrative-based medicine

Patient stories: 'The experience of a range of potential storytellers, communicating for difference reasons with a range of different audiences'[23]
Patient narratives: defined as predominantly factual, whereas stories are reflective, creative and value laden, usually revealing something important about the human condition[24]

BOX 10.2 **Models of public involvement**

Focus groups . . .
- involve six to eight participants with a common experience
- help to gauge levels of patient satisfaction with existing services and redesign
- last around 90 minutes
- detailed structured outline of questioning is facilitated and data analysed.

Citizens' juries . . .
- involve 12–16 ordinary people in decisions that affect their communities
- address issues important to planning or policy
- sit for up to 4 days and are assisted by independent moderators
- conclusions are compiled in a report that is submitted to commissioners.

Deliberative opinion poll . . .
- involves 250–600 participants reflecting baseline opinion and demography
- measures informed opinion on an issue after considering the evidence
- deliberate in smaller groups for 2–4 days
- compose questions to be put to commissioning bodies in plenary discussion.

Standing panels . . .
- may be a research panel or an interactive panel
- health panel consists of around 12 members of the public
- meet three times a year to discuss topics set by the commissioning body
- recruited by quota sampling to cover range of demographic characteristics.

Community issue groups . . .
- combination of focus group and citizen's jury
- consists of between 8 and 12 people
- meet for around 2 to 2½ hours on several occasions
- discuss designated issues in depth and revisit the discussion.

Consensus conferences . . .
- 10–20 volunteers recruited from advertisements
- steering committee chosen by conference organisers
- attend 2 preparatory weekends where they are briefed and they identify questions
- 3- to 4-day conference open to the public, where the panel retires and prepares a report.

contract, such as the GP Access Questionnaire and the Practitioner Profile Questionnaire, were designed as outcome measures to assess practice perform-ance. However, experts and others have their doubts about the full validity of conclusions derived from patient feedback.

While there are reports that some differences between practices can be detected using questionnaire data, the results may be attributable more to patient characteristics and random error than to differences between practices and variation between doctors.[31] Organisational differences such as access are reported to be a notable exception, where more than 20% of variance can be apportioned to differences in the time patients have to wait for appointments. One way to reduce error may be to combine patient experience with other sources of quality information, such as those within the clinical and organisa-tional domains of the Quality and Outcomes Framework to obtain a composite score, which identifies outlier practices and areas for personal development through GP appraisal.[32]

Patient-Reported Outcome Measures

Currently, Patient-Reported Outcome Measures (PROMS)[33] assess the quality in the delivery and outcomes (health gains) of four hospital-based clinical pro-cedures (varicose veins, groin hernia, hip replacements and knee replacement) from the patient perspective using pre- and post-operative surveys in England. It is intended that PROMS will be extended to GP practices and clinical com-missioning groups in England. However, hospital pilots using PROMS have provided inconsistent results and their use should be applied with caution.[34]

Medical revalidation

Revalidation for doctors was introduced in 2013 in the UK to enable doctors to demonstrate their 'fitness to practise' to the medical regulator, the GMC. Central to the revalidation process is feedback from patients, logging a record of complaints, significant event analysis and evidence of satisfactory comple-tion of annual appraisal. The value of patient feedback within revalidation is controversial. In a GMC-commissioned study of around 1065 doctors, patients valued seeing their 'usual doctor', highlighting the importance of continuity of care. Doctors' age, gender and ethnic background were of less importance than other variables such as where a doctor had obtained his or her medical degrees.[35] According to the British Medical Association, the implications of this bias are that 5% of GPs may consistently fall below the mean average for patient satisfaction.

PATIENT AND PUBLIC INVOLVEMENT AND PRIMARY CARE

It is recognised that pursuing the strategy for greater PPI will have significant implications for the funding of primary care, particularly its impact on GPs' consultation time. However, there is a need for greater clarity at national level about explicit roles and responsibilities, ethical professional practice and budgeting decisions if much greater patient involvement is to become a reality. Shared decision-making in the patient–doctor relationship requires more research, including regarding its impact on GP specialty training.[36] A number of potential barriers to implementation (*see* Box 10.3) will also have to be considered and overcome if PPI is to be incorporated effectively into primary care.

BOX 10.3 Barriers to patient and public involvement in primary care

- Lack of understanding of the purpose of involvement
- Insufficient evidence of effectiveness
- Patients and public representatives are self-selected with their 'own agendas'
- Health professions' negative attitudes and lack of skills
- Patients lack of information and training to make objective decisions
- Inadequate validated mechanisms for involvement
- Concerns about unrealistic expectations of healthcare
- Patient-centred decisions not based on evidence, quality and cost
- Inverse care law and inequity: 'those who shout the most get the most'
- Patient experience conflicts with targets in primary care (e.g. HbA_{1c})
- Patient involvement resists switches to cheaper treatment drugs, as they are perceived as being less effective
- Patient harm may result from self-care or self-monitoring
- Health professionals' anxiety and defensive practice
- Manipulation by patients (e.g. benefits, insurance, medico-legal claims)
- More litigation

Note: a P3 virtual network member provided patient feedback on this chapter.

REFERENCES

1. Department of Health. *Equity and Excellence: liberating the NHS*. London: The Stationery Office; 2010.
2. NHS Scotland. *The Healthcare Quality Strategy for NHSScotland*. Edinburgh: Scottish Government; 2010.
3. Department of Health. *The NHS Outcomes Framework 2013/2014*. London: Department of Health; 2012.
4. Coulter A, Ellins J. Effectiveness of strategies for informing, educating, and involving patients. *BMJ*. 2007; **335**(7609): 24.
5. Health Foundation. *Involving Patients in Improving Safety*. London: Health Foundation; 2013.
6. Darzi A. *High Quality Care for All: NHS next stage review final report*. London: Department of Health; 2008.
7. National Institute for Health and Care Excellence. *Patient Experience in Adult NHS Services: improving the experience of care for people using adult NHS services. NICE guideline 138*. London: NICE: 2012. Available at: http://guidance.nice.org.uk/CG138 (accessed 6 March 2013).

8. Royal College of General Practitioners. *P3 Carers Resource*. London: RCGP. Available at: www.rcgp.org.uk/policy/rcgp-policy-areas/patient-engagement-patient-partnership-group-ppg/p3-carers-resource.aspx (accessed 6 March 2013).

9. www.patients-association.com

10. www.scotlandpatients.com

11. Oliver S. Patient involvement in setting research agendas. *Eur J Gasteroenterol Hepatol*. 2006; **18**(9): 935–8.

12. Royal College of General Practitioners. *Patient Online*. London: RCGP; 2013. Available at: www.rcgp.org.uk/clinical-and-research/practice-management-resources/health-informatics-group/patient-online.aspx (accessed 10 February 2014).

13. Quality Compliance Systems. *GP Surgeries: welcome*. London: Quality Compliance Systems. Available at: www.ukqcs.co.uk/cqc-gp/registration-for-gp-practices/ (accessed 10 February 2014).

14. www.napp.org.uk

15. Murie J, Hanlon P, McEwen J, *et al*. Needs assessment in primary care: general practitioners' perceptions and implications for the future. *Br J Gen Pract*. 2000; **50**(450): 17–20.

16. Department of Health. *Liberating the NHS: no decision about me, without me – consultation*. London: Department of Health; 2012.

17. www.chooseandbook.nhs.uk

18. Balint M. *The Doctor, his Patient and the Illness*. London: Pitman Medical; 1964.

19. Sackett DL, Rosenberg W, Gray JA, *et al*. Evidence based medicine: what it is and what it isn't. *BMJ*. 1996; **312**(7023): 71–2.

20. Haynes RB, Taylor DW, Sackett DL, editors. *Compliance in Health Care*. London: John Hopkins University Press; 1979.

21. Barofsky I. Compliance, adherence and the therapeutic alliance: steps in the development of self-care. *Soc Sci Med*. 1978; **12**(5A): 369–76.

22. Royal Pharmaceutical Society of Great Britain. *From Compliance to Concordance: towards shared goals in medicine taking*. London: Royal Pharmaceutical Society of Great Britain; 1997.

23. 1000 Lives Plus. *Learning to Use Patient Stories*. NHS Wales; 2010. Available at: www.1000livesplus.wales.nhs.uk/sitesplus/documents/1011/T4I%20%286%29%20Learning%20to%20use%20Patient%20stories%20%28Feb%202011%29%20Web.pdf (accessed 31 July 2013).

24. Haigh C, Hardy P. Tell me a story: a conceptual exploration of storytelling in healthcare education. *Nurse Educ Today*. 2011; **31**(4): 408–11.

25. Murray J, Tapson J, Tumbull L, *et al*. Listening to local voices: adapting rapid appraisal to assess health and social needs in general practice. *BMJ*. 1994; **308**(6930): 698–700.

26. Paddison CA, Abel GA, Roland MO, *et al*. Drivers of overall satisfaction with primary care: evidence from the English General Practice Patient Survey. *Health Expect*. Epub 2013 May 30.

27. Howie J, Heaney D, Maxwell M. Quality, core values and the general practice consultation: issues of definition, measurement and delivery. *Fam Pract*. 2004; **21**(4): 458–68.

28. Mercer S, Howie J. CQI-2-a new measure of holistic interpersonal care in primary care consultations. *Br J Gen Pract*. 2006; **56**(525): 262–8.

29. Little P, Everitt H, Williamson I, *et al*. Observational study of effect of patient centred-

ness and positive approach on outcomes of general practice consultations. *BMJ*. 2001; **323**(7318): 908–11.

30. General Medical Council. *Patient Questionnaire*. Available at: www.gmc-uk.org/patient_questionnaire.pdf_48210488.pdf (accessed 7 June 2013).

31. Haggerty JL. Are measures of patient satisfaction hopelessly flawed? *BMJ*. 2010; **341**(7318): c478.

32. Sahota N, Hood A, Shankar A, *et al*. Developing performance indicators for primary care: Walsall's experience. *Br J Gen Pract*. 2008; **58**(557): 856–61.

33. Health and Social Care Information Centre. *Patient Reported Outcome Measures*. Available at: www.ic.nhs.uk/proms (accessed 30 July 2013).

34. Appelby J. Patient reported outcome measures: how are we feeling today? *BMJ*. 2012; **344**(7839): d8191.

35. Davies P. Should patients be able to control their own records? *BMJ*. 2012; **345**(7871): e4095.

36. Is patient involvement possible when decisions involve scarce resources? A qualitative study of decision-making in primary care. *Soc Sci Med*. 2004; **59**(1): 93–102.

Part II

People and Improvement

CHAPTER 11

Patient and public involvement: part 2

Jill Murie & Julie Ferguson

In this second chapter on patient and public involvement (PPI), some of the practical implications of this strategy are explored from the perspectives of healthcare professionals and patients. Consideration is given to the potential educational value and impact of PPI for the individual clinician before discussing a number of interlinked issues of importance: (a) consent, (b) complaints and effective communication of risk, (c) compliance, adherence and concordance, and (d) patient access to their personal health records. The chapter concludes by reflecting on the importance of shared decision-making as a means to enhance the quality and experience of healthcare.

PATIENT AND PUBLIC INVOLVEMENT AND MEDICAL EDUCATION
Undergraduate and postgraduate training

Patients have always been central to medical education.[1] However, the role was initially a passive one, where the patient was used to illustrate medical conditions, rather than an active role where the patient is directly involved in teaching, assessment or curriculum development. The role of patients as formal educators in primary care in the UK was not fully recognised until the early 1970s with the advent of vocational training for general practice. This notion was consolidated by the Postgraduate Medical Education and Training Board in 2004.[2] However, while patients perceive their contribution to medical teaching positively,[3] a recent literature review concluded that active patient involvement in education lacked evidence that was based on robust theoretical models.[4]

The British Medical Association publication *The Role of the Patient in Medical Education* provides an overview of patients, real and simulated, in undergraduate and postgraduate medical education.[1] Patient contact may take place in a variety of educational activities including lecture demonstrations, tutorials, face-to-face discussion and simulated exercises such as the Objective Structured Clinical Examination. This grounding in patient interaction is reported to add value to the assessment of communication skills, empathy and examination techniques.[5]

In general practice, specialty trainees' communication and consultation skills are rigorously evaluated using workplace-based assessment tools including the consultation observation tool (*see* Box 11.1) and patient satisfaction questionnaires.

BOX 11.1 Specific communication skills of general practitioner trainees assessed by the consultation observation tool

A. Discovers the reasons for the patient's attendance
1. Encourages the patient's contribution
2. Responds to cues
3. Places complaint in appropriate psychosocial context
4. Explores patient's health understanding

B. Defines the clinical problem
5. Includes or excludes likely relevant significant condition
6. Appropriate physical or mental state examination
7. Makes an appropriate working diagnosis

C. Explains the problem to the patient
8. Explains the problem in appropriate language

D. Addresses the patient's problem
9. Seeks to confirm the patient's understanding
10. Appropriate management plan
11. Patient is given the opportunity to be involved in significant management decisions

E. Makes effective use of the consultation
12. Makes effective use of resources
13. Conditions and interval for follow-up are specified

Continuing professional development

All primary care clinicians must participate in regular continuing development as a means to uphold and improve upon professional standards. Continuing professional development (CPD) is defined as:

> a process of lifelong learning for all individuals and teams, which enables professionals to expand and fulfill their potential and which also meets the needs of patients and delivers the health and health care priorities of the NHS.[6]

In 2004, the General Medical Council previously stated that

> CPD should take into account the needs and wishes of patients and public in developing CPD schemes, setting standards and monitoring.[7]

However, in June 2012 this guidance went further, emphasising that current guidance

> will also help patients and the public understand what we expect doctors to do to stay up to date and improve the safety and quality of care they provide. It may also encourage patients to give feedback to doctors about areas where CPD may benefit their care.[8]

Appraisal and revalidation

General practitioner (GP) appraisal began in 2004 as a formative, developmental and educational process.[9] In 2013, satisfactory annual appraisal is a requirement of revalidation and licensing with the General Medical Council. Supporting information for appraisal and revalidation includes CPD, which shows GPs are keeping 'up to date' with evidence-based practice. A review of complaints and compliments is provided every year and a patient satisfaction questionnaire every 5 years. For each category of supporting information, GPs should provide evidence of reflection on their practice, learning and implementation of learning in practice. Case reports provide evidence of reflection and the patient perspective.[10,11] The Royal College of General Practitioners (RCGP) has recommended that GPs aggregate 50 CPD 'credits' annually (250 in a 5-year revalidation cycle). In practice, 'credits' are difficult to verify, particularly in terms of the impact on patient care or patient feedback arising from CPD.[12]

BOX 11.2 Potential ways to demonstrate effective communication skills for general practitioner appraisal

- Attend a consultation skills course and reflect on this
- Undergo a peer review of videotaped consultations, and reflect on the feedback
- Discuss a videotaped surgery with a colleague trained to give consultation skills feedback
- Undertake a simulated surgery with feedback, and reflect on the results – this might be helpful for a small study group, particularly for sessional doctors
- Out-of-hours treatment centres normally record all telephone conversations with patients and these may be used to review and reflect on telephone communication skills, preferably with a peer group or trained facilitator

The consultation process in general practice is fundamental to the doctor–patient relationship and a platform on which the quality of care is judged. Communication with patients involves verbal, non-verbal language and paralanguage such as appropriate silence, eye contact and body posture, as well as providing information and checking understanding. Potential ways to demonstrate effective communication skills for general practice appraisal purposes are shown in Box 11.2.[13]

CONSENT

Eliciting informed consent constitutes active shared decision-making, where the impact of a 'wrong' decision may be significant for the health and well-being of the patient. In reality, consent is often implicit, verbal and applies to common interventions in primary care, such as routine investigations and treatment. Explicit written consent is elicited, where there is risk and uncertainty. Importantly, consent applies not just to investigation and treatment but also to non-clinical areas such as audio recordings, photographs and other visual images of patients,[14] as well as consent for journal publication[15] and clinical research.[16]

Clinicians may be unable to elicit informed consent for routine health procedures, such as screening, when a patient lacks capacity owing to severe mental illness or learning difficulties.[17] In that event, independent advocacy is required and the Adults with Incapacity Act (Scotland) 2000[18] or the Mental Capacity Act 2005[19] may be invoked. These acts enable appropriate sharing of confidential information with a legal representative. An 'advanced directive' may be also put in place, and 'power of attorney' granted, when the patient is sufficiently well enough to provide informed consent – for example, in dementia cases. The development of KIS (Key Information Summary)[20] in NHS Scotland combines a patient's emergency care summary for out-of-hours care, Palliative Care Summary and Anticipatory Care form. KIS will enable information that a patient consents to share to be available to other services delivering care to him or her.[20]

COMPLAINTS

The number of complaints against doctors has increased by 18% between 2009 and 2010. There are many factors that may account for this, including increased consumerism, greater expectations of professional accountability, the changing doctor–patient relationship, advertising by solicitors, and the growth of a perceived 'victim' or 'blame' culture in wider society.

Complaints may be reduced or avoided by considering the salient lessons from the recent inquiry into high infant mortality rates after cardiac surgery at Bristol Royal Infirmary (Box 11.3).[21] In addition, identifying and addressing poor communication skills can reduce complaints against doctors if corrected early in their career.[22] A specific subject that can be very difficult to communicate clearly to patients is the concept of 'risk'. Risk communication is defined as 'The open, two-way exchange of information and opinion about risk, leading to a better understanding of the risk in question, and promoting better clinical decisions about management'.[23] There are a number of key principles when discussing the risks and benefits of treatment with patients (Box 11.4).[24]

BOX 11.3 Strategies to reduce complaints (lessons from the Bristol inquiry)

- Involve patients (or their parents) in decisions
- Keep patients (or parents) informed
- Improve communication with patients (or parents)
- Provide patients (or parents) with counselling and support
- Gain informed consent for all procedures and processes
- Elicit feedback from patients (or parents) and listen to their views
- Be open and candid where adverse events occur

BOX 11.4 Strategies for effective communication of 'risk' to patients*

- Personalise risks and benefits as far as possible
- Use absolute rather than relative risk
- Use natural frequency rather than a percentage (e.g. 10 in 100 rather than 10%) and be consistent with the population base when comparing risks
- Define the period of time to which the risk applies (e.g. for cardiovascular risk assessment, 10 years)
- Use positive and negative framing
- Avoid terms such as rare, uncommon and common and use numerical data if possible
- Use a combination of numerical and pictorial formats
- Offer support and make sure the patient is aware of the risks, benefits and consequences of the options available
- Provide patients with suitable shared decision-making aids

The following imaginary clinical example illustrates some of the key concepts of 'risk'. Two chemotherapy treatments are available, drugs A and B. The 5-year survival of 100 patients with drugs A and B is 92/100 and 94/100, respectively. The absolute benefit of drug A over drug B is 2/100 (2%) and the relative benefit is 2/8 (25%). Risk can also be expressed graphically (e.g. by using a hazard pictogram). For example, Figure 11.1 depicts the likely reduction of cardiovascular events from 49/100 to 31/100 as a result of a patient stopping smoking.

---

* Adapted from the National Institute for Health and Care Excellence.

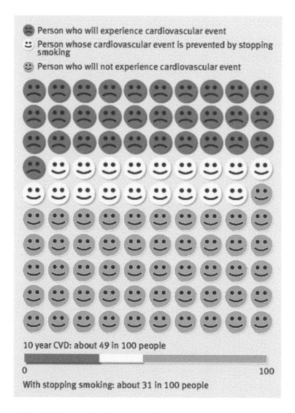

FIGURE 11.1 Example of a hazard pictogram*

COMPLIANCE, ADHERENCE AND CONCORDANCE

Clinicians and patients typically overestimate compliance with medication.[25] For example, approximately 20%–30% of patients taking daily or weekly medication for osteoporosis discontinue therapy after 6–12 months of treatment.[26] The financial implications of non-adherence – the extent to which the patient's behaviour matches agreed recommendations from the prescriber – for the health service are considerable.

While the patient perspective on adherence is not well understood, most compliance is selective, targeted and partial. Patients take drug 'holidays' and may be overly compliant before review appointments ('white coat' adherence). Rather than being incompetent in following instructions or deviant, patients make reasoned decisions, even if their reasoning is different to those of their doctors. Methods to improve concordance (e.g. mutually agreed prescribing) are shown in Box 11.5.

---

* Adapted with permission from the Institute of Health and Society, Newcastle University.

BOX 11.5 **Strategies to improve concordance**

Identify barriers

- Difficulty swallowing
- Physical problems (poor vision, hearing and manual dexterity)
- Polypharmacy
- Unsuitable presentation (e.g. child-resistant packaging)

Anticipate problems

- Advise on side effects
- Provide written as well as oral instructions for patients, carers and/or family
- Avoid frequent dose regimens and consider once-daily fixed combinations
- Prescribe 'forgiving' drugs (e.g. those with a long half-life, such as amlodipine)
- Provide pillboxes

Agree

- Involvement of prescriber in patients' model of illness
- Shared goals in treatment decision-making
- Development of a 'prescribing alliance'

Consider

- Low socio-economic status and educational attainment
- Depression or memory impairment and substance misuse
- Lack of social support
- Multiple co-morbidity

Monitor concordance

- Repeated motivational interviewing at review appointments
- Telephone consultation, text messages asking about compliance
- Structured patient adherence questionnaires
- Prescription refills and pill counts; look at pill-taking pattern
- 'Virtual ward'
- Measure drug concentration in serum
- Electronic medicines counting (electronic pillbox – patient must be told)
- Outcomes of treatment

PATIENT ACCESS TO RECORDS

The Data Protection Act 1998[27] allows all UK citizens access to all data held about them electronically. All patient records are officially owned by the government and are the property of neither the practice nor the patient. The Access to Health Records Act 1990[28] allows patients access to medical information stored in non-computerised format.

Potential benefits of allowing patients access to their records are summarised in Box 11.6. Provisos include the removal of third-party correspondence and harmful information, with annotations indicating where information has been removed. If patients consider their records to be inaccurate they may add comments, but are not able to erase information. This is potentially a very time-consuming process. However, patients may ask questions as a result of reading their records, thus increasing their responsibility for self-management and reducing the demand for consultations.

BOX 11.6 Potential benefits of patients having access to their records

- Clarifies a sometimes obscure medical process to patients
- Balances the equality of access to personal information
- Patients are enabled to participate in their own management
- Doctors' rationale and clinical management are understood
- Patients' understanding of their illnesses is enhanced
- Communication between patients and their doctors is more open
- Patients can better participate in their own management plans
- Inaccuracies in patients' records are identified and amended
- Inappropriate language or incorrect statements are avoided
- Potential litigation may be reduced
- May help to manage the demand for consultations

The RCGP has demonstrated its commitment to patient ownership of data by announcing plans to deliver patient online services and access to their medical records within a safe and secure governance structure.[29] The Department of Health Information Strategy *The Power of Information*[30] has stated that, by 2015, all general practices will be expected to make available electronic booking and cancelling of appointments, requesting of repeat prescriptions, viewing of clinical investigation results, all communications with the practice and full access to records.

Giving patients greater online access to clinical information may have negative consequences including the increased use of health professionals' time to explain records to worried patients and an unrealistic expectation of GPs' email response time. Doctors may feel the need to use lay language and omit information such as differential diagnoses, which may add to the distress patients suffer. This would diminish the usefulness of the patient's record and raise serious medico-legal issues.

SHARED DECISION-MAKING

Shared decision-making (SDM) is an interactive process in which clinicians and patients plan healthcare within a relationship of mutual understanding and respect. However, patients' care preferences may be 'misdiagnosed'. SDM maximises the potential to incorporate patients' values and preferences and evidence-based practice into clinical decision-making.

The OPTION (observing patient involvement) scale was developed to reliably assess SDM in the consultation[31] and has been used in reviewing videotapes for the Membership of the Royal College of General Practitioners examination.[32] While the aim of the RCGP is to treat patients as 'partners' or 'equals with different expertise', the concept of 'partnership' remains unclear and controversial.[33,34] Training health professionals in adopting patient-centred approaches is reported to improve patient satisfaction,[35] but barriers do exist and include time constraints and being affected by differing patient characteristics and the context or complexity of the clinical situation.[36]

Patient characteristics include the extent to which they want to become involved, their familiarity with the condition, their age and educational attainment.[36] While some patients seek a high level of autonomy, to burden others may be highly inappropriate.[37,38] Their involvement needs to be carefully gauged, discretionary and flexible and needs to reflect their needs and preferences.[38] There are also clinical situations in which SDM may not be possible – for example, in accident and emergency, severe mental illness and paediatrics.

To make SDM easier, a range of 'patient-mediated interventions' have been devised to encourage active participation. These patient decision aids are detailed, personal tools informing patients of options and outcomes. Examples include shared care record cards for amiodarone monitoring,[39,40] a tailored programme for proton pump prescribing[41] and an online resource for adolescent mental health promotion.[42]

CONCLUSIONS

PPI has always been and continues to be a key priority in the National Health Service. It potentially affects all aspects of healthcare from planning, design and development, through delivery and finally evaluation and improvement. However, the way in which PPI is translated and enacted in the day-to-day practice of healthcare professionals and the experiences of patients continues to evolve. While much is expected of PPI, and it is thought to confer many potential benefits, there is still a lack of rigorous evidence of its acceptability, feasibility and impact – that is, its overall utility as a method that can contribute to improving the patient experience, capturing learning and making healthcare safer and more efficient.

Both this chapter and the previous chapter by necessity have provided a brief overview of the key principles of PPI, illustrated by a potpourri of practical examples in the National Health Service. Important aspects of PPI unfortunately had to be excluded. However, it is hoped that the selected content helped to provide a flavour of the PPI agenda and its importance, and that it also demonstrated how intertwined PPI is with the vision for high-quality primary care.

REFERENCES

1. British Medical Association, Medical Education Subcommittee. *Role of the Patient in Medical Education.* London: British Medical Association; 2008. Available at: http://bma.org.uk/-/media/Files/PDFs/Developing%20your%20career/Becoming%20a%20doctor/Role%20of%20patient.pdf (accessed 2 March 2014).
2. Postgraduate Medical Education and Training Board. *Patients' Role in Healthcare: the future relationship between patient and doctor.* London: PMETB; 2008.
3. Lucas B, Pearson D. Patient perceptions of their role in undergraduate medical education within a primary care teaching practice. *Educ Prim Care.* 2012; **23**(4): 277–85.
4. Towle A, Bainbridge L, Godolphin W, *et al.* Active patient involvement in the education of health professionals. *Med Educ.* 2010; **44**(1): 64–74.
5. Ahuja AS. Involve patients and carers in training health professionals. *Educ Prim Care.* 2011; **22**(3): 195.
6. Chief Medical Officer. *A Review of CPD in General Practice.* Leeds: Department of Health; 1998.
7. General Medical Council. *Continuing Professional Development.* London: GMC; 2004.
8. General Medical Council. *Continuing Professional Development: guidance for all doctors.* Manchester: GMC; 2012.
9. Murie J. GP appraisal recruitment in Scotland 2005. *BMJ Careers.* 2005; **331**(7512): 59–60.
10. Murie J. Medical case reports: a modern tradition. *Scott Med J.* 2010; **55**(3): 2–3.
11. de Wet C, Murie J. Lamb pays lip service: two cases of ecthyma contagiosum. *Scott Med J.* 2011; **56**(1): 57.
12. Murie J, Wakeling J. Verification of 'Learning Credits' by GP appraisers: judging supporting information for revalidation. *Educ Prim Care.* 2011; **22**(6): 369–76.
13. NHS Education for Scotland. *SOAR Scottish Appraisal Online Resource: Relationships with Patients.* Available at: http://gp.appraisal.nes.scot.nhs.uk/resources.aspx (accessed 6 March 2013).
14. General Medical Council. *Making and Using Visual and Audio Recordings of Patients.* London: GMC; 1997.
15. Smith J. Patient confidentiality and consent to publication. *BMJ.* 2008; **337**: a1572.
16. General Medical Council. *Good Practice in Research and Consent to Research.* London: GMC, 2010. Available at: www.gmc-uk.org/Research_guidance_FINAL.pdf_31379258.pdf (accessed 30 July 2013).
17. Murie J. Feasibility of screening for and treating vitamin D deficiency in forensic psychiatric inpatients. *J Forensic Leg Med.* 2012; **19**(8): 457–64.
18. Adults with Incapacity (Scotland) Act 2000. Edinburgh: Crown Copyright; 2000.
19. Mental Capacity Act 2005. London: HMSO; 2005.
20. National Information Systems Group. *Key Information Summary (KIS).* Edinburgh: National Information Systems Group, NHS National Services Scotland. Available at: www.nisg.scot.nhs.uk/why-nisg/our-services/project-management/key-information-summary-kis (accessed 14 November 2011).
21. Coulter A. After Bristol: putting patients at the centre. *BMJ.* 2002; **324**(7338): 648–51.
22. Kinnersley P, Edwards A. Complaints against doctors. *BMJ.* 2008; **336**(7649): 841–2.
23. Ahl AS, Acree JA, Gipson PS, *et al.* Standardisation of nomenclature for animal health risk analysis. *Rev Sci Tech.* 1993; **12**(4): 1045–53.

24. Flynn N, Staniszewska S. Improving the experience of care for people using the NHS services: summary of NICE guidance. *BMJ*. 2012; **344**(7851): d6422.

25. Zeller A, Ramseier E, Teagtmeyer A, *et al*. Patients' self-reported adherence to cardio-vascular medication using electronic monitors as comparators. *Hypertens Res*. 2008; **31**(11): 2037–43.

26. Papaioannou A, Kennedy CC, Dolovich L, *et al*. Patient adherence with osteoporosis medications: problems, consequences and management strategies. *Drugs Aging*. 2007; **24**(1): 37–55.

27. Cabinet Office. Data Protection Act 1998. London: HMSO.

28. Cabinet Office. Access to Health Records Act 1990. London: HMSO.

29. Royal College of General Practitioners. *Patient Online*. London: RCGP; 2013. Available at: www.rcgp.org.uk/clinical-and-research/practice-management-resources/health-informatics-group/patient-online.aspx (accessed 30 July 2013).

30. Department of Health. *The Power of Information: putting all of us in control of the health and care information we need*. London: Department of Health; 2012.

31. Elwyn G, Edwards A, Kinnersley P, *et al*. Shared decision making and the concept of equipoise: the competences of involving patients in healthcare choices. *Br J Gen Pract*. 2000; **50**(460): 892–9.

32. Siriwardena AN, Edwards AG, Campion P, *et al*. Involve the patient and pass the MRCGP: investigating shared decision making in a consulting skills examination using a validated instrument. *Br J Gen Pract*. 2006; **56**(532): 857–62.

33. Wirtz V, Cribb A, Barber N. Patient-doctor decision-making about treatment within the consultation: a critical analysis of models. *Soc Sci Med*. 2006; **62**(1): 116–24.

34. Entwistle VA, Watt IS. Patient involvement in treatment decision-making: the case for a broader conceptual framework. *Patient Educ Couns*. 2006; **63**(3): 268–78.

35. Lewin SA, Skea ZC, Entwistle V, *et al*. Interventions for providers to promote a patient-centred approach in clinical consultations. *Cochrane Database Syst Rev*. 2001; **10**: CD003267.

36. Légaré F, Ratté S, Gravel K, *et al*. Barriers and facilitators to implementing shared decision-making in clinical practice: update of a systematic review of health profes-sionals' perceptions. *Patient Educ Couns*. 2008; **73**(3): 526–35.

37. Deber RB, Kraetschmer N, Urowitz S, *et al*. Do people want to be autonomous patients? Preferred roles in treatment decision-making in several patient populations. *Health Expect*. 2007; **10**(3): 248–58.

38. Thompson AG. The meaning of patient involvement and participation in health care consultations: a taxonomy. *Soc Sci Med*. 2007; **64**(6): 1297–310.

39. Murie J. Amiodorone monitoring: involving patients in risk management. *Br J Cardiol*. 2003; **10**(1): 70–2.

40. Murie J. Developing an evaluated patient-mediated intervention for monitoring amio-darone therapy. *Br J Cardiol*. 2005; **12**(1): 71–3.

41. Murie J, de Wet C, Simmonds R, *et al*. Glad you brought it up: a patient-centred pro-gramme to reduce PPI prescribing in general practice. *Qual Prim Care*. 2012; **20**(2): 141–8.

42. Murie J, Dickson A. Think Positive: a mental health promotion website for 12 to 18 year olds. *Int J Mental Health Promot*. 2012; **4**(1): 26–33.

CHAPTER 12

Clinician engagement

Steven Wilson

INTRODUCTION

It may seem self-evident but the people who are best placed to make significant improvements to the quality of patient care are the front-line clinical teams who actually deliver it. The active engagement of these clinicians is essential to the successful implementation of healthcare quality improvement.[1] However, engendering meaningful engagement that empowers clinicians to play an integral role in safety and improvement initiatives is not an easy task. Davies *et al.*[1] identified the non-engagement of clinicians as a 'long-standing, multi-factorial and international problem'. The published literature shows a number of recurring barriers and challenges to clinical engagement, including lack of time and resources, limited knowledge and skills, and organisational impediments.[2] Overcoming these barriers requires a planned and concerted effort with strong commitment from primary care leaders and managers. Without this a lot of effort can be wasted, despite the best of intentions. This article describes what is meant by clinical engagement, and why it is so important, and sets out four key areas to be addressed when engaging primary care clinicians in efforts to make patient care safer and improve service quality.

What do we mean by clinical engagement?

There is no one clear definition of clinical engagement. It is variously described in the literature as an attitude, a behaviour, an outcome or sometimes a combination of all three. The degree or level of clinical engagement can fall anywhere along a continuum ranging from disaffection, through passive involvement to active collaborative engagement. Good clinical engagement requires a shift from merely informing and consulting to that of collaborating with and empowering clinicians. Effectively it's the difference between '*done with*' rather than '*done to*'. Understandably, clinicians actively resist hectoring, lecturing, criticism and data judging their performance. Previous negative experiences have left many clinicians cynical or at best apathetic to engagement in quality improvement initiatives. In this age of integrated team working, where quality improvement initiatives transcend primary and secondary care, it is important to emphasise that the engagement of all clinicians is essential. Done well, clinical engagement creates a common cause and a climate of shared commitment to quality improvement (QI) initiatives.

Why is clinical engagement important?

Given the increasing pressures on healthcare organisations to improve the quality and safety of patient care, the need to engage clinicians in QI is crucial. Alongside time, resources, information and skills there is increasing evidence that the active participation of clinicians in any improvement initiative dramatically improves its chances of success.[3] Effective clinical engagement has the potential, therefore, to improve healthcare delivery; enhance the patient's experience and outcomes; increase employee satisfaction; and aid recruitment and retention.

Clinical engagement enables shared accountability and improved collaboration between clinicians and managers. Organisations where clinicians are fully engaged with managers in strategic planning and decision-making perform better than those where clinicians are alienated from strategic processes of the organisation.[4] Conversely, evidence shows a lack of meaningful clinical engagement in such initiatives may significantly harm its chances of success.[5]

How do I engage clinicians?

Clinical engagement is catalysed by a combination of processes. There are four key areas to be addressed in order to build and sustain clinician engagement in safety and quality improvement:
1. know your audience (explore)
2. make it easy to get involved (enable)
3. stimulate the desire (encourage)
4. lead by example (exemplify).

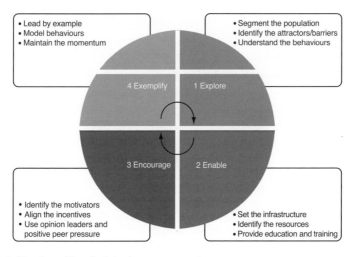

FIGURE 12.1 The four E's of clinical engagement

EXPLORE

Clinicians are not a single homogeneous group and therefore a 'one size fits all' approach to clinical engagement is not an option. It is essential to know your audience and their context well and to tailor your engagement efforts to that audience's needs. For this reason, an important early step in the engagement process is to determine who the key stakeholders are and how they will be involved. Stakeholder engagement is a process of relationship management that seeks to enhance understanding and alignment between organisations and their stakeholders. In the case of clinical engagement, stakeholder mapping and segmentation techniques[6] are very helpful in identifying the following.

- Audience type:
  — medical, nursing, allied health professional
  — primary, secondary, tertiary care
  — senior, junior grade staff
  — location, base
- Appropriate channels and messages for different clinical groups
- Clinical groups with the greatest influence and interest in specific topics
- Disengaged or hostile clinical groups who need extra effort to reach and convince
- Educational and/or emotional gaps that may exist

The power structures in healthcare are complex and constantly changing. Understanding the hidden power and influence of stakeholders is critical to engagement.[7] A clear understanding of the nature of their expectations, interests, power and influence will help to avoid conflict and to forge positive relationships.

ENABLE

There may be underlying, compelling reasons why clinicians are not able to engage in QI and safety initiatives. Managers need to recognise and address the practical and structural barriers and make it easy for clinicians to get engaged. Any attempts to encourage engagement that do not recognise these contextual factors are likely to breed frustration only.

The necessary physical and technological infrastructure must also be in place to support planning, coordination and leadership of QI activities. Information technology is not the 'silver bullet' solution but it is increasingly recognised as an important tool for data collection, analysis and interpretation. To secure engagement it is essential that clinicians have robust data/information available in the right format and at the right time to identify areas that need improvement and to systematically assess progress.

Healthcare organisations are often dealing with an educational deficit where many clinicians do not understand QI and its importance, which contributes to their reluctance to participate. Research by Davies *et al.*[1] found that clinicians have 'a limited understanding of the latest concepts and methods underlying quality improvement'.

Clearly clinicians' time is limited, particularly in primary care, so it is important to look for innovative, timely and cost-effective ways of building their knowledge and skills in methods of QI. Related knowledge needs to be embedded into undergraduate education, training, professional development and appraisal. Revalidation has the potential to act as a powerful incentive for medical engagement, with all doctors now being required to provide evidence in their annual appraisal that they are actively engaging in meaningful QI.

ENCOURAGE

The established approaches to encourage and influence clinician behaviour change (education, regulation and information) are not effective on their own. Clinicians' experiences, beliefs, and needs are crucial to engagement, and emotional associations can powerfully shape their actions. Clinician behaviour is determined by the complex interplay between extrinsic and intrinsic motivation. However, it is the intrinsic intangible motivators that must be leveraged to really engage clinicians. Plsek and Kilo[8] believe we need to 'change the attractors, or tap into existing ones better'. The power of intrinsic motivation can be harnessed for safety and quality improvement by:

- making it salient – attention is drawn to what is novel and relevant
- speaking their language – use stories and personal encounters to bring safety and quality improvement to life
- understanding the attractor patterns – for clinicians these are mastery, autonomy, affiliation, accomplishment, and so forth
- celebrating success and providing regular positive feedback
- making it easy to get involved – breaking down the organisational barriers to engagement.

Each audience has different information needs and ways that it prefers to receive communication. We are strongly influenced by who communicates the information and how credible they are to the users.[9] Identifying and using local opinion leaders to promote QI and safety is one successful way to build engagement.[10] Opinion leaders are respected individuals with extensive interpersonal networks whose opinion is influential when changing practice or introducing new ways of working. Locock *et al.*[11] have reviewed the evidence on the use of opinion leaders and shown that their expertise, interpersonal skills and understanding of local practice can have a significant positive role in influencing uptake in safety improvement.

There is good evidence from social science that people's behaviour is strongly influenced by the actions of those who are like them.[12] Dawson *et al.*[13] suggest the influence of colleagues is one of 'multiple cues' identified by clinicians as significant factors affecting their practice. Peer influence is a powerful yet greatly underused resource in building engagement and spreading behaviour. Positive peer pressure can strongly influence attitudes and behaviours. When peers share a mutual respect, they will listen to, learn from and support one another in ways that can foster engagement, shape opinions and generate energy for change.

EXEMPLIFY

When it comes to safety improvement, evidence shows that senior clinicians must lead by example and model the behaviour they want to see from others.[10] A visible commitment by senior clinicians and managers can bring the necessary credibility and sustainability to QI initiatives.[14] If senior leaders are not engaged in the initiatives they are encouraging others to participate in, this could act against clinicians' desire for reciprocity and fairness. To build the enthusiasm and energy needed for effective clinical engagement, senior clinicians and managers should strive to create an organisational culture in which all clinicians are supported to be involved in continuous improvement efforts.

Attitudes and situations will change and the goalposts will be constantly shifted. Engagement needs continuous effort, focus and time to maintain the initial momentum and enthusiasm that has been established.[15] Continuous review of engagement feedback, tackling disengagement and addressing engagement burnout are important ongoing tasks for embedding a sustainable culture of improvement.

CONCLUSIONS

Traditionally, clinical engagement has tended to focus on those few doctors who hold highly visible positional roles (e.g. medical director or clinical director). Although institutional and service leaders have greater overall responsibility, it is the front-line clinicians who ultimately hold the key to success, by using their day-to-day experience to inform constant improvement of services. For effective and sustainable improvements in the safety and quality of patient care, we must build and nurture an inclusive culture where clinicians at all levels across primary and secondary care are actively engaged in improvement activities. This requires clinicians and managers working in partnerships to bring together the expertise and capacity of all parties involved. It is imperative that clinicians and managers build trust in their collective ability to identify solutions.

The value of early and sustained clinical engagement in quality and safety initiatives cannot be overstated. However, the time and effort involved in building effective sustainable clinical engagement should not be underestimated. It is a long-standing problem that is acknowledged to be one of the more challenging aspects of healthcare quality improvement. The active engagement of primary care in safety improvement initiatives is essential but, as yet, only very partially realised, although the National Health Service for Scotland via the general medical services contract has started down that path.[16] By taking a more considered approach to engagement that draws on general theories of change management, marketing and motivation we can support and address the undoubted challenges that lie ahead.

REFERENCES

1. Davies H, Powell A, Rushmer R. *Healthcare Professionals' Views on Clinician Engagement in Quality Improvement: a literature review.* London: Health Foundation; 2007. Available at: www.health.org.uk/publications/engaging-clinicians-report/ (accessed 5 November 2013).
2. The King's Fund. *Improving the Quality of Care in General Practice: independent inquiry into the quality of care in general practice in England.* London: The King's Fund; 2011.
3. Ham C. Improving the performance of health services: the role of clinical leadership. *Lancet.* 2003; **361**(9373): 1978–80.
4. NHS Institute for Innovation and Improvement and the Academy of Medical Royal Colleges. *Engaging Doctors: what can we learn from trusts with high levels of medical engagement – key findings from seven trusts.* Coventry: NHS Institute for Innovation and Improvement; 2011.
5. Stern Z. The future of quality leadership. *Int J Qual Health Care.* 2002; **14**(2): 85–6.
6. Scholes K, Johnson G. Stakeholder mapping: a tool for public sector managers. In: *Exploring Public Sector Strategy.* London: Financial Times/Prentice Hall; 2000. pp. 165–85.
7. Bourne L, Walker DHT. Visualising and mapping stakeholder influence. *Management Decision.* 2000; **43**(5): 649–60.
8. Plsek PE, Kilo CM. From resistance to attraction: a different approach to change. (Positively Influencing Physicians). *Physician Executive.* 1999; **25**(6): 6–46.
9. Lavis JN, Robertson D, Woodside JM, *et al.* How can research organizations more effectively transfer research knowledge to decision makers? *Milbank Q.* 2003; **81**(2): 221–48.
10. Ovretveit J. Leading improvement. *J Health Organ Manag.* 2005; **19**(6): 413–30.
11. Locock L, Dopson S, Chambers D, *et al.* Understanding the role of opinion leaders in improving clinical effectiveness. *Soc Sci Med.* 2001; **53**(6): 745–57.
12. Griskevicius V, Cialdini RB, Goldstein NJ. Applying (and resisting) peer influence. *MIT Sloan Manage Rev.* 2008; **49**(2): 84–8.
13. Dawson S, Sutherland K, Dopson S, *et al. The Relationship between R&D and Clinical Practice in Primary and Secondary Care: cases of adult asthma and glue ear in children.* Final Report. Cambridge and Oxford: Judge Institute of Management Studies, University of Cambridge; Saïd Business School, University of Oxford; 1998.
14. Wiener BJ, Shortell SM, Alexander J. Promoting clinical involvement in hospital quality improvement efforts: the effects of top management, board and physician leadership. *Health Serv Res.* 1997; **32**: 491–510.
15. Siriwardena, A Niroshan. Engaging clinicians in quality improvement initiatives: art or science? *Qual Prim Care.* 2009; **17**(5): 303–5.
16. www.scottishpatientsafetyprogramme.scot.nhs.uk/

CHAPTER 13

Professionalism

Niall Cameron

This chapter will explore how current concepts of medical professionalism fit in with the desire to embed a patient safety and quality improvement culture in primary healthcare. It will examine how the concept of medical professionalism has been defined and developed and the processes and events that have influenced this development. Additionally it will examine why consideration of the nature of medical professionalism is pivotal to addressing this issue, the barriers that exist to achieving this aim and how these challenges can be met.

WHY IS PROFESSIONALISM IMPORTANT?

Other chapters of this book describe and explore a range of resources and methods that can support the development of a safety and improvement culture. A number of these focus on innovations in analysing and interpreting available information; others focus on the methodologies and resources that can be developed and employed to support this aim. However, a common theme through many of them is implicit recognition that to achieve success will require active and meaningful engagement with these processes by health professionals. This has been accompanied by explicit acknowledgement and identification of the human factors that influence individual engagement in this area. A distinction has been drawn between personal human factors and system-led human factors in patient safety.[1] While it may be assumed that professionalism should extend into both areas and would inevitably increase the likelihood of health professionals 'doing the right thing', it can be argued that the existing culture of medical professionalism can also inhibit this aim.

This is clearly a complex issue and it follows that this problem will not be solved simply by the creation of guidelines, the availability of accurate and timely information, the provision of education or expertise in evidence-based medicine and patient safety methods alone. It is therefore necessary to examine the aspects of professionalism that can be harnessed to drive this change and also those aspects of the culture of professionalism that may act as barriers to meeting these aspirations.

WHAT IS PROFESSIONALISM?

Medicine has long been accepted as embodying the key elements of professionalism. These include a requirement for specialised training resulting in the attainment of particular skills and the possession of specialised knowledge. They also include the right to be self-regulating, including setting the standards for admission to the profession, the right to set the ethical and clinical standards required of its members and the right to govern the behaviour of its members.[2]

As a consequence of these rights, a set of corresponding duties were recognised that included adherence to the established code of conduct and a duty to provide a service that promoted the best interests of patients and valued the interests of patients over self-interest.[3] Therefore it would appear implicit that even from the requirement of *primum non nocere* that acceptance of these conditions would necessarily imply a commitment to a safety and improvement culture that by now should be an established element of medical professionalism.

OLD PROFESSIONALISM: OLD PROBLEMS

Although many would still view medicine as a paradigm profession, the rapid advances in medical science, knowledge and technology of the late twentieth century were matched by societal changes and a correspondingly increasingly critical analysis of the existing culture of medical professionalism.[4] Medicine stood accused of operating an elitist, paternalistic, secretive cabal that was accountable only to itself, protecting the interests of its members over that of the public good.[5] These negative characteristics and the tribalistic behaviour they engendered were clearly unlikely to foster transparency and meaningful engagement in processes that some regarded as undermining the status and professional autonomy they enjoyed.

The growing scepticism about the nature of medical professionalism and whether the values it espoused remained fit for purpose was accompanied by discussion and debate within the medical community itself. In 1994 Calman[6] reflected these concerns when he argued it was an appropriate time to attempt to redefine professionalism. This was followed in 1995 by the publication of *Good Medical Practice* by the General Medical Council (GMC), which outlined seven headings of 'Good Medical Practice' (GMP) and the 'Duties of a Doctor'.[7] Both publications highlighted the requirement for a tangible commitment to delivering good clinical care and maintaining professional standards.

A more seismic shift followed the reaction to the publication of the Kennedy Report into the Bristol heart surgery scandal[8] and the wide reporting of several other high-profile scandals, including the results of Dame Janet Smith's Shipman Inquiry.[9] Together they served to portray an image of a profession that had lost its way and was complicit in putting patients at risk by failing to address concerns about patient safety that were known or should have been known. Specifically, Dame Janet described the GMC as 'an organisation designed to look after the interests of doctors, not patients'.[9]

'NEW PROFESSIONALISM'

To be fair, the profession itself had not stood still in the years leading up to and following the publication of the Kennedy report and the results of the Shipman Inquiry. Like other traditional professions, the medical workforce had undergone a significant change in demographics and had begun to reflect societal changes that saw its members becoming more representative of the general population. This generation of doctors had to address many challenges including consumerism, the increasing complexity of medicine itself and the ethical questions new technologies and changing attitudes raised. This led to a willingness on the part of the profession to examine its values and how these should be defined and demonstrated. A flurry of activity reflected the growth of almost a cottage industry in this area and resulted in the publication of a number of charters that attempted to define a 'new medical professionalism'.[10] One unifying feature of these statements was a firm emphasis on 'patient-centredness' as a founding principle and a desire to minimise the 'doctor-centred' nature of previous definitions of professionalism.[11]

Even if it is accepted that previous definitions of professionalism were too narrow and outdated, the attempt to reflect the complexity of modern healthcare and the desire to address identified concerns resulted in charters that detailed an increasingly long list of attributes that doctors should demonstrate in their professional behaviour. The duties of a doctor as outlined in GMP has grown from 46 separate criteria in the 1995 edition to the 80 areas covered by the most recent edition of GMP, which now even includes instructions regarding the use of social media.[12] The GMC guidance now also makes it explicit that a doctor's responsibilities go beyond providing good clinical care and maintaining his or her skills; the doctor must take a lead in ensuring patients receive high-quality care, are treated with dignity and the doctor has duties (to whistle-blow) if these criteria are not met.

In addition recent events in the UK have turned the spotlight onto not just doctors but all those who work in the health service. The Francis report into events that took place in the Mid-Staffordshire Hospital Trust outlines the duty all health professionals have, to understand and accept their responsibilities for patient safety and quality of care, and to act if they encounter unacceptable examples.[13] Regrettably, the events in the Mid-Staffordshire Hospital Trust would appear to suggest that despite the seemingly continuous endeavour to stratify and codify professionalism, very little has changed in ensuring patient safety apart from the production of an arsenal of statements and policy documents.

While the comprehensive nature of such guidance can be admired there is a danger that the desire to address all concerns results in a bureaucratic, determinist process that attempts to objectify values and behaviours that are at their heart subjective and resistant to definition and measurement. It is a familiar philosophical problem that the greater the attempt to define something in absolute terms the further the resulting description dilutes the essence of what is understood.

NEW PROFESSIONALISM: NEW PROBLEMS

It is perhaps not surprising that given the onerous nature of the responsibilities expected of doctors that the profession has struggled to demonstrate their compliance with and embrace all that is now expected of them. Health professionals have not only to meet the expectations of their regulators but are faced with increasingly onerous national and local contractual obligations. While responding to the call to respect and maximise the autonomy of the individual, health professionals are not only expected to act as gatekeepers, utilising finite resources effectively while improving access to care but, in addition, to take on responsibility for minimising risk and promoting a 'quality agenda' in the health service.[14] It is not surprising that 'what would you like me to stop doing so I can do this' has become a familiar complaint of a profession who sees itself as being presented with an ever-increasing range of responsibilities. Although the patient safety and quality improvement agenda would appear to be at the heart of GMP, further efforts have to be made to overcome the perception that this represents yet another unattractive add-on in a list of professional responsibilities.[15]

It is also appropriate to question how these aims can truly flourish in the face of a conflict between a desire to promote best practice and the increasing awareness of resource limitations. It appears self-evident that when resource issues dominate, greater value will be placed on those areas that lend themselves to measurement; consequently, there will be less inclination to dedicate resources to developing processes that explore more qualitative aspects of healthcare, such as the culture of an organisation and the behaviours of its workforce.[15]

Many commentators have emphasised the need to develop a culture of support in order to embed quality improvement processes. However, one unintentional consequence of the desire to promote transparency and accountability has been the creation of a perception that health professionals are now working in a culture of suspicion and scrutiny. Health professionals may be seen as being the solution to minimising risk and promoting safety but also fear being made the scapegoat and perhaps vilified in the media when problems arise. The effect of this loss of trust is impossible to quantify but it has been pointed out that although an obvious consequence is to erode the regard the public has for health professionals, patients themselves are also likely to be disadvantaged.[16] Patients may further suffer if this loss of confidence leads to a preference for a 'safety first' culture where health professionals seek to avoid all possible risk. Although accepting the tenet of *primum non nocere* may seem to be a key step in developing a safety culture, a bland endorsement ignores the issue that competing harms may exist where choosing not to intervene to minimise risk may not be in the best interests of the patient.

In 2006 the chief medical officer for NHS England acknowledged that: 'Much more of the harm caused to patients stems from error in unsafe systems than from incompetent or negligent doctors'.[17] He went on to suggest that one solution in assuring the quality of care was the availability of reliable information to support clinical activity and the provision of a robust and timely analysis of the results of that activity. However worthy an aspiration, the reality is that the systems to support such a process are at best patchy and inconsistent and risk ignoring the needs of clinical situations that do not lend themselves to measurement. Additionally, even with the most effective supporting infrastructure, there has to be a motivation for the workforce to make best use of available resources.

Medical educationalists have outlined the concerns they have about the 'Generation X and Y' of doctors. These doctors are described as representing a generation of health professionals that although familiar with technology and throughout their training are schooled in the methodologies of a safety and quality culture are considered to lack a previous generation's altruism and motivation, which may pose a greater threat to the quality of clinical care. This may lead to a laissez-faire attitude that acknowledges that the risk of unintentional harm is inherent in clinical practice and therefore accepts that there is little that an individual can do to alter this.[18]

MOVING FORWARDS: ACHIEVING ENGAGEMENT

However, the challenges that this particular issue raises for healthcare professionals are not peculiar to it alone and there is much to learn from a critical analysis of previous experience. If attitude is accepted as being of paramount importance, a useful starting point is to explore what attributes and behaviours are desirable.

All too often, innovation in medicine and the advancement of the quality of care is represented by the introduction of new technology or methods. However, this risks ignoring that it is how these techniques are employed that makes the real difference. The introduction of new systems can appear very top-down and may often conflict with individual aspirations. The greatest chance of successful integration may lie in ensuring that they build on existing work, and while addressing contractual requirements, are clearly underpinned by recognised and shared professional values. There is therefore a need to be equally innovative in considering how the medical workforce is supported to address this challenge and to explore how these aspirations can fit in with and enhance existing models of professional behaviour.[19]

The experience gained from coaching and mentoring schemes for health professionals may offer one way forwards. The benefits of such schemes have been identified and importantly they allow the opportunity for health professionals to focus on flaws in their existing practice and receive support to improve performance. Many of these schemes have focused on health professionals who are at the beginning of their careers but it is illogical to infer that experience assures performance or decreases the value of targeted support. In fact, experience may be accompanied by a heightened challenge in admitting difficulties or concerns particularly when faced with new methodologies.[20]

The introduction of annual appraisal for all doctors represents a sea change in how health professionals demonstrate their commitment to continuing professional development. Although participation in appraisal is a key part of revalidation, appraisal is designed to be a supportive and developmental process that addresses the full scope of a doctor's clinical practice. As part of this process all doctors have to provide supporting information about their practice in a number of areas including significant event analysis, complaints, information about their participation in continuing professional development activities, and the quality improvement activities they have undertaken, with reflection on how all of these have affected their practice. Importantly, it also offers doctors the opportunity to discuss any concerns they have about their health with a colleague in a confidential setting and to analyse feedback on their behaviour from colleagues and patients. To encourage objectivity and transparency trained appraisers are randomly appointed to appraise a colleague and cross specialty appraisal is encouraged. When I have discussed the introduction of the appraisal process with non-health professionals, their only surprise has been that our profession has taken so long to put such a system in place.

The benefits and impact of an effective appraisal process have been high-lighted before,[21] but appraisal also offers the opportunity to gather and share information about areas of practice that can promote the safety and quality agenda. What it has revealed is that doctors are and have been making a sustained contribution to this agenda, but with some exceptions often their efforts are uncoordinated, not shared and do not receive the recognition they deserve (including from themselves). Involvement in this process has high-lighted that many health professionals do not fully understand what is meant by a 'safety and quality improvement culture' and do not realise that invariably they already are, at some level, making a contribution to its development. The emphasis on quantitative audit and the introduction of mystifying arrays of poorly understood quality improvement models has led to confusion and risks stifling engagement.

Peer review of supporting information such as significant event analyses and criterion audit activity has been shown to be useful in facilitating the appraisal discussion. It has the advantage of providing objective feedback while maintaining the focus on the individual, reflecting existing and accepted models of professional behaviour. There is a need to improve the collation and dissemination of such potentially valuable information and to provide and develop the resources to support health professionals in these activities.[22]

The need for professional leadership in promoting and coordinating this agenda is clear. Changes in working practices and structural reconfiguration of the health service have led to the creation of a fractionalised and dislocated system where individual elements strive to meet multiple and disparate targets. While this may result in compliance with targets, it is questionable whether this will ensure thoughtful and consistent professional engagement with a safety and improvement culture. Although these issues and the variety of platforms available appear to attract no shortage of commentators, much of what is written appears to be reactive, reinforcing the challenges rather than offering a proactive solution. There is a need for positive leadership and a clear and consistent manifesto to provide direction and stimulus. The absence of consistent medical leadership in the patient safety agenda and the risks involved in neglecting the influence of professional cultures has been highlighted.[23] There are notable exceptions, particularly from the United States, where Gawande[24] has been able to demonstrate an understanding of the complexity and changing nature of medical professionalism and sought to offer leadership in embedding this agenda. More recently, in the UK a number of programmes have been established to provide the resources and support necessary to develop leadership among National Health Service staff.[25]

Professionalism is now a taught subject on medical curriculums; however, assessment may only demonstrate a student's knowledge of professional codes rather than an understanding of how this translates into professional behaviours. It has been suggested that the daunting nature of ensuring adherence to all the desired individual attributes could be aided by encouraging students to develop a broader understanding of professionalism. Rather than concentrating on securing a statistical evidence base for our behaviour, greater influence in healthcare may come from encouraging students and health professionals to reflect on the work of writers such as Toon[26] who have explored professionalism from a vocational and ethical perspective.

The research that has been done in this area can also offer organisations who seek to engage with professionals valuable insights in how this can be achieved. In 2012 The King's Fund published a discussion paper that explored the view that it was critical to ensure medical engagement in management, leadership and service improvement in order to maintain and improve performance.[27]

One successful example cited described the following principles:
- ask doctors to lead – the mantra is 'physician-led, data-driven, evidence-based'
- ask doctors what they want to work on
- make it easy for doctors to lead and to participate – optimise the time
- provide resources
- provide recognition
- support medical staff leaders with courage – where they meet with resistance
- provide opportunities to learn and grow.

This study emphasised that change in healthcare can be achieved by recognising the positive aspects of medical professionalism and developing a strategy that reflects the aims of the organisation but allows and supports health professionals to engage with one another to drive learning, quality and professional satisfaction. Although focused on medical leadership, it appears to offer a useful framework that could be employed to foster the meaningful professional engagement that is necessary for the patient safety agenda to prosper. Health professionals have much to contribute to the patient safety culture. Effective engagement can represent a tangible demonstration of the principles of professionalism and may achieve more in terms of enhancing these professional values. It is also likely to lead to a wider appreciation and recognition of these values than any complex and abstract set of criteria. It is also clear that health professionals have much to lose from failing to engage positively in supporting this process. Appearing to be seen as a group either motivated by self-interest or as passive cogs will inevitably erode both the development and wider public perception of medical professionalism.

REFERENCES

1. Flin R, Winter J, Sarac C, *et al. Human Factors Review.* Geneva: World Health Organization; 2009. Available at: www.who.int/patientsafety/research/methods_measures/human_factors/en/ (accessed 10 November 2013).
2. Thistlewaite J, Spencer J. *Professionalism in Medicine.* Oxford: Radcliffe Publishing; 2008.
3. Irvine D. Time for hard decisions on patient centred professionaliasm. *Med J Aust.* 2004; **181**(50): 271–4.
4. Freidson E. *Professional Dominance: the social structure of medical care.* Chicago, IL: Aldine; 1970.
5. Illich I. *Limits to Medicine. Medical nemesis: the expropriation of health.* Harmondsworth: Penguin; 1976.
6. Calman K. The profession of medicine. *BMJ.* 1994; **309**(6962): 1140–4.
7. General Medical Council. *Duties of a Doctor.* London: GMC; 1995.
8. Smith R. All changed, changed utterly. *BMJ.* 1998; **316**(7149): 1917–18.
9. Shipman Inquiry. *Safeguarding Patients: lessons from the past – proposals for the future.* (2004) Available at: http://webarchive.nationalarchives.gov.uk/20090808154959/http:/www.the-shipman-inquiry.org.uk/reports.asp (accessed 10 November 2013).
10. Chisolm A, Ashkam J. *A Review of Codes and Standards for Doctors in the UK, USA and Canada.* Oxford: Picker Institute Europe; 2006. Available at: www.pickereurope.org/item/documemnt/59 (accessed 10 November 2013).
11. Ashkam J, Chishol A. *Patient-Centred Medical Professionalism: towards an agenda for research and action.* Oxford: Picker Institute Europe; 2006.
12. General Medical Council. *Good Medical Practice.* London: GMC; 2013. Available at: www.gmc-uk.org/guidance/good_medical_practice.asp (accessed 10 November 2013).
13. Francis R. *Robert Francis Inquiry Report into Mid-Staffordshire NHS Foundation Trust.* London: The Stationery Office; 2010.
14. ABIM Foundation, American Board of Internal Medicine; ACP-ASIM Foundation, American College of Physicians-American Society of Internal Medicine; European Federation of Internal Medicine. Medical professionalism in the new millennium: a physician charter project of the ABIM Foundation. *Ann Intern Med.* 2002; **136**(3): 243–6.
15. Waring J. Beyond blame: cultural barriers to medical incident reporting. *Soc Sci Med.* 2005; **60**(9): 1927–35.
16. O'Neill O. *Reith Lectures 2002: A Question of Trust.* London: BBC Radio 4; 2002. Available at: www.bbc.co.uk/radio4/reith2002/ (accessed 6 March 2014).
17. Chief Medical Officer. *Good Doctors, Safer Patients.* London: Department of Health; 2006.

18. Roland M, Rao SR, Sibbald B, *et al*. Professional values and reported behaviours of doctors in the USA and UK: quantitative survey. *BML Qual Saf*. 2011; **20**(6): 515–21.

19. Lester HE, Hannon KL, Campbell SM. Identifying unintended consequences of quality indicators: a qualitative study. *BMJ Qual Saf*. 2011; **20**(12): 1057–61.

20. Steven A, Oxley J, Fleming WG. Mentoring for NHS doctors: perceived benefits across the professional and personal interface. *J R Soc Med*. 2008; **101**(11): 552–7.

21. West M. How can good performance among doctors be maintained? *BMJ*. 2002; **325**(7366): 669.

22. Bowie P, Cameron N, Staples I, *et al*. Verifying appraisal evidence using feedback from trained peers: views and experiences of Scottish GP appraisers. *Br J Gen Pract*. 2009; **59**(564): 484–9.

23. Lamont T. *Where are the Doctors in Patient Safety Research?* [Blog]. London: BMJ Group; 2012. Available at: http://blogs.bmj.com/bmj/2012/09/24/tara-lamont-where-are-the-doctors-in-patient-safety-research/ (accessed 6 march 2014).

24. Gawande A. Personal best: top athletes and singers have coaches. Should you? *New Yorker*. 2011 Oct 3. Available at: www.newyorker.com/reporting/2011/10/03/111003fa_fact_gawande?currentPage=all (accessed 10 November 2013).

25. NHS Education for Scotland. Leadership and Management. Available at: www.nes.scot.nhs.uk/education-and-training/by-theme-initiative/leadership-and-management.aspx (accessed 10 November 2013).

26. Toon PD. Towards a philosophy of general practice: a study of the virtuous practitioner. *Occas Pap R Coll Gen Pract*. 1999; (78): iii–vii, 1–69.

27. The King's Fund. *Exploring Medical Leadership and Engagement*. London: The King's Fund, 2012. Available at: www.kingsfund.org.uk/projects/review/leadership-nhs/exploring-medical-leadership-and-engagement (accessed 10 November 2013).

CHAPTER 14

Peer review

Paul Bowie & John McKay

The overall objective of peer review is to improve patient safety and health outcomes.[1]

In this chapter the concept of peer review is defined and the multiplicity of roles it plays in healthcare education and practice is outlined, together with the contribution it can make to improve the quality and safety of primary care. The latter contribution is demonstrated via a particular focus on describing the underlying theory, development, operation and research outputs of a successful and long-established Scottish peer feedback model for general practice.

INTRODUCTION

The concept of peer review is well established in healthcare education and clinical practice. In its broadest sense it describes the evaluation of specific aspects of a person's performance by a peer or group of peers.[2] Making a determination on individual performance inevitably involves making some form of professional judgement. In primary care, until recently, peer review (if thought about at all) was probably most commonly associated with the process by which manuscripts submitted to medical journals were assessed for scientific rigour and suitability for publication.

Now, however, systems of peer review play an active role in contributing to the evaluation of a range of performance and care quality issues in the United Kingdom (*see* Box 14.1) and internationally – despite it undoubtedly being a 'threatening prospect' for most doctors and clinicians in general.[3] It is clear that peer feedback, therefore, is potentially well placed to play a key role in informing professional learning and making a significant contribution to improving the quality and safety of primary care. Indeed, a recent systematic review of the published evidence demonstrated the broad purpose and primary rationale for devising and implementing peer-review processes (*see* Box 14.2).

> **BOX 14.1 Examples of peer-review systems in primary care**
>
> - Compliance monitoring of the Quality and Outcomes Framework contract by peer visitors
> - Specialty training practice assessment and accreditation visits by peers
> - Annual appraisal of a GP by a trained GP peer appraiser
> - Scottish Prospective GP Educational Supervisors submission of quality improvement activities for peer review
> - Royal College of General Practitioners Quality Practice Accreditation is assessed and awarded by peers
> - Underperforming GPs undergo peer review of aspects of clinical work (e.g. prescribing and referrals)

Defining peer review

Despite its long-standing and increasing use in healthcare, accurately defining peer review is actually problematic because of the different variations of approach. The term 'peer' followed by 'review', 'assessment', 'feedback' and 'appraisal' are used interchangeably in the literature.[1] It is also complicated by the underlying intention of the review process and whether this is formal (e.g. awarding research funding or granting specialty training accreditation) or informal (e.g. patient case conferences or seeking out feedback from a trusted colleague on a specific work issue).

The purpose of peer review can also differ in terms of professional importance, ranging from a 'low stakes' reflective discussion on a clinician's practice at one end of the spectrum, to an external 'high stakes' evaluation of performance for re-licensure to practise medicine at the other.[1-3] Arguably, most clinicians would recognise the concept in terms of its simple and frequent application between colleagues as a 'voluntary, informal, and collaborative' means of giving feedback on a professional or clinical issue. The following definition is perhaps best placed, therefore, to capture the full range of meanings attributed to this important educational and improvement method:

> The evaluation by a practitioner of creative work or performance by other practitioners in the same field in order to assure, maintain and/or enhance the quality of work or performance.[1]

Adequately defining a 'peer' is also a difficult task depending on the context, purpose and mode of feedback or assessment being provided in a peer-to-peer relationship. For example, is a young, newly qualified doctor with little professional or clinical experience equally matched as a 'peer' to a much more experienced and expert, older doctor? Many diverse definitions exist but the description of a peer as 'a health practitioner with relevant clinical experience in similar health service environments who also has the knowledge and skills to contribute to the review of other health practitioners' performance'[1] is arguably closest to how most clinicians would understand and recognise this concept. However, depending on the nature of the specific issue under review (e.g. significant event analysis (SEA) or consultation skill), possessing appropriate clinical experience does not necessarily inculcate an individual with the necessary knowledge and skills to properly review a practitioner's performance in this specific area.

For the learner (or recipient of feedback) there is an expectation that peer reviewers will be professionally credible and acceptable. A summary of the literature on this topic reported that peer review would appear to be particularly effective if, among other factors, it is provided by colleagues who are respected by the learner.[4] The credibility of the reviewer is also known to be important to individual practitioners in their perception and acceptance of feedback.[5] Grol and Lawrence[4] reported that in their experience, doctors who take part in peer review undergo an educational process that allows them to adopt a self-critical stance with regard to their professionalism. Effectively, they need to undertake 'critical thinking,' which is described as a disposition to carefully consider problems that present in practice and then be able to act on feedback given.[6]

BOX 14.2 Systematic literature review: primary purpose of peer-review activity uncovered[1]

- Assessment of the clinician's domains of professional practice
- Assessment of delivery of care in accordance with clinical guidelines
- Assessment of organisational quality of care
- Peer review as a requirement for continuing professional development
- Assessment of significant events
- Quality assurance of clinical laboratory practices
- Peer review for the purposes of credentialing healthcare providers
- Assessment of suspected underperforming of the healthcare provider

---

ABOUT THE NHS EDUCATION FOR SCOTLAND PEER FEEDBACK MODEL

In the west of Scotland, a well-established educational model[7] aims to provide GPs with informed, objective, confidential and independent feedback from trained peers on the standard of three quality improvement (QI) activities that are also core elements informing medical appraisal[8] and revalidation – videoed consultations, criterion-based audit and SEA. The peer feedback model is coordinated by NHS Education for Scotland (NES) and is used on a voluntary basis by GPs as part of regional arrangements for participating in continuing professional development activity. It was initially developed as a means of promoting and enhancing educational understanding and practical skills related to quality improvement techniques and the doctor–patient consultation. A key driver, however, was the provision of external and independent judgements, verification and feedback on the quality of an educational process

that is performed by a practitioner and which ultimately had important implications for improving patient safety.

More recently, the purpose of the model has moved beyond the confines
of continuing professional development, and is now being used as a development aid as part of the national prospective GP educational supervisors
course, whereby participants must submit a consultation video and SEA for
peer review as part of the qualification process. Additionally, a large west of
Scotland health authority has used the system to provide developmental feedback on the quality of SEAs submitted by GP teams as part of the Quality and
Outcomes Framework contract arrangements,[9] thereby gaining insights into
patient safety-related learning needs at an organisational level – this is an
important learning development given the virtual non-engagement by general
practice teams in the formal reporting of patient safety incidents to established
regional and national systems.[10]

The novel aspect of the NES peer feedback model is that it appears to be
the only one reported in the literature that utilises GP peers who are specifically trained to review and provide developmental feedback – using structured
assessment methods – on the aforementioned QI and appraisal activities outlined. Importantly, the model adheres robustly to the five key educational
principles of an effective peer-review system (*see* Box 14.3). To date, around
50% of west of Scotland GP principals (approximately 1000) have submitted at least one piece of QI evidence for peer review since its inception in the
late 1990s. The model has since been adapted by general practice managers
and the pharmacy and dental professionals for review of SEAs as one way of
demonstrating an explicit contribution to the growing patient safety agenda
in primary care.[11]

BOX 14.3 Principles of effective peer-review systems[1]

- The governing body of a health services organisation and its leadership have
  a responsibility to support effective peer review
- Healthcare professionals have a professional responsibility to regularly and
  actively engage in peer review
- Peer review should produce valid and reliable information
- Processes for peer review must be transparent, fair and equitable, and legally
  and ethically robust
- The outcomes of peer review should be applied ultimately to improve patient
  care

'New' definition of peer review

As a direct consequence of how the model has evolved, the existing definitions of a 'peer' and 'peer review' previously discussed have been adapted to
align with its unique and very specific purpose. Within this context, a peer
is described as an 'informed, independent GP who has received appropriate

training in the areas on which they are asked to review and provide formative, constructive feedback to colleagues'.[7,11] This definition recognises the
expectation that a peer who is tasked with providing feedback to professional colleagues should at least have undergone related training in order that
feedback is constructive and delivered within an acceptable educational framework,[12] thereby reducing the risk of poorly delivered negative feedback being
given to individual practitioners.

Similarly, 'peer review' is defined very specifically and deliberately as the
'evaluation of one element of an individual's performance by trained colleagues
using a validated review instrument to facilitate developmental feedback'.[7,11]
Although 'validation' is only one of the psychometric properties of the 'instrument' that requires to be considered in such a model,[13] the definition signifies
that the assessment content of the instrument would at least be relevant having
been subjected to a robust development process and also endorsed by 'users'
and 'experts'. Compared with other systems of peer review, therefore, key differences with this model are the recruitment and training of external peer
reviewers and the use of psychometrically developed and tested instruments
to facilitate feedback by these peers.[14-16]

How the model works

The model works as follows: Individual clinicians and managers submit their
SEA or audit reports or videoed consultations in standard formats to the NES
office (see Figure 14.1). The reports are screened for confidentiality issues before

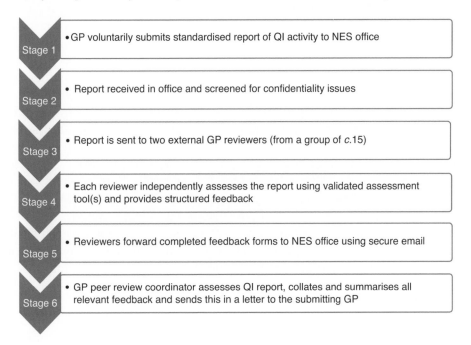

Stage 1 • GP voluntarily submits standardised report of QI activity to NES office

Stage 2 • Report received in office and screened for confidentiality issues

Stage 3 • Report is sent to two external GP reviewers (from a group of c.15)

Stage 4 • Each reviewer independently assesses the report using validated assessment tool(s) and provides structured feedback

Stage 5 • Reviewers forward completed feedback forms to NES office using secure email

Stage 6 • GP peer review coordinator assesses QI report, collates and summarises all relevant feedback and sends this in a letter to the submitting GP

FIGURE 14.1 NHS Education for Scotland (NES) peer feedback system for the submission
of significant event analysis or criterion audit reports

being sent to two members of a trained peer group. Each peer assesses them independently and the aforementioned assessment instruments are completed (providing numerical and narrative-based feedback). Constructive, developmental, and confidential comments on the standard of the completed activity are returned to a GP peer-review coordinator who collates all of the feedback, then compiles a written report summary and passes this to the submitting individual. Typically, the feedback will confirm good standards of practice and/or highlight potential areas for improving the application of the technique or skill and also suggestions for making patient care safer, where judged appropriate. In the case of videoed consultations, the feedback is provided on a written basis, unless consultation performance is judged to be unsafe or gives cause for concern and then a face-to-face meeting is arranged to explore the issues highlighted by the reviewers.

Educational theory

The underlying principles of the model are based on an adaptation of cognitive continuum theory.[17] This framework aids understanding of the thinking used in performing a range of tasks. The aim is to improve the quality of reflection on particular tasks. How this is done is described in one of six 'modes of practice' ranging from the highly structured scientific experiment (mode 1) to intuitive judgements (mode 6). Peer review sits between modes 4 (system-aided judgement) and 5 (peer-aided judgement) and is designed to minimise the probability of a mode 6 judgement (self-assessment) leading to invalid conclusions on decisions made.

Given the increasing importance being accorded to the links between medical appraisal and revalidation in the United Kingdom,[18,19] more attention will inevitably be paid to the standard of supporting evidence (e.g. SEAs) being submitted. Ultimately, someone has to make a judgement as to whether it is 'good enough'. GP appraisers have consistently voiced their discomfort at being given this task.[20,21] This external peer-review system allows the judgements to be made prior to an appraisal with a built-in sampling process of 'quality control' ensuring fairness across the country – that is, a national standard. However, the feasibility of a national external peer-review system to support appraisal (or other improvement intervention that can be enhanced by peer review) is open to question. For such a system to function, additional resources will be required. One option is to consider the vision that all GPs are potential peer reviewers – with appropriate training – with local 'experts' taking on the role of quality assuring the process. If it is to be practicable, much wider discussion is needed. The status quo, however, may not be an option if revalidation is to be a robust process.

Some may question the need for peer review of this type. However, the literature on the very limited value of self-assessment in healthcare education is clear.[22] The benefit, therefore, of providing additional peer review should not only be desirable but – given the potential stakes – essential. The adaptation of the Hammond model of cognitive continuum theory[17] underpins this justification by encouraging a more rational (rather than merely intuitive) approach to decision-making on material submitted for appraisal – or for specialty training or clinical governance purposes – which is then included in a revalidation folder.

Recruitment and training of peer reviewers

One important aspect of the feasibility of any peer-review model is the ability to recruit individuals who are prepared to participate as professional reviewers of aspects of their colleagues' performance and provide appropriate feedback. This will depend on factors such as whether reviewers need to be local, national or international, the degree of 'expertise' required, and the acceptability of the process to the proposed reviewers. Where difficulties in recruitment have been experienced, suggested methods of recruiting reviewers include inviting professionals who are known to organisers or administrators of the model, and requesting participants to suggest reviewers or contacting existing reviewers to nominate other professional colleagues.[1]

Within the context of healthcare education, it is desirable that anyone who is involved in giving feedback should be skilled in the process. Schroter and Groves[23] outlined four aims for any process used in the training of peer reviewers for medical journals. Three of these could be applied to most models of medical peer review: (1) to make clear what constitutes a fair, specific and constructive review for the learner; (2) to understand what matters to those commissioning the review; and (3) to produce reviews that reflect the qualities desired from training.

It is highly important, therefore, that reviewers are trained in the principles of effective feedback, which were described by Wood:[24]

- helping clarify what is good performance
- facilitating the development of reflection in learning
- delivering high-quality information to the participant about his or her learning
- encouraging reviewer and peer dialogue around learning
- encouraging positive motivational beliefs and self-esteem
- providing opportunities to close the gap between current and desired performance
- peer reviewers need to be chosen appropriately and trained in delivering appropriate feedback.

The importance of each of these elements of feedback will vary depending on the type and purpose of the feedback model, but it would seem essential that reviewers are not only trained but also updated in the elements of good feedback practice. This may not always be achieved. In their review of peer assessment instruments used for judging professional performance, Evans *et al.*[25] found that none of the studies described rater training when developing the instrument. Guidance, if given, consisted only of short written instructions.

Primary care safety, improvement and governance

The NES model described is underpinned by a growing research evidence base[7,11,14–16,26–33] and is valued by participants (*see* Box 14.4). Aligning the concept of peer review with the evaluation of QI activities provides 'added value' to the methods applied and the results generated, thereby enhancing their contribution to making patient care safer for all those with a stake in the quality of the healthcare system. Examples are as follows.

- *For patients and the public*: it provides reassurance that healthcare teams take patient safety seriously and are learning from error-related systems failure. Additional independent review of SEA, criterion audit and consultation skills acts as a 'double-check' on standards and may be useful for making judgements, particularly where providing evidence of participation in these improvement activities attracts public funding.
- *For healthcare professionals and teams*: it facilitates the identification of learning needs and opportunities for rapid improvement in patient safety with external review acting as an independent feedback mechanism and offering additional developmental insights by colleagues trained in the process.
- *For NHS board leaders and educational specialists*: it validates and enhances the purported value and role of SEA, criterion audit and consultation skill in education, learning and patient safety.
- *Leading on criterion audit or SEA or seeking to improve consultation skill all contributes to organisational learning and helps build a safety culture*: embedding these activities as part of accreditation, appraisal and educational initiatives has enabled healthcare teams to learn from, for example, patient safety incidents or improvement outcomes, which previously might not have been prioritised or dealt with adequately.
- *Independent review of SEA and criterion audit is a key improvement mechanism*: feedback on these QI activities from trained peer colleagues has provided important input into further system changes and improvements that were necessary to minimise the risk of future hazards and harm to patients.
- *Greater understanding and evidence of learning and improvement*: it has led to research on submitted SEA reports that has provided a more informed understanding of what goes wrong in different healthcare settings; why safety incidents may occur; the range of individual and healthcare team learning needs identified; the types of system changes that are necessary; and insights into the potential sustainability of improvements.

Currently in the United Kingdom, medical revalidation is based on the recommendation of the local 'responsible officer' (RO) to the General Medical Council.[34] This recommendation is based on a doctor's appraisal over 5 years. As part of the supporting information for appraisal, GPs are expected to provide two SEA reports and one quality improvement report (such as a criterion audit) per appraisal. Current review of these activities is by a single appraiser. External verification of these activities by the peer-review model discussed would enhance the objectivity of a doctor's evidence and inform appraisal leads and ROs when making decisions and recommendations based on the evidence presented. In addition, where underperformance of a doctor is being addressed by ROs a valid and reliable external peer review can help chart progress in remediation efforts.

BOX 14.4 Examples of feedback on the feedback from participants

'I found the whole process very rewarding and I am glad I took part. External peer review is very useful as it is completely unbiased with no personal feelings towards the person doing the work'. (*Practice Manager*)	'It's not just the public; it is anyone outside the practice. It is just a little bit too cosy to just mention your errors to one person and expect that to necessarily promote things forward . . . I can see for the general public you know, if you want things to have any kind of rigour then you want outside comments'. (*GP*)
'. . . the SEA report, where you look at what conclusions have been drawn and you go whoa, whoa – you just really missed the point here.' (*GP Peer Reviewer*)	'GP Appraisers might not be quite as honest and quite as frank as someone completely independent'. (*GP*)

CONCLUSIONS

The basic concept of peer review is well established in many primary care systems and is largely based on sound educational principles and theory. However, the NES peer feedback model described in this chapter potentially adds much-needed value to the concept and, as such, is well placed as a method of external and independent review that can enhance the standard of improvement activities undertaken by primary care clinicians and managers, while also offering an element of professional and organisational accountability. Its transferability to other healthcare settings has yet to be tested, but the same principles and practices should apply. In one sense, it is arguably the QI method with the greatest potential impact in terms of the wide-ranging improvement contribution it can make at different levels (patient, individual practitioner, organisational and regulatory) of healthcare practice simultaneously.

REFERENCES

1. Australian Commission on Safety and Quality in Healthcare. *Peer Review of Health Care Professionals: a systematic literature of the literature.* Melbourne: Australian Commission on Safety and Quality in Healthcare; 2009.

2. Helfer RE. Peer evaluation: its potential usefulness in medical education. *Br J Med Educ.* 1972; **6**(3): 224–31.

3. Grol R. Peer review in primary care. *Qual Assur Health Care.* 1990; **2**(2): 119–26.

4. Grol R, Lawrence M. *Quality Improvement by Peer Review.* Oxford General Practice Series, 32. Oxford: Oxford University Press; 1995.

5. Sargeant J, Mann K, Ferrier S. Exploring family physicians' reactions to multisource feedback: perceptions of credibility and usefulness. *Med Educ.* 2005; **39**(5): 497–504.

6. Greco PJ, Eisenberg JM. Changing physicians' practices. *N Engl J Med.* 1993 Oct 21; **329**(17): 1271–3.

7. Bowie P, Cameron N, Staples I, *et al.* Verifying appraisal evidence using feedback from trained peers: views and experiences of Scottish GP appraisers. *Br J Gen Pract.* 2009; **59**: 484–9.

8. Scottish Executive, NHS Education for Scotland, Royal College of General Practitioners (Scotland) and British Medical Association (Scotland). *GP Appraisal Scheme: a brief guide.* Edinburgh: Scottish Executive; 2003. Available at: www.sehd.scot.nhs.uk/publications/gpabg/gpabg-00.htm (accessed 2 June 2013).

9. Department of Health. *New GMS Contract 2006/7.* London: The Stationery Office; 2006.

10. McKay J, Bowie P, Murray L, *et al.* Levels of agreement on the grading, analysis and reporting of significant events by general practitioners: a cross sectional study. *Qual Saf Health Care.* 2008; **17**: 339–45.

11. Bowie P, Quinn P, Power A. Independent feedback on clinical audit performance: a multi-professional pilot study. *Clin Govern Int J.* 2009; **14**(3): 198–214.

12. Pendleton D, Scofield T, Tate P, *et al. The Consultation: an approach to learning and teaching.* Oxford: Oxford University Press; 1984.

13. Van der Vleuten CPM. The assessment of professional competence: developments, research and practical implications. *Adv Health Sci Educ.* 1996; **1**(1): 41–67.

14. Cameron N, McMillan R. Enhancing communication skills by peer review of consultation videos. *Educ Prim Care.* 2006; **17**(1): 40–8.

15. Lough JRM, McKay J, Murray TS. Audit and summative assessment: a criterion-referenced marking schedule. *Br J Gen Pract.* 1995; **45**(400): 607–9.

16. McKay J, Murphy D, Bowie P, *et al.* Development and testing of an assessment instrument for the formative peer review of significant event analyses. *Qual Saf Health Care.* 2007; **16**(2): 150–3.

17. Hammond KR. Towards increasing competence of thought in public policy formation. In: Hammond KR, editor. *Judgement and Decision in Public Policy Formation.* Boulder, CO: Westview Press; 1978. pp. 11–32.

18. Secretary of State for Health. *Trust, Assurance and Safety: the regulation of health professionals in the 21st century.* White Paper presented to Parliament by the Secretary of State for Health by Command of Her Majesty. London: The Stationery Office; 2007.

19. Department of Health. *Good Doctors, Safer Patients: proposals to strengthen the system to assure and improve the performance of doctors and to protect the safety of patients. A report by the Chief Medical Officer.* London: Department of Health; 2006.

20. Jelley D, van Zwanenberg T. Peer appraisal in general practice: descriptive study in the Northern Deanery. *Educ Gen Pract.* 2001; **11**(1): 281–7.

21. Lewis M, Welwyn G, Wood F. Appraisal of family doctors: an evaluation study. *Br J Gen Pract.* 2003; **53**(491): 454–60.

22. Colthart I, Bagnall G, Evans A, Allbutt H, Haig A, Illing J, and McKinstry B. *Medical Teacher*. 2008; **30**(2): 124–45.

23. Schroter S, Groves T. BMJ training for peer reviewers. *BMJ*. 2004; **328**: 658.

24. Wood D. *Formative Assessment*. Understanding Medical Education Series. Association for the Study of Medical Education (ASME), Edinburgh 2007.

25. Evans R, Elwyn G, Edwards A. Review of instruments for peer assessment of physicians. *BMJ*. 2004; **328**(7458): 1240–3.

26. Bowie P, McCoy S, McKay J, *et al*. Learning issues raised by the educational peer review of significant event analyses in general practice. *Qual Prim Care*. 2005; **13**(2): 75–84.

27. McKay J, Bowie P, Lough M. Variations in the ability of general medical practitioners in applying two methods of clinical audit: a five-year study of assessment by peer review. *J Eval Clin Pract*. 2006; **12**(6): 622–9.

28. Bowie P, McKay J, Dalgetty E, *et al*. A qualitative study of why general practitioners may participate in significant event analysis and educational peer review. *Qual Saf Health Care*. 2005; **14**(3): 185–9.

29. McKay J, Shepherd A, Bowie P, *et al*. Acceptability and educational impact of a peer feedback model for significant event analysis. *Med Educ*. 2008; **42**(12): 1210–17.

30. McKay J, Pope L, Bowie P, *et al*. Peer feedback in general practice: a focus group study of trained reviewers of significant event analyses. *J Eval Clin Pract*. 2009; **15**(1): 142–7.

31. Murie J, McCrae J, Bowie P. The peer review pilot project: a potential system to support GP appraisal in NHS Scotland. *Educ Prim Care*. 2009; **20**: 34–40.

32. McMillan R, Cameron N. Factors influencing the submission of videotaped consultations by general practitioners for peer review and educational feedback. *Qual Prim Care*. 2006; **14**(2): 85–9.

33. Bowie P, Cooke S, Lo P, *et al*. The assessment of criterion audit cycles by external peer review: when is an audit not an audit? *J Eval Clin Pract*. 2007; **13**(3): 352–7.

34. Shepherd A, Cameron N. What are the concerns of prospective responsible officers about their role in medical revalidation? *J Eval Clin Pract*. 2010; **16**(3): 655–60.

CHAPTER 15

Professional appraisal

Ian Staples, Niall Cameron & Carl de Wet

This chapter begins with a contextual overview of appraisal before describing the general practitioner (GP) appraisal system in Scotland and its potential value for participants. The effective characteristics of an appraisal meeting are also considered before the chapter concludes with examples of how the GP appraisal process is being supported in practice.

BACKGROUND

The origins of appraisal in the workplace can be traced back to the early 1940s in the United States.[1] It was initially introduced with the expectation that it would help to increase the productivity of the workforce, but the scope of appraisal expanded in the 1980s in some industries to include the professional development of employees. Since then, the reasons for conducting appraisals have evolved further, so that it is now increasingly used as a performance management tool.

In this capacity, line managers (the 'appraisers') typically assess employees (the 'appraisees'), grading their performance. The results of this assessment have significant implications for the employee, who may receive financial (and other) rewards for success but may, conversely, be demoted or face redundancy or a range of other disciplinary sanctions for perceived failure. It is therefore hardly surprising that, when appraisal is used as a performance management tool, it has been found to paradoxically de-incentivise employees and thereby reduce organisational efficiency.[2] Similarly, it can lead to protracted and expensive legal challenges of organisational decisions about redundancies and promotions that were based only on the results of an appraisal.[3]

Therefore, it seems reasonable, and potentially more useful, to adopt a developmental approach in preference to a performance management approach for appraisal. In this model, the appraiser (a line manager or a peer) assists the appraisee to reflect on and assess his or her own performance and experiences in order to identify learning needs and whether there is a need for further personal, professional or performance improvement.[4] However, there is still a lack of suitably robust evidence to support the effectiveness of this reflective approach to appraisal in the healthcare sector.[5-7]

Today, appraisal is ubiquitous in the public sector in the United Kingdom (UK) and typically combines elements of personal development and performance management. For example, the national agreement on pay and conditions of service for National Health Service staff outlined in the *Agenda for Change* handbook includes the requirement that all non-medical staff have annual Knowledge and Skills Framework reviews by their line managers.[8] The main aim of these review meetings is to determine the employee's current level of development in relation to the key skills required to perform his or her role effectively. It also seeks to identify and prioritise resultant learning needs and to agree an action plan to address these needs within a specific timescale (typically the next 12-month period).

During the 1990s a series of high-profile patient safety incidents were widely reported in the media in the UK and presented as national scandals. This shocked the confidence of the UK public in the medical profession in general and raised concerns about the profession's ability to self-regulate effectively.[9] In response, the General Medical Council published a draft policy on revalidation in 1997 in which it recommended that annual appraisal of all doctors should be introduced.[10] Subsequently, a system of appraisal for all GPs was introduced in Scotland in 2003.

THE GENERAL PRACTITIONER APPRAISAL SYSTEM IN SCOTLAND

There were two main tasks that required immediate attention after the decision to implement a national system of GP appraisal in 2003. The first task was to agree the formal content, format and processes of appraisal. This was achieved through consensus-building methods involving the major stakeholder: the Royal College of General Practitioners, senior leaders from the different health boards, the Scottish Executive, the British Medical Association and NHS Education for Scotland (NES). The second task was the recruitment and training of potential GP appraisers. This was achieved during a period of 18 months and laid the foundation for all further developments.

A key principle guiding the design of the system was that appraisal should encourage GPs to focus on their own learning needs. To help achieve this aim, five core categories were developed:
1. Prescribing
2. Criterion audit
3. Communication
4. Significant event analysis
5. Referrals.

The annual appraisal process includes a formal, scheduled meeting between the GP (appraisee) and the trained appraiser at a mutually convenient time and venue. At present all appraisers are also GPs, but it has been suggested that suitably trained clinicians and managers from other professions may in future also be recruited for this role.

Appraisees self-select one of the five core categories each year in advance of their appraisal meeting, aiming to cover all five categories over a 5-year cycle. During the year they collect evidence of their performance relevant to this category and submit it electronically for review in advance of the scheduled meeting with their named appraiser. The aim of the meeting is to review all aspects of the appraisee's professional work, identify and consider his or her learning needs and devise and agree a plan to address them according to the perceived priority over the course of the following year. During the meeting the core category is discussed in detail but the appraisee is also encouraged to reflect on *all* aspects of the *Good Medical Practice* framework as it relates to his or her work. The main discussion points and agreed outcomes of the meeting are recorded by the appraiser and 'signed off' by the appraisee. The report helps to feed a virtuous cycle where improvement activity is followed by critical reflection, which in turn leads to further improvement and so on.

The relationship and interactions between the appraiser and appraisee is a key determinant of the success of the appraisal process. More research is required to determine which appraiser and appraisee characteristics and behaviour are conducive to success and whether that can be distilled into an educational resource. However, there is already a rich body of evidence from interview techniques and counselling skills that may be applicable and transferable to the appraisal meeting.[11] A selection of the desired characteristics of an appraiser and appraisal meeting is shown in Table 15.1.

TABLE 15.1 Characteristics of an effective appraiser and appraisal meeting

Appraisal meeting	Appraiser
Structured	• Agree an agenda at the beginning of the meeting
	• Signpost areas for discussion as well as the beginning and end of the meeting and its different components
	• The appraiser manages the interview effectively and summarises the discussion regularly
A safe and supportive experience	• Clarify confidentiality boundaries
	• Develops rapport through the use of reflective and empathic interventions
	• Works cooperatively with the appraisee and checks for understanding and agreement with suggestions
Provides 'space' for the appraisee to talk and reflect on his or her performance	• Avoids inappropriate interruption or 'blocking' the appraisee.
	• Interventions are meaningful and designed to encourage further reflection, deeper understanding and learning
	• Tolerate and use silence constructively during the meeting

(*continued*)

Appraisal meeting	Appraiser
Provides opportunities for appraisees to address emotional issues (if any) resulting from their work	• Sensitive to and aware of the potential emotional components of the material the appraisee discusses (explicit and implicit) • Makes non-collusive, empathic interventions and encourages the appraisee to freely express his or her feelings • Accepts the expression of emotions (anger, sadness, grief) and responds appropriately
Challenges the appraisee to consider how he or she might improve patient care	• Asks appropriately probing open questions • Asks the appraisee to think about what he or she could do to develop and improve his or her work • Helps the appraisee to formulate an action plan to implement identified improvements
Develop a specific, measurable, achievable, realistic and timely personal development plan	• Helps the appraisee to identify his or her learning needs • Challenges the appraisee to look at his or her learning in a balanced manner in terms of personal interests, needs as a professional practitioner and the needs of the wider department or service within which he or she works. • Encourages the appraisee to think about how he or she could collect evidence of improvement in his or her performance as a result of participation in personal development and quality improvement activities
Meaningfully explore probity issues	• Alert to issues of probity (ethical issues) that are implicit or explicit in the material the appraisee submits, expresses or infers • Asks exploratory, open questions about any probity issues • Encourages the appraisee to reflect on and to identify any potential probity issues
Meaningfully explore any ongoing health problems or concerns	• Alert to issues about the appraisee's (implicit or explicit) in the submitted material or expressed or inferred during the meeting • Asks exploratory open questions about any health issues • Encourages the appraisee to reflect and to identify potential health issues • Refrains from a clinical role in relation to any health issues identified

POTENTIAL VALUE OF APPRAISAL

Appraisal, and specifically the quality of appraisal, has been positively associated with improved patient care outcomes in secondary care.[12] In Scotland, GPs were surveyed in 2006 to determine their perceptions of the relevance and impact of the GP appraisal system at that time. As a result of appraisal, 47% of respondents indicated altering their educational activity, 33% undertook additional training, 14% reflected on their own health and 13% reported a positive impact on their career development.[13] While self-reported data is useful, further research is required to objectively determine whether changes in GPs' behaviour has a tangible impact on the quality and safety of patient care.

Appraisal has good potential as a safety improvement intervention and there is an expectation that GPs will submit evidence in this domain. The appraisal meeting provides opportunity for GPs to reflect on safety-critical aspects of their work in a structured, facilitated and focused manner. Between meetings, GPs are encouraged to actively consider opportunities for improvement by asking, 'Is this something I could include in my appraisal folder or my continuous professional development log book for this year's appraisal meeting?' The core categories naturally dovetail with care quality expectations – criterion audit, significant event analysis and reviewing patient referrals are well-recognised and widely promoted quality and safety improvement methods.

Finally, the group of appraisers themselves is potentially a very useful resource. Because of their interactions with a large number of GPs (approximately 22 appraisal meetings a year) from different practices, they gain valuable experiences and insights that can help to 'pollinate' good practice or a new innovation across a region.

SUPPORT FOR GENERAL PRACTITIONER APPRAISAL

NES provides a GP Appraisal Toolkit – an educational resource that is freely available to all appraisees. It is hosted on the Scottish Online Appraisal Resource website. The toolkit provides practical examples, 'how to' guides and information about a wide range of quality improvement tools, methods and approaches commonly used by GPs in Scotland. There is information about effective clinical audits, significant event analysis, prescribing reviews and audits, reviews of referrals, methods for looking at communication skills with patients (including the use of video) and methods for assessing teamwork and communication skills with colleagues (including multi-source feedback). The toolkit includes advice and suggestions for GPs working in less-traditional capacities (sessional, out-of-hours, forensic) about ideas for quality improvement projects and ways they can adapt the tools to make them relevant to their circumstances.

The toolkit is updated and revised regularly. For example, the trigger review method was added in 2013 after a number of pilot studies demonstrated its potential as a learning and improvement tool. The trigger review method allows GPs to screen random samples of high-risk patient records for evidence of previously undetected patient safety incidents and a standardised report pro forma encourages reflection, learning and action on the findings.[14]

The 'right' attitude, knowledge and skills are essential in an appraiser to ensure the effectiveness of the appraisal process.[15] As a result, NES invests significant resources and time in training new and existing appraisers. The new GP appraiser course is one example of this investment. The course was initially information based, but has evolved to include skill-based learning and would-be appraisers' competencies are now also formally evaluated.[16] The success of the course has been such that, for the last 2 years, it has also been offered to aspiring appraisers from secondary care settings who attend with GP recruits. Participants have reported significant perceived benefits from these cross-specialty 'mini' appraisals during the training process, which has helped them to develop a more objective and generic approach to appraisal. Existing appraisers from general practice (and more recently also secondary care) can attend a 1-day 'Further Intensive Skills course' for additional training or as an update.[17]

RECOMMENDATIONS FOR CREATING AN EFFECTIVE APPRAISAL SYSTEM

- Use information technology to support all aspects of the appraisal process (appointment scheduling; uploading evidence and supporting materials; formal reports, feedback and evaluation).
- Design and disseminate a toolkit of quality improvement methods and tools (with practical examples and 'how to' guides) for the use of appraisees. Ideally, the resource should be free and easily accessible.
- Invest in the recruitment, training and support of appraisers.
- Evaluate the quality of your system regularly through, for example, informal feedback from appraisees, formal documentation and quality indicators.
- Conduct an annual performance review at least annually with your appraisers and invite input from the appraisees (look at appraisee feedback, summary forms and other quality indicators with them).

FURTHER READING

To learn more about medical appraisal in Scotland, please visit the Scottish Online Appraisal Resource website (www.scottishappraisal.scot.nhs.uk).

REFERENCES

1. Wiese DS, Buckley RM. The evolution of the performance appraisal process. *J Manage Hist.* 1998; **4**(3): 223–49.
2. Ingraham PW. Of pigs in pokes and policy diffusion: another look at pay-for-performance. *Public Admin Rev.* 1993; **53**(4): 348–56.
3. Martin DC, Bartol KM, Kehoe PE. The legal ramifications of performance appraisal: the growing significance. *Public Pers Manage.* 2000; **29**(3): 379–405.
4. Kolb DA. *Experiential Learning: experience as the source of learning and development.* Englewood Cliffs, NJ: Prentice Hall; 1984.
5. Mann K, Gordon J, MacLeod A. Reflection and reflective practice in health professions education: a systematic review. *Adv Health Sci Educ Theory Pract.* 2009; **14**(4): 595–621.
6. Wald HS, Borkan JM, Taylor JS, *et al.* Fostering and evaluating reflective capacity in medical education: developing the REFLECT rubric for assessing reflective writing. *Acad Med.* 2012; **87**(1): 41–50.
7. Chivers G. Utilising reflective practice interviews in professional development. *J Eur Ind Train.* 2003; **27**(1): 5–15.
8. NHS Employers. *Appraisal and Simplified KSF.* Leeds: NHS Employers. Available at:

www.nhsemployers.org/PAYANDCONTRACTS/AGENDAFORCHANGE/KSF/Pages/
Appraisal-and-simplified-KSF.aspx (accessed 11 November 2013).

9. Hunter C, Blaney D, McKintry B, *et al.* GP appraisal: a Scottish solution. *Educ Prim Care.* 2005; **16**(4): 434–9.

10. Department of Health. *The new NHS: modern, dependable.* London: Stationery Office, 1997.

11. Heron J. *Helping the Client: a creative practical guide.* London: Sage Publications; 2001.

12. West MA, Borrill C, Dawson J, *et al.* The link between management of employees and patient mortality in acute hospitals. *Int J Hum Resour Man.* 2002; **13**(8): 1299–310.

13. Colthart I, Cameron N, McKinstry B, *et al.* What do doctors really think about the relevance and impact of GP appraisal 3 years on? *Br J Gen Pract.* 2008; **58**(547): 82–7.

14. de Wet C, Bowie P. Screening electronic patient records to detect preventable harm: a trigger tool for primary care. *Qual Prim Care.* 2011; **19**(2): 115–25.

15. NHS Revalidation Support Team. *Quality Assurance of Medical Appraisers: recruitment, training, support and review of medical appraisers in England.* Available at: www.gmc-uk.org/static/documents/content/RST4.pdf (accessed 12 November 2013).

16. Law S, Haman H, Cameron N, *et al.* GP peer appraisal in Scotland: an ongoing and developing exercise in quality. *Educ Prim Care.* 2009; **20**(2): 99–105.

17. Staples I, Wakeling J, Cameron N. A review of further training for GP appraisers in Scotland. *Educ Prim Care.* 2010; **21**(1): 25–37.

CHAPTER 16

Multi-source feedback

Annabel Shepherd

Multi-source feedback (MSF) is a novel method of assessing healthcare professionals that has gained increasing credibility in the past decade. In this chapter the relevance of MSF as a method for assessing professional behaviours in healthcare is explored along with the evidence supporting its usefulness. The MSF programme developed by NHS Education for Scotland (NES) is described alongside the lessons learned and how these can inform the design and implementation of MSF processes which contribute to improving the quality and safety of healthcare. The chapter concludes with a description of the method's advantages and limitations.

WHAT IS MULTI-SOURCE FEEDBACK?

MSF is a method of assessment that, instead of placing the individual under examination conditions, relies on a number of raters (e.g. immediate colleagues) to make judgements about an individual's *workplace* behaviour as part of a healthcare team.[1] Raters are asked to rate and comment on simple and complex tasks they have observed an individual performing as they interacted with the individual in the course of his or her day-to-day work. These judgements can relate to interpersonal behaviours such as communication skills and other behaviours such as clinical skills, which are important elements in providing safe patient care.

The MSF process is flexible and can be adapted in different ways. For example, raters can be colleagues, employees, managers or even health service users and the process can be paper-based or electronic. MSF can also be administered for a variety of purposes that range from providing the individual with developmental feedback to making judgements about their ability to progress and work in a particular field. The four typical steps of the process are shown in Figure 16.1.

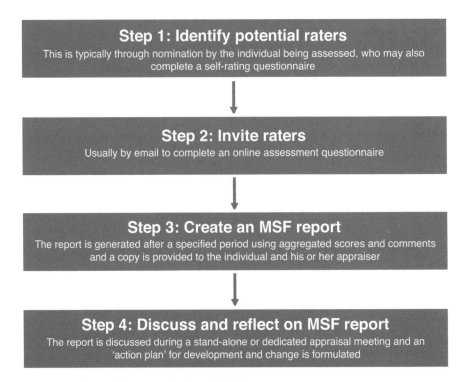

FIGURE 16.1 The multi-source feedback (MSF) process

MSF is promoted as a method to improve patient safety and enhance quality in a number of healthcare settings. Ramsey *et al.*[2] first published data concerning the question of how reliable MSF is as an assessment for healthcare professionals in the United States in 1989. Since then, MSF has been implemented in many other healthcare settings. For example, MSF has been used as a method for the recertification of physicians in Canada since 1999,[3-6] it is used to provide formative feedback to post-graduate trainees in Australia[7] and in the United Kingdom (UK) it is part of the assessment process of trainees in all the medical specialties. Since 2003 it has been one of the core components of the annual appraisal of general practitioners (GPs) in Scotland.[8] More recently, the General Medical Council (GMC), the UK medical regulator, included it as an essential component of medical revalidation[9] and has published criteria to support MSF questionnaire development.[10]

DESIGN AND IMPLEMENTATION OF THE NES MULTI-SOURCE FEEDBACK PROGRAMME

The aim of GP appraisal in Scotland is to enhance the ability of the general practice workforce to successfully meet the different challenges they face.[8] GPs collect evidence and information about their performance over the course of a year and reflect on and assess their ability to fulfil their different roles while successfully functioning as part of a team. This information is used to formulate and agree a personal development plan for the GP during the appraisal interview. In support of this process, NES has included MSF as a component of annual appraisal for GPs since 2003. As a result, the design and implementation of an MSF programme was commissioned. This, in turn, required the design and development of the 'What is a good GP?' questionnaire.

A number of questions have been identified that should be considered when developing, designing and implementing an MSF programme in any healthcare setting (*see* Box 16.1).[1,11,12] These questions are essential to ensure the MSF method is in fact the right choice for an organisation's purposes and that it is adapted and implemented appropriately. The growing understanding of the role of assessment methods such as MSF has led to greater consideration of their purpose and design, and the consequences for the delivery of healthcare services.[13,14] When choosing to implement MSF we must bear in mind that an inadequate appreciation of the complex competencies required by a healthcare staff group could impact on service delivery.[15,16] A poorly conceived MSF process could be ultimately detrimental to individual and team performance.[17,18]

BOX 16.1 Questions to consider when designing and implementing a multi-source feedback programme

- What is the *purpose* of introducing a multi-source feedback programme?
- *Who* is being assessed and by whom? In other words, who are the raters and how will they be nominated?
- Is there already a suitable questionnaire for this setting and programme purpose? *What* is being assessed and what questions are being asked?
- Is adequate and clear information and/or training available (if relevant) for prospective participants, raters and facilitators (people providing feedback)?
- How will the questionnaires be administered?
- How will reports be generated and disseminated?
- How will the reports be used? For example, will feedback be provided? If yes, by whom, when and where? Will facilitators require additional training? What resources are currently available or may be required to implement the programme and provide appropriate support for participants and facilitators?
- What are the expected programme outcomes and will they be evaluated?

In the UK, MSF questionnaires have typically been developed by mapping questionnaire items to established GMC standards for clinical practice.[19,20] The 'What is a good GP?' questionnaire used a similar approach but widened its development strategy to include qualitative methods and close partnership working with a range of clinical and non-clinical front-line staff. This design choice was made deliberately because of the assumption that primary healthcare teams' insight into qualities important for 'the good GP' may identify additional aspects reflective of the role of GPs as members of a multidisciplinary team.

Primary healthcare teams from selected west of Scotland general medical practices were recruited and asked to provide comments in response to the question: 'What is a good GP?' After 1588 responses were gathered the data were reduced and coded to create a 37-item questionnaire with six domains (categories). In order to establish content validity, primary care team members were asked to rate each item for relevance to the overall domain and comment on the wording of the statements. The final validated 'What is a good GP?' MSF questionnaire is shown in Box 16.2. While it has overlapping themes with the GMC's document *Good Medical Practice*[21] and the GMC's working framework for appraisal and assessment,[22] there are a number of additional items, while some items relate to different domains (categories).

BOX 16.2 The six domains and individual questions of the 'what is a good GP?' MSF questionnaire

1. Professional values

How much do you agree that the doctor is:
a. honest and trustworthy?
b. able to demonstrate respect for confidentiality?
c. able to maintain a healthy work–life balance?
d. able to maintain good health while doing the work of a GP?
e. sensitive to cultural issues?

2. Communication skills

How much do you agree that the doctor is:
a. able to put patients at ease?
b. willing to listen to patients, colleagues and staff?
c. able to record his or her consultations consistently and accurately?
d. able to write legibly?
e. able to use a computer at a level deemed appropriate by the practice?
f. able to use email as deemed appropriate by the practice?
g. committed to using the telephones as deemed appropriate by the practice?
h. is able to speak good English?

3. Clinical care

How much do you agree that the doctor is:
a. up to date with his or her clinical knowledge?
b. diagnostically astute?
c. able to make appropriate decisions?
d. a safe prescriber, particularly with dangerous drugs?
e. an appropriate user of the referral system?
f. willing to care effectively for a dying patient (e.g. terminal care)?
g. able to handle the uncertainty of general practice?

---

4. Working with colleagues

How much do you agree that the doctor is:

a. able to value colleagues' contributions?
b. willing to implement agreed changes?
c. committed to the whole practice team?

5. Personality issues

How much do you agree that the doctor is:

a. approachable?
b. polite to patients and staff?
c. enthusiastic about the job?
d. willing to compromise where appropriate?
e. calm under pressure?
f. of professional appearance?
g. able to demonstrate a sense of humour where appropriate?

6. Duties and responsibilities

How much do you agree that the doctor is:

a. willing to take responsibility for getting his or her share of the work done?
b. willing to take responsibility for follow-up of patients where necessary?
c. committed to continuing his or her personal learning?
d. willing to learn from mistakes and recognises his or her limitations?
e. well organised?
f. easily accessible and able to be contacted when necessary?

Overall

How much do you agree that this doctor is a good GP?

A MSF programme with the main purpose of ensuring professionals meet a minimum competence level will predominantly use numerical rating scales. However, the NES MSF programme had the additional aims of informing continuing personal development and to provide educational feedback to participants. To help facilitate these aims, raters were asked to provide additional free text information in addition to numerical ratings. Feedback in the form of free text narrative comments can be particularly powerful mediators of change, especially when they relate to behaviour.[23] However, it is important to remember that narrative comments may infringe rater anonymity[1] and some participants have been found to be overly preoccupied by them.[24] The 'what is a good GP?' report combines both these approaches, as demonstrated in the extract from a fictional case study shown in Figure 16.2.

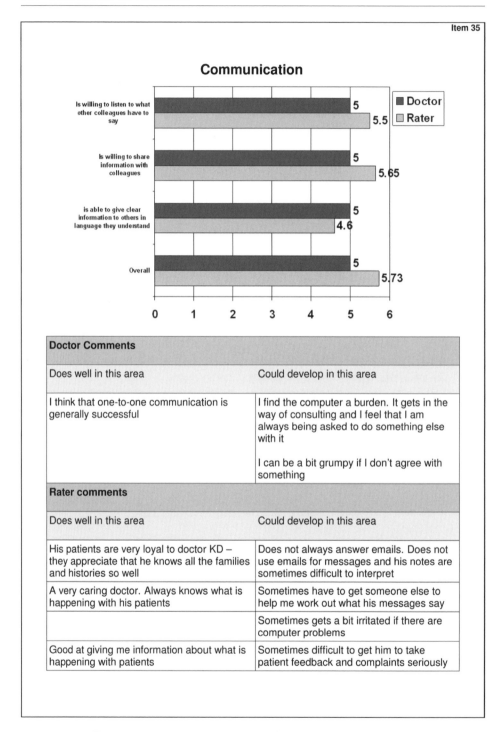

Item 35

Communication

	Doctor	Rater
Is willing to listen to what other colleagues have to say	5	5.5
Is willing to share information with colleagues	5	5.65
is able to give clear information to others in language they understand	5	4.6
Overall	5	5.73

Doctor Comments

Does well in this area	Could develop in this area
I think that one-to-one communication is generally successful	I find the computer a burden. It gets in the way of consulting and I feel that I am always being asked to do something else with it
	I can be a bit grumpy if I don't agree with something

Rater comments

Does well in this area	Could develop in this area
His patients are very loyal to doctor KD – they appreciate that he knows all the families and histories so well	Does not always answer emails. Does not use emails for messages and his notes are sometimes difficult to interpret
A very caring doctor. Always knows what is happening with his patients	Sometimes have to get someone else to help me work out what his messages say
	Sometimes gets a bit irritated if there are computer problems
Good at giving me information about what is happening with patients	Sometimes difficult to get him to take patient feedback and complaints seriously

FIGURE 16.2 Extract from a 'What is a good GP?' multi-source feedback report

In order to ensure that the questionnaires were completed and interpreted as intended, information leaflets for participants and potential raters were developed to explain the purpose and practical application of the MSF method and distributed as paper copies and electronically. While there were initial concerns that providing too many instructions to raters could compromise the validity of results,[19] there is emerging evidence that providing information may improve response rates,[25] ensure anonymity and improve feedback quality.[11]

A website was also developed to ensure that participants were provided with sufficient information that questionnaires were completed appropriately and that related reports were used and interpreted as intended. The website enabled GPs to register for MSF, initiate the process, nominate raters and eventually download reports and feedback provided by colleagues. In this programme, the appropriate use of information technology streamlined the MSF process and was linked with improved feasibility and acceptability. It reduced related administration to a minimum, assured the anonymity of raters and reports, providing information about aggregated rating scores and comments that were electronically assembled and automatically forwarded.[1]

The choice of raters, the method of feedback and the frequency of participation in an MSF process is dictated by the intended purpose of the process and informs decisions regarding its administration. In the NES MSF programme GPs are encouraged to select raters from a range of staff groups including non-clinical staff. This reflects the purpose of providing GPs with feedback from a wide range of multidisciplinary team members and on the broad range of their professional practices, rather than simply focus in one particular area (e.g. perceived clinical skills).

Openness and transparency about the aims and outcomes of an MSF process is very important. The NES MSF programme ensures that clarity about how the results will be made available to participants and the possible outcomes of participation are made abundantly clear. In contrast with some MSF processes developed for doctors in the UK, the NES programme makes the MSF report available to the GP before the facilitated feedback meeting with his or her appraiser. This allows the GP time for self-reflection on the findings, which is known to vary in timing and depth between individuals.[26]

POTENTIAL ADVANTAGES, LIMITATIONS AND USEFULNESS OF MULTI-SOURCE FEEDBACK

In the last decade, MSF has gained credibility in medical education because of changes in the way assessment is used in healthcare. It is now understood that the method and content of assessments articulate what knowledge and skills are required and should, therefore, be prioritised by the learner.[27-30] As the imperative to robustly demonstrate competence in the workplace increases, there has been a move towards assessments that try to adequately reflect the personal and professional attributes required of staff groups rather than testing arguably more abstract notions of knowledge and skills.[15,31] MSF is a type of work-based assessment, focusing on the 'does' level of the psychologist George Miller's[32] framework that describes clinical competence and has a number of important advantages – but also limitations – when compared with more traditional assessment methods.

The main advantage of MSF is that the assessments reflect individuals' 'on the job' performance rather than performance under test conditions.[33] MSF encapsulates the competency required to fulfil the role, therefore, rather than focusing on artificially developed criteria. Moreover MSF can be used to assess aspects of team working such as communication skills, which are difficult to assess using traditional methods.[11,24] MSF's greatest potential may therefore derive from the fact that it provides an assessment of, and feedback about, the way individuals work with others.[11] MSF may also help to build and promote a culture of 'team learning' within which it is acceptable (even expected) to provide feedback to members in your team and be involved in their personal and professional development.[1] A final advantage is that the administration of MSF processes is demonstrated to be feasible and acceptable to many participants.[1,3,5,6,19,20]

While many MSF questionnaires have construct validity[6] there is still uncertainty about the reliability of the results. By its very nature MSF is applied in non-examination conditions and there are numerous potential factors that may influence the method's reliability. Traditionally, one assessor using an objective, structured pro forma would examine several students. With the MSF method several raters, with variable levels of training, experience and opportunities to observe the person being assessed, complete their assessments without any prior calibration.[1] Their ratings are also more likely to be influenced (biased) by personal relationship issues, the negative impact of hierarchy and the fact that they typically have little or no experience of providing feedback in a developmental manner, when compared to medical educationalists.[11] Between eight and ten raters are required to improve the likelihood of MSF results being reliable[20] but difficulties achieving these numbers are also described.[19] This may be especially relevant for healthcare workers who operate in small teams and certain staff groups such as sessional healthcare workers.

The tendency towards leniency and overcritical feedback is well documented in the field of assessment but may be magnified in MSF, since the raters are not subjected to ongoing calibration training.[1] Issues such as use of patient raters in specific clinical areas (e.g. psychiatry) are also important considerations, while other specialties (e.g. medicine of the elderly) may be unduly impacted by factors influencing case mix or the demographics of the patient group as a whole.[34]

The aim of any assessment process, however, should be to assure and also raise standards.[31] It is unclear whether this is the case as the association between MSF scores and clinical performance is unclear. The potential (if any) of MSF to improve patient outcomes[35-37] or its educational value for individuals and teams[38] has also not been demonstrated. It has recently been suggested that the MSF method provides only limited summative information.[11] Although MSF scores for individuals have a tendency to improve over time, resulting changes in behaviour are described as small to moderate, with calls for further research to explore the learning potential of MSF for individuals and teams.[38]

Despite evidence that a range of barriers to the acceptance of MSF feedback may exist, the evaluation of the NES MSF programme found early changes in professional practices from those participating. However, the use of trained facilitators within a strong national GP appraisal support network may also have accounted for some of the positive responses encountered in the evaluation.[37-42] Overall it is recognised that more work is required to establish the parameters for enhancing the educational impact of MSF and demonstrating more effectively how this assessment method contributes to improving the quality and safety of primary care.

CHAPTER SUMMARY

- MSF is a method of assessment which relies on a number of raters (e.g. immediate colleagues) to make judgements about an individual's *workplace* behaviour as part of a healthcare team.
- It is important to clarify the intended purpose of an MSF programme before implementing it – is it to assess fitness to practise, assess team working or for continuing personal development requirements? This influences the administration process, nomination of raters, format and method of feedback and choice of questionnaire.
- There are a number of different MSF questionnaires available commercially. The 'What is a good GP?' MSF questionnaire was developed in partnership with front-line staff and is used in the NES MSF programme for general practice.
- The majority of participants in the NES MSF programme found the method acceptable, feasible and useful.

REFERENCES

1. Shepherd A, Lough M. What is a good general practitioner (GP)? The development and evaluation of a multi-source feedback instrument for GP appraisal. *Educ Prim Care*. 2010; **21**: 149–64.
2. Ramsey P, Carline JD, Inui TS, *et al*. Predictive validity of certification by the American Board of Internal Medicine. *Ann Intern Med*. 1989; **110**(9): 719–26.
3. Hall W, Violato C, Lewkonia R, *et al*. Assessment of physician performance in Alberta: the physician achievement review. *CMAJ*. 1999; **161**(1): 52–7.
4. www.nspar.ca/
5. Violato C, Marini A, Toews J, *et al*. Feasibility and psychometric properties of using peers, consulting physicians, co-workers, and patients to assess physicians. *Acad Med*. 1997; **72**(10 Suppl. 1): S82–4.
6. Lockyer J. Multisource feedback in the assessment of physician competencies. *J Contin Educ Health Prof*. 2003; **23**(1): 4–12.
7. The Royal Australasian College of Physicians. *PREP Basic Training*. Sydney: RACP. Available at: www.racp.edu.au/page/educational-and-professional-development/prep-basic-training (accessed 6 November 2013).
8. www.scottishappraisal.scot.nhs.uk/home.aspx

9. Department of Health. *Medical Revalidation – Principles and Next Steps: the report of the Chief Medical Officer for England's Working Group.* London: Department of Health; 2008. Available at: http://webarchive.nationalarchives.gov.uk/+/www.dh.gov.uk/en/publicationsandstatistics/publications/publicationspolicyandguidance/dh_086430 (accessed 6 November 2013).

10. General Medical Council. *Revalidation: the way ahead.* London: GMC; 2010. Available at: www.gmc-uk.org/Revalidation_The_Way_Ahead.pdf_32040275.pdf (accessed 6 November 2013).

11. Bracken D, Timmreck CW, Church AH. *The Handbook of Multi-source Feedback: the comprehensive resource for designing and implementing MSF processes.* Illustrated ed. John Wiley & Sons, New Jersey; 2001.

12. Wood L, Hassell A, Whitehouse A, *et al.* A literature review of multi-source feedback systems within and without health services, leading to 10 tips for their successful design. *Med Teach.* 2006; **28**(7): e185–91.

13. Wiggins G. *Assessing Student Performance: exploring the purpose and limits of testing.* Jossey-Bass, San Francisco; 1993.

14. Messick S. *Validity of Psychological Assessment: validation of inferences from persons' responses and performances as scientific inquiry into score meaning.* Research Report RR-94-45. Princeton, NJ: Educational Testing Service; 1994.

15. Gonczi A. Competency based assessment in the professions in Australia. *Assess Educ Princ Pol Pract.* 1994; **1**(1): 27–44.

16. Wolf A. *Competence-Based Assessment.* Buckingham, England: Open University Press; 1995.

17. Messick S. Consequences of test interpretation and use: the fusion of validity and values in psychological assessment. Princeton, NJ: Educational Testing Service; 1998.

18. Boud D. Assessment and the promotion of academic values. *Stud High Educ.* 1990; **15**: 101–11.

19. Campbell JL, Richards SH, Dickens A, *et al.* Assessing the professional performance of UK doctors: an evaluation of the utility of the General Medical Council patient and colleague questionnaires. *Qual Saf Health Care.* 2008; **17**(3): 187–93.

20. Archer JC, Norcini J, Davies HA. Use of SPRAT for peer review of paediatricians in training. *BMJ.* 2005; **330**(7502): 1251–3.

21. General Medical Council. *Good Medical Practice (2013).* London: GMC; 2013. Available at: www.gmc-uk.org/guidance/good_medical_practice.asp (accessed 6 November 2013).

22. General Medical Council. *GMP Framework for Appraisal and Revalidation.* London: GMC; 2013. Available at: www.gmc-uk.org/doctors/revalidation/revalidation_gmp_framework.asp (accessed 6 November 2013).

23. Smither JW, Walker AG. Are the characteristics of narrative comments related to improvement in multirater feedback ratings over time? *J Appl Psychol.* 2004; **89**(3): 575–81.

24. Hersen M, Thomas J. *Comprehensive Handbook of Psychological Assessment: industrial and organizational assessment.* Illustrated ed. John Wiley & Sons, New Jersey; 2004.

25. Gray A, Lewis A, Fletcher C, *et al. 360 Degree Feedback Best Practice Guidelines.* London: British Psychological Society; 2007.

26. Sargeant JM, Mann KV, van der Vleuten CP, *et al.* Reflection: a link between receiving

and using assessment feedback. *Adv Health Sci Educ Theory Pract.* 2009; **14**(3): 399–410.

27. Ben-David MF. The role of assessment in expanding professional horizons. *Med Teach* 2000; **22**(5): 472–7.

28. Van der Vleuten CPM, Dolmans DM, Scherpbier AA. The need for evidence in education. *Med Teach.* 2000; **22**(3): 246–50.

29. Wood T. Assessment not only drives learning, it may also help learning. *Med Educ.* 2009; **43**(1): 5–6.

30. Frederiksen N. The real test bias: influences of testing on teaching and learning. *Am Psychol.* 1984; **39**(3): 193–202.

31. Cox M, Irby DM, Epstein RM. Assessment in medical education. *N Engl J Med.* 2007; **356**(4): 387–96.

32. Miller GE. The assessment of clinical skills/competence/performance. *Acad Med.* 1990; **65**(9): S63–7.

33. Norcini JJ. Work based assessment. *BMJ.* 2003; **326**(7392): 753–5.

34. Shepherd A, Cameron N. What are the concerns of prospective responsible officers about their role in medical revalidation? *J Eval Clin Pract.* 2010; **16**(3): 655–60.

35. Lockyer J, Violato C, Fidler H. Likelihood of change: a study assessing surgeon use of multisource feedback data. *Teach Learn Med.* 2003; **15**(3): 168–74.

36. Smither JW, London M, Reilly RR. Does performance improve following multisource feedback? A theoretical model, meta-analysis and review of empirical findings. *Pers Psychol.* 2005; **58**(1): 33–66.

37. Overeem K, Faber MJ, Arah OA, *et al.* Doctor performance assessment in daily practise: does it help doctors or not? A systematic review. *Med Educ.* 2007; **41**(11): 1039–49.

38. Violato C, Lockyer JM, Fidler H. Changes in performance: a 5-year longitudinal study of participants in a multi-source feedback programme. *Med Educ.* 2008; **42**(10): 1007–13.

39. Sargeant J, Mann K, Sinclair D, *et al.* Understanding the influence of emotions and reflection upon multi-source feedback acceptance and use. *Adv Health Sci Educ Theory Pract.* 2008; **13**(3): 275–88.

40. Owens J. Is multi-source feedback (MSF) seen as a useful educational tool in primary care? A qualitative study. *Educ Prim Care.* 2010; **21**: 180–5.

41. Fidler H, Lockyer JM, Toews J, *et al.* Changing physicians' practices: the effect of individual feedback. *Acad Med.* 1999; **74**(6): 702–14.

42. Sargeant JM, Mann KV, Ferrier SN, *et al.* Responses of rural family physicians and their colleague and coworker raters to a multi-source feedback process: a pilot study. *Acad Med.* 2003; **78**(10 Suppl.): S42–4.

CHAPTER 17

Practice management

Marion Macleod

INTRODUCTION

The independent contractor status of general practice in the United Kingdom (UK) requires that the practice business be managed, and most general practitioner (GP) partnerships now employ a practice manager (PM) to do this on their behalf. Managers come to general practice from a variety of backgrounds and with an array of past experiences and qualifications. Many have had no previous experience of working in a healthcare environment, while others have developed their managerial skills on the job while working within a general practice. There is no nationally defined PM role and so the managerial duties and responsibilities to be undertaken are usually those that are desired by the GPs.

This chapter starts with an overview of the history of practice management as context for the decision to create the Practice Managers' Network in Scotland. Three important initiatives that affect the role of PMs and on improving the quality of patient care are then discussed: (1) a vocational training scheme (VTS) for PMs, (2) appraisal and (3) continuous professional development (CPD).

THE HISTORY OF PRACTICE MANAGEMENT

In 1948 when the UK National Health Service (NHS) came into being, the role of PM did not exist. The vast majority of GPs were male and worked single-handed. They worked from home and either their wife or their housekeeper answered the telephone and dealt with the calls from patients and relatives. There were no appointment systems and many requests for house visits to review patients.

The landscape of general practice changed significantly in 1966 as a result of 'The Family Doctor Charter'. Because it entitled practices to claim back up to 70% reimbursement of staff costs, large numbers of administrative staff and nurses were appointed, and a small number of forward-thinking practices began employing PMs to manage the staff.[1] The 1990 'General Practice in the National Health Service' contract required GPs to provide core medical services, and offered a range of financial incentives to those who met health promotion and screening targets. This led to many more practices employing a PM to ensure their financial profits were maximised.

Two years into the contract, a survey about the state of practice management in Scotland recognised that there was no clearly defined role for PMs, that there were 'wide variations in the range of responsibilities and tasks', and that the PM's role 'probably evolved in response to individual practice circumstances.'[2]

Therefore, it is hardly surprising that standards across practices varied considerably. Baker,[3] seeking to explain this variation in 1992, noted:

> after training practice status a practice manager is the most important variable in explaining the level of practice development . . . every practice could have a designated manager, and this study suggests that they should.

Even though the value of the role of PM was gaining greater recognition, there was still a need to redefine both the GP and the PM role within many practices. It was conceivable that this would be a challenging task and that 'in order to do this GPs will have to acquire an appreciation of the complexity of practice management without the need to interfere in its day-to-day workings.'[4] A qualitative study of the roles of PMs in Aberdeen recognised that

> the influential role of the practice manager and the transfer of administrative responsibilities from partners to the manager has altered general practitioners' perceptions of managers. This, along with the increasing employment of managers with experience from different sectors, has led to an increase in the professional status of managers.[5]

An increase in the number of practices adopting 'fundholding' status further bolstered the recruitment of PMs and, in turn, the informal recognition of the value good management added to a practice. The importance of practice management was formally recognised with the *New General Medical Services Contract: Investing in General Practice 2003*, with Annex C describing a competency framework for practice management encompassing three types of management activities: administrative, managerial and strategic.[6] These three activities are interrelated and part of a continuum along which PMs function on a daily basis. The 2003 contract made provision for practices to be rewarded for achieving quality targets related to good practice organisation and management. With that, the role of the PM entered a new era.

PRACTICE MANAGERS' NETWORK

At around the same time as the introduction of the 2003 GP contract, the then Scottish Executive Health Department funded the development of a national learning network for practice managers. A full-time national coordinator was appointed to lead and develop the network and local coordinators (nominated by their practice manager peers) were appointed in each regional health board area to support this development and to ensure engagement of PMs in their areas.

The initial objectives of the coordinators were to:

- increase PMs' awareness of important local and national issues and developments
- improve standards of care by providing a forum for PMs to share good practice in their health board area and across Scotland
- support PMs and provide opportunities for them and their teams to develop the necessary skills to meet new challenges (at that time, the new contract)
- identify PMs' training needs and encourage them to engage with CPD.

From the beginning, the national coordinator worked closely with the officers of the Scottish Executive Health Department to ensure invitations to various national strategic working groups as the representative of PMs. They also recognised that PMs were ideally placed to provide strategic leadership and would have a key role in the future modernisation of primary care. For the first time, PMs had a voice and some influence at the highest levels of Scottish government and healthcare.

The local coordinators are experienced PMs who are funded on a sessional basis to support the national coordinator. They have many responsibilities, including ensuring that information and best practice is spread by organising meetings, learning events and road shows and providing networking opportunities to minimise isolation, offering support and mentoring to new PMs. They also regularly work in partnership with the primary care division of their local health board to provide a PM perspective, when invited to do so.

One of the first actions of the new national coordinator was to survey Scottish PMs to determine their learning and development needs. Three areas were identified as priorities: (1) strategic management, (2) financial management and (3) employment law. In response, a series of regional 'roadshows' was delivered to address the identified learning needs. PMs were very positive about the perceived value of these events and greatly appreciated the fact that their CPD needs were being recognised for the first time, and at least partially funded. At present, the national and local coordinators continue to actively identify the learning needs of their PM colleagues through a mixture of methods, including networking, horizon scanning and feedback during appraisal interviews.

VOCATIONAL TRAINING SCHEME FOR PRACTICE MANAGERS

In recognition of the importance of the PM role, and the need to build capacity in order to improve the business of general practice, the Scottish Government Health Department (SGHD) agreed to fund a VTS for PMs for an initial 2-year period from 2005. Since then, NHS Education for Scotland (NES) has continued to fund the scheme because they recognise the importance and value of having appropriately trained managers within general practice.

The aim of the scheme is to produce PMs with the required competencies, knowledge, attributes and behaviours for a successful career in general practice management. In other words, the aim of the VTS is to produce strategic business managers with the necessary acumen to 'helicopter' (see the bigger picture), and identify and lead change to improve patient safety and service quality and minimise risk.

The scheme's design is modelled on the successful GP Specialty Training scheme in which trainees are linked with and work alongside an experienced GP (the educational supervisor). Following a rigorous selection process, PM trainees are geographically paired with an educational facilitator – a PM with a special interest in training and development. The educational facilitator's role is a challenging one and requires excellent communication and interpersonal skills together with a high level of emotional intelligence. They have to know when to adapt their approach between acting as *mentor* – offering the trainee support and guidance; *coach* – encouraging the trainee to reflect on his or her work experiences and find the answer to his or her own questions; and *teacher* – challenging the trainee's attitudes, beliefs and behaviours to help him or her see things from a different perspective.

The VTS programme provides both an operational and strategic view of practice management. For example, the residential training event programme includes a review of current SGHD policies, business strategy, leadership and management, change management, patient safety, risk management, significant event analysis and quality improvement methods – the strategic elements of general practice management. The operational aspects of practice management are addressed via a programme of one to one tutorials delivered by the trainees' educational facilitators. Their individual learning needs are identified from an online 'menu' for practice management development. The menu is regularly updated throughout the year to provide links to the relevant SGHD publications. It provides a themed directory of the skills and expertise relevant to the PM role, all electronically linked to the relevant documentation and contractual information.

Trainee applications are invited from new PMs and aspiring PMs with supervisory or management experience within general practice. As part of the assessment strategy, trainees take the lead in delivering a service improvement project within the practice, providing them the opportunity to put the management theory learned on the programme into action. Trainees subsequently write this up as a management report, demonstrating how their project has benefitted patients. They are subsequently required to submit a portfolio of reflective evidence and attend a viva voce. The programme is accredited at the undergraduate level by the University of the West of Scotland. Trainees from across all corners of Scotland – from Shetland to the Borders and from the Western Isles to Fraserburgh – have now completed the VTS.

APPRAISAL

The new General Medical Services contract (2003) required that PMs be appraised. However, few GPs had been trained in, or knew how to conduct, performance appraisals of their managers and many PMs found the appraisal process to be neither positive nor supportive. Following a workshop on appraisal at their 2004 annual PM networking conference, PMs continued to convey enthusiasm for effective appraisal by their GP employers or with a PM peer. The introduction of GP peer appraisal in 2003 had been a driver in taking peer appraisal forwards for PMs. A handbook, *Appraisal for Practice Managers in Scotland*, which supported both employer and peer appraisal, was subsequently developed in 2005 by the network and disseminated to every GP practice in Scotland.

PMs continued to express a desire for peer appraisal. They wanted the same opportunity GPs had been given – for example, to meet with a trained PM appraiser who understood their job and with whom they could discuss their development needs and construct a personal development plan. In 2008, funding was identified to run a peer appraisal pilot across four health board areas. The PM peer appraisers undertook the same intensive training programme as GP appraisers. The pilot was independently evaluated and it demonstrated 'that a peer appraisal system for Managers in General Practice is an effective tool for promoting professional development and meets an important unmet need within the NHS'.* Given this positive finding, peer appraisal training was extended nationally across Scotland. Post-appraisal feedback remains positive and there is an existing but unmet demand for more appraisal; however, limited funding continues to preclude a wider role out of the scheme.

CONTINUING PROFESSIONAL DEVELOPMENT

Practice managers in Scotland are privileged that NES – a special health board with a remit to promote learning and education for NHS staff – invests so much in their CPD. The benefit of CPD to both the individual and his or her employing organisation has long been recognised, both in developing new skills and knowledge and in ensuring healthcare professionals are kept up to date. A 2011 report from the NHS Future Forum concluded that all staff within the NHS must have access to CPD to help develop flexibility and deliver the health service of the future by enabling them to respond to changing healthcare needs, new technology and ways of delivering care. Furthermore, CPD needs to be regarded seriously, adequately resourced and prioritised and should be linked to staff appraisals.[7]

The General Medical Council, while considering the CPD needs of medical staff, acknowledged in 2011 that to be effective CPD must be embedded in appraisal and personal development plans and 'must be directed towards improving and maintaining practice'.[8] The Future Forum accepted that 'CPD

---

*   Peer appraisal pilot of managers in general practice (NHS Education for Scotland), unpublished report.

is a crucial part of good management and effective clinical governance. The issues around provision of CPD are complex, including issues around funding and staffing cover'.[9]

The issues relating to CPD provision and its funding within general practice are equally complex. Little has been written on the subject of practice management development or the availability of appropriate CPD. NHS Education South Central, part of the South Central Strategic Health Authority in England, conducted a project to scope the availability and relevance of CPD opportunities, networking or professional support for PMs across Oxfordshire and the Isle of Wight. They found 'little and varied formal common professional development support . . . [for PMs in] . . . a professionally isolating role . . . that provides huge changes and challenges in the current NHS'.[10] The project conclusions were that PMs needed a supportive network, induction into their role, learning opportunities and resources, appraisal and personal development plans. Their recommendations included further work to explore the possibility of piloting the Scottish practice manager's appraisal system and competency framework.[10]

McLaren *et al.*'s[11] study of PM engagement with CPD in the south of England identified that they tend to make the most of opportunities to keep up to date and develop and maintain their skills in the operational management of the practice. Perceived benefits of CPD were enhanced skills, motivation, confidence, workforce and role development and patient benefit through service enhancement. Participation of PMs in CPD activities was limited by 'negative attitudes, time pressures, lack of finance, and awareness of inclusivity in wider CPD policies'.[11] They concluded that such resistance must be overcome if PMs are to expand their role to meet the challenges of delivering the primary care services of the future.

A subsequent paper, *Development Needs of Practice Managers in Primary Care*, concluded in 2010 that

> there is an extending and expanding role for the practice manager. The factors which will influence future development of the practice manager workforce are complex and diverse. Whilst it would be undesirable to lose some of the benefits of the diversity of the role, it is clear that a structure for professional development is required.[12]

While the importance and benefits of CPD are recognised across the home countries of the UK, lack of funding and the structures to support CPD for PMs could have a significant negative impact in some areas. PMs in Scotland are fortunate that PM development and CPD is supported and at least partially funded by NES via the Scottish Practice Management Development Network.

FURTHER READING

For more information and an overview of support and educational opportunities for managers based in GP practices across Scotland, please visit:

- www.nes.scot.nhs.uk/education-and-training/by-discipline/medicine/general-practice/practice-manager-development.aspx (*Practice Manager Development*).
- Practice Manager Patient Safety Education Scenario: www.nes.scot.nhs.uk/media/961112/practice_management_development_network.pdf

REFERENCES

1. Pollock AM. *NHS Plc: the privatisation of our healthcare*. London: Verso Books; 2005.
2. Grimshaw J, Youngs H. Towards better practice management: a national survey of Scottish general practice management. *J Manage Med*. 1994; **8**(2): 56–64.
3. Baker R. General practice in Gloucester, Avon and Somerset: explaining variations in standards. *Br J Gen Pract*. 1992; **42**(363): 415–18.
4. Harrison J, Burns P. Expectations of general practice gateways and bridges. *Health Manpow Manage*. 1994; **20**(1): 21–6.
5. Westland J, Grimshaw J, Maitland J, *et al.* Understanding practice management: a qualitative study in general practice. *J Manage Med*. 1996; **10**(5): 29–37.
6. Department of Health National Health Services. *Investing in General Practice: the new General Medical Services Contract. Annex C: competency framework for practice management*. Available at: www.nhsemployers.org/SiteCollectionDocuments/gms_contract_cd_130209.pdf (accessed 10 November 2013).
7. Department of Health NHS Future Forum. *Education and Training: a report from the NHS Future Forum*. 2011. Available at: www.gov.uk/government/uploads/system/uploads/attachment_data/file/213751/dh_127543.pdf (accessed 10 November 2013).
8. General Medical Council. *Review of the GMC's Role in Doctors' Continuing Professional Development: final report*. London: GMC; 2011. Available at: www.gmc-uk.org/Final_Report_on_review_of_CPD_14_Oct_2011_web_version.pdf_44813249.pdf (accessed 10 November 2013).
9. Department of Health NHS National Future Forum. *Clinical Advice and Leadership: a report from the NHS Future Forum*. 2011. Available at: www.gov.uk/government/uploads/system/uploads/attachment_data/file/213750/dh_127542.pdf (accessed 10 November 2013).
10. NHS Education South Central. *An exploratory project scoping the development needs of practice managers across Oxfordshire and the Isle of Wight at February 2009*. NHS Education South Central; 2009. Available at: www.oxforddeanery.nhs.uk/pdf/NESC_PCTF_Practice_Managers_Educational_Report.pdf (accessed 10 November 2013).
11. McLaren S, Woods L, Boudioni M, *et al.* Developing the general practice manager role: managers' experiences of engagement in continuing professional development. *Qual Prim Care*. 2007; **15**: 85–91.
12. McCall J, McKay M, Stone L. Development needs of practice managers in primary care. *Educ Prim Care*. 2010; **21**(3): 141–2.

CHAPTER 18

General practice nursing

Susan Kennedy

The contribution that practice nurses have made to the delivery of quality primary care services has been considerable.[1]

INTRODUCTION

General practice nurses (GPNs) deliver highly skilled, evidence-based care to the patient populations of the general practices that employ them. They work in collaboration with other professions and agencies, and in partnership with patients, families and carers. The responsibilities of the GPN role include anticipating health needs, promoting self-care and self-management, enabling patients to be as healthy and independent as possible, and providing holistic support and care for long-term conditions.

GPNs are a group of clinical practitioners who often work independently and in isolation. They enter general practice with widely different levels of experience and capabilities and are expected to fulfil roles tailored to the individual needs of their employers. As a result, GPNs' continuing professional development (CPD) typically depends on *them* identifying and addressing their personal learning needs as they relate to their context and specific roles. Despite GPNs' increasing desire and need for a wide range of CPD resources there is still very limited organisational structures to support them on a national basis in the United Kingdom (UK).[2] In addition, the roles and responsibilities of GPNs continue to increase in response to the rising demands of modern primary care, posing a number of important challenges that have to be considered and addressed to ensure that quality nursing care continues to be delivered in a safe, effective and person-centred manner.

This chapter begins with a brief description of the history, evolution and increasingly important role of the general practice nurse in Scotland. The recruitment and learning needs of new GPNs are then considered, followed by a focus on developments in the CPD and appraisal of existing GPNs. The chapter concludes by reflecting on a number of potential challenges and opportunities for further developing nursing in the general practice setting.

THE EVOLUTION OF THE GENERAL PRACTICE NURSE

Since the inception of the UK National Health Service (NHS) in 1948, and possibly even before that, general practitioners (GPs) have employed nurses.[3] In the 1980s the nature of the role of GPN was challenged[4] and it was argued that they should be integrated into community nursing teams because of the many similarities between their responsibilities (e.g. wound care and vaccination). However, around the same time the responsibilities of GPNs were beginning to extend (e.g. cervical cytology screening) and expand (e.g. supporting people with long-term conditions) and the distinct role of the GPN as a healthcare professional providing wide-ranging nursing care to all age groups from a base in general medical practices became clear and indisputable.

In 1990, new legislation provided practices with financial incentives for employing GPNs to deliver health promotion policies, which led to a significant increase in their numbers.[5] GPNs gained confidence and experience of consulting as the first point of contact with patients and some started prescribing independently (after undergoing additional and required training), which allowed them to complete clinical encounters and manage chronic medical conditions.[6] It is estimated that GPNs now conduct more than a third of all consultations in general practice in Scotland.[7]

National nursing regulatory bodies exist to protect the public, ensure that all registered nurses exceed the minimum training and practice standards and issue the required licences for nurses, including GPNs, to legally work. In the UK, the Nursing and Midwifery Council (NMC) fulfils these responsibilities.[8] It stipulates that in order to maintain their registration and licence all nurses must, among other things:
- possess the necessary knowledge and skills to practise in a safe and effective manner without direct supervision
- recognise and work within the limits of their competence
- keep their knowledge and skills up to date throughout their working life
- participate in appropriate learning events in order to maintain and further develop their professional competence.

RECRUITMENT AND TRAINING FOR NEW GENERAL PRACTICE NURSES

There are approximately 3700 whole-time equivalent GPs and 1400 GPNs serving Scotland's estimated population of 5.2 million.[7] The majority of GPNs are aged 45 years or over, each typically with more than 2 decades' experience and training (usually self-directed and self-funded). The ageing workforce and increasing demand for more GPNs are powerful incentives to recruit and train more staff, but this will only happen through strong leadership and the provision of adequate resources.[9]

At present, there is no shortage of interested applicants for vacant GPN positions. The main recruitment challenge, however, is to find and match candidates with the *right* skills-set required for specific GPN roles. One of the main reasons for this is that pre-registration training programmes do not equip nurses with all of the necessary skills and knowledge for a GPN role.[10] This deficiency was noted as early as the 1980s: 'Practice nurses need special training to extend knowledge and skills well beyond those of general professional training in order to function competently, with assurance, and with safety.'[11] For example, cervical screening and management of long-term conditions are not taught.

Newly employed GPNs therefore require robust transitional support mechanisms and have to adopt experiential learning styles.[12] Potential strategies to achieve this aim may include:

- providing general practice placements for student nurses
- creating career pathways to allow progression and promotion
- distance-based, part-time diploma and degree courses
- development of nationally recognised vocational GPN programmes.

GPN leaders lobbied the NMC for GPN to be recognised as a specialised practice with an academic programme. Few universities now deliver this; this is most likely because of a combination of limited curriculum relevance, the substantial investment in time and money required and the programme not being a mandatory requirement for practice.

Recognising these difficulties, and the importance to support and train new GPNs, NHS Education for Scotland (NES) subsequently developed a 1-year practice-based educational programme specifically tailored to this professional group. The programme involves the following components:

- regular tutorials with trained GPN educational supervisors
- workshops delivered on dedicated study days
- provision of and access to e-learning educational resources
- documenting, evidencing and reflecting on learning via an e-portfolio.

Participants are assessed through simulated consultations, direct observation of clinical skills demonstration, case-based discussions, significant event analysis, reflection and evidence-based essays. The aim is to continue to develop this programme into a national training programme for GPNs, with a target of 80% of all new GPNs to complete this within 5 years suggested for England.[9]

CONTINUED PROFESSIONAL DEVELOPMENT

GPNs should continue to learn, develop and update their knowledge and skills throughout their careers. This is usually left to the discretion of the individual GPNs. There are learning opportunities, including short, generic preparatory programmes, specialist courses, study days devoted to specific skills and academic higher education programmes. There is also growing recognition of the importance of GPN career pathways and personal learning plans.

NES has adopted a 'Career & Development Framework for General Practice Nursing'.[13] The framework describes different GPN levels (practitioner, senior practitioner, advanced practitioner and consultant practitioner) and is based on four educational pillars:

1. Clinical practice
2. Facilitation of learning
3. Leadership
4. Evidence, research and development.

Professional networks

One of the major recognised barriers to effective CPD is professional isolation. For example, a recent survey of GPNs found an association between increased feelings of isolation and reduced learning, less productive appraisals and decreased likelihood to remain in their jobs.[14] Because of the independent GP model for delivering primary care in the UK, GPNs are especially likely to be isolated, as they tend to work alone or in very small groups. Being part of a professional network has been shown to reduce isolation, strengthen professional identities and increase healthcare professionals' confidence and functioning within multidisciplinary teams.[15] GPNs are also more likely to incorporate new evidence into practice if they are exposed to it while part of a trusted group.[16]

Local and national GPN networks were formed in the UK in the 1990s with the aims of providing peer support and educational resources and promoting the profession. NES successfully piloted a GPN professional network in 2006. Subsequently, a post was created for a national coordinator to manage the network on a national level, with the assistance of a number of newly recruited sessional GPN educational advisors at regional level. The network's aims are to promote accessible national quality assured education, build capacity and capability and improve communication about GPN-related issues.

Shared learning opportunities

Protected learning time and problem-based small group learning (PBSGL) are two examples of methods (opportunities) for CPD and learning to be shared by different professional groups. Inter-professional learning should not be confused with multi-professional education. The latter is simply the passive sharing of learning. Inter-professional learning, on the other hand, has the following potential benefits:

- increased confidence
- promotion of reflective practice
- improved communication between different healthcare professionals
- enhanced understanding of different professional roles.[17]

In Scotland, GPNs are encouraged to participate in PBSGL. A recent qualitative study found this method was feasible and acceptable for GPNs and could increase their likelihood of implementing new evidence in their practice.[18] However, some GPNs may not value facilitated and shared learning as much as other team members.[19] It is unclear whether this is because of the existence of professional hierarchies, lack of prior experience with this approach, personal preference for didactic learning, or for more practical reasons such as lack of time. Evaluation of the value of PBSGL continues, but early results indicate more experienced GPNs are generally enthusiastic about the method.

APPRAISAL

The implication of professional self-regulation for GPNs is that they have a responsibility to be accountable for their own professional performance and competence and be able to clearly demonstrate this. However, according to the General Medical Services contract: 'All practice employed nurses [should] have Personal Learning Plans which have been reviewed at annual appraisal'.[20] A recent online survey of 1161 GPNs found 86% had been appraised overall (dropping to 74% of GPNs working in a practice with a single GP partner).[21] Of these, only a third was supported in developing a personal development plan. In Scotland, a survey of GPNs in a single health board area found 79% of responders had an appraisal in the last year, with 19% describing it as being of no benefit.[22] The results suggest there is ample room for improvement, but that they are comparable with those of a NHS England staff survey in which 77% of respondents reported being appraised and only 34% described the appraisal process as well structured.[23]

Peer review has been suggested as a potential way for GPNs to develop more effective PDPs through formative feedback and by providing a more objective, external perception. Combing peer review with a criterion-based performance assessment tool has been found to further improve GPNs' practice.[24]

Following a small study that explored peer GPN appraisal,[25] in 2012 NES evaluated a training programme for GPN appraisers and the feasibility of each conducting up to five peer appraisals over a 3-month period. Appraisees were invited to take part by submitting a standardised NES form based on the four 'pillars' in the Career and Development Framework with supporting evidence such as criterion audit, significant event analysis or case reflections. These methods were chosen because they allow GPNs to learn from patient safety incidents and offer support and guidance to help implement the necessary improvements to prevent harm to patients in the future.[26] These tools are most effective when used within a strong and positive safety culture that supports changing attitudes and altered professional behaviours.

GPN appraisers were trained to conduct 2-hour interviews with the aim of supporting appraisees to develop and agree PDPs. Appraisees described this process as more valuable than any other previous appraisal. The implication may be that peer appraisal would better support GPNs than the current model, especially with pending NMC revalidation guidance.

POTENTIAL CHALLENGES AND OPPORTUNITIES

There have recently been calls to shift the primary care skills mix even further from GPs to GPNs. This is based, in part, on findings that general practices that employ more GPNs perform better in some areas of the Quality and Outcomes

Framework.[27] This shift is not only about the overall workforce capacity but also the scope of their roles. The Quality and Outcomes Framework incentivises the expansion of GPNs' roles and, in the process, create new opportunities, including GPNs becoming partners in their practices. However, a large part of GPNs' work is now linked to clinical algorithms and the management of long-term conditions. While important, prioritising this aspect of practice can be detrimental to their professional development and retaining the skills required for a more generalist, holistic approach to care. Conversely, GPs may potentially become de-skilled in managing common long-term conditions.

There have also been concerns that with GPNs requiring traditional medical skills and responsibilities, there is a gradual blurring of professional roles.[28,29] However, a recent study found nurses and allied health professionals still rated their professional identities lower when compared with those of GPs and pharmacists.[30] If GPNs are to maintain their professional identity, it is important that the acquisition of any new skills has to be accompanied by a simultaneous infusion of the core values outlined by their NMC code.[29]

The key factors that determine the degree and speed with which the role of GPNs expand are the expectations and perceptions of nurses and their employers.[31] Proactive nurses welcome and seek out new challenges to further develop their roles, which usually benefits the practices. Conversely, more reactive nurses may be a barrier to change and differences in perceptions of their roles can cause conflict within practice teams.

Finally, it is worth remembering that leadership is one of the four pillars of quality nursing care. In areas with dedicated GPN leaders there are usually planned strategic approaches to learning that support innovation and change to improve patient care. Unfortunately, this model of leadership is uncommon. At the national level, GPN representation is rare and there are only a few GPN leaders in positions with any real influence. The appointment of sessional NES GPN educational advisors has made it possible to support a variety of professional networks and to promote the exchange of knowledge, skills and resources. However, there is much more that can be done. At the practice level, GPNs can be leaders in innovation and quality improvement by being role models and could also reasonably be expected to take responsibility for some clinical governance issues.

CONCLUSION

GPN is a vibrant and exciting career choice that should be considered by any nurse. It allows many opportunities to develop clinical and decision-making skills with the scope for autonomous practice and a wide range of potential further role development possibilities. However, inherent in the role is the responsibility to reflect on the quality and safety of the delivered care. This requires a commitment to CPD and appraisal and providing evidence-informed interventions and using consultation approaches that place the person at the centre. Learning opportunities to prepare nurses new to GPN are therefore essential and should emphasise a practice-based curriculum that adequately reflects the dynamic nature of the role. Networking and inter-professional learning opportunities are valuable for established GPNs and should be integrated with effective appraisal processes.

KEY POINTS

- The role of GPNs continue to expand and evolve, with increasing responsibilities but also exciting new opportunities.
- A national, structured approach to prepare candidates for GPN is needed.
- GPNs require structured support, a range of educational resources and peer appraisal for effective CPD.
- The potential value of inter-professional approaches to learning, such as PBSGL, should be investigated further.

REFERENCES

1. Gupta K. Who is the practice nurse? In: Carey L, editor. *Practice Nursing*. London: Bailliere Tindall; 2000.
2. Stephenson J. Practice nurses under 'additional pressure'. *Nursing Times*. 2011 March 4. Available at: www.nursingtimes.net/nursing-practice/clinical-zones/practice-nursing/practice-nurses-under-additional-pressure/5026670.article (accessed 22 November 2013).
3. Marsh GN. Group practice nurse: an analysis and comment on six months' work. *BMJ*. 1967; **1**: 489–91.
4. Hockey L. Is the practice nurse a good idea? *Br J Gen Pract*. 1984; **34**(259): 102–3.
5. Hoare K, Mills J, Francis K. The role of government policy in supporting nurse-led care in general practice in the United Kingdom, New Zealand and Australia: an adapted realist review. *J Adv Nurs*. 2011; **68**(5): 963–80.
6. Department of Health. Improving patients' access to medicines: a guide to implementing nurse and pharmacist independent prescribing within the NHS in England. London: Department of Health; 2006. Available at: http://webarchive.nationalarchives.gov.uk/+/www.dh.gov.uk/en/PublicationsandStatistics/Publications/PublicationsPolicyandGuidance/DH_4133743 (accessed 22 November 2013).
7. Information Services Division, NHS National Services Scotland. *Primary Care Workforce Survey 2013*. Edinburgh: ISD. Available at: www.isdscotland.org/Health-Topics/General-Practice/GPs-and-Other-Practice-Workforce/primary-care-workforce-survey-2013.asp (accessed 29 November 2013).
8. Nursing and Midwifery Council. *The Code: standards of conduct, performance and ethics for nurses and midwives*. London: NMC; 2008.
9. Aston J. General practice workforce. *Independent Nurse*. November, 2013.
10. Sykes C, Urquhart C. Pre-registration nurse placements in general practice: an evaluation. *Pract Nurs*. 2012; **23**(8): 413–18.
11. Mourin K. A practice nurses' course: content and evaluation. *J R Coll Gen Pract*. 1980; **30**: 78–84.

12. Bowers-Lanier B. Professional development: a lifelong investment and journey with curricular milepost. *Nurs Educ.* 2009; **48**(5): 235–6.

13. NHS Education for Scotland. *Career & Development Framework for General Practice Nursing.* Edinburgh: NHS Education for Scotland; 2011. Available at: www.mnic.nes. scot.nhs.uk/media/52579/gp_nursing_framework_final.pdf (accessed 29 November 2013).

14. O'Donnell C, Jabereen H, Watt G. Practice nurses' workload, carer intentions and the impact of professional isolation: a cross-sectional survey. *BMC Nurs.* 2010; **9**: 2.

15. Gopee N. The role of peer assessment and peer review in nursing. *Br J Nurs.* 2001; **10**(2): 115–21.

16. Doran DM, Mylopoulos J, Kushniruk A, *et al.* Evidence in the palm of your hand: development of an outcomes-focused knowledge translation intervention. *Worldviews Evid Based Nurs.* 2007; **4**(2): 69–77.

17. Hale C. Interprofessional education: the way to a successful workforce? *Br J Ther Rehabil.* 2003; **10**(3): 122–7.

18. Overton GK, McCalister P, Kelly D, *et al.* Practice-based small group learning: how health professionals view their intention to change and the process of implementing change in practice. *Med Teach.* 2009; **31**: 514–20.

19. Bunnies S, Gray F, Kelly D. Collective learning, change and improvement in health care: trialling a facilitated learning initiative with general practice teams. *J Eval Clin Pract.* 2011; **18**(3): 630–6.

20. British Medical Association. *Quality and Outcomes Framework for 2012/13: guidance for PCOs and practices.* London: NHS Employers; 2012. Available at: www.google.co.uk/url?sa=t&rct=j&q=&esrc=s&frm=1&source=web&cd=6&ved=0CE8QFjAF&url=http%3A%2F%2Fbma.org.uk%2F-%2Fmedia%2FFiles%2FPDFs%2FPractical%2520advice%2520at%2520work%2FContracts%2Fgpqofguidance20122013.pdf&ei=Hl6PUoe4LuyV7AbbyIHABQ&usg=AFQjCNHFyDNQXXJ9QfGB8QymVDnN8Sj6Jg (accessed 22 November 2013).

21. Crossman S. *The WiPP 'SNAPshot' Survey. Supporting nurses and practice: a national survey investigating employment conditions and professional development support for nurses in general practice in the UK.* May 2008. Available at: www.wipp.org.uk/uploads/GPN/Final%20SNAPshot%20Survey%20Report%20SC.pdf (accessed 22 November 2013).

22. Cochrane A, Cowan C. *NHSGGC Practice Nurse 2010 Survey: workforce trends and development needs.* NHS Greater Glasgow and Clyde; (unpublished report) Glasgow, 2011.

23. NHS Employers. *Appraisal and Simplified KSF.* Leeds: NHS Employers; 2011. Available at: www.nhsemployers.org/PayAndContracts/AgendaForChange/KSF/Pages/Appraisal-and-simplified-KSF.aspx (accessed 22 November 2013).

24. Scarpa R, Connelly PE. Innovations in performance assessment: a criterion based performance assessment for advanced practice. *Nurs Adm Q.* 2011; **35**(2): 164–73.

25. Murie J, Wilson A, Cerinus M. Practice nurse appraisal: evaluation report. *Educ Prim Care.* 2009; **20**(4): 291–7.

26. Bowie P. Reporting and learning from harmful incidents. *Pract Nurse.* 2010; **40**(9): 38–41.

27. National Nursing Research Unit, King's College London. Do we need more practice nurses? *Policy Plus Evidence, Issues and Opinions in Healthcare.* 2010; **23**: 60–61. Available at: www.kcl.ac.uk/nursing/research/nnru/publications/Policy-plus-Review.pdf (accessed 22 November 2013).

28. Charles-Jones H, Latimer J, May C. Transforming general practice: the redistribution of medical work in primary care. *Soc Health Illness*. 2003; **25**(1): 71–92.

29. Carey L, Jones M. Autonomy in practice: is it a reality. In: Carey L, editor. *Practice Nursing*. London: Baillière Tindall; 2000. pp. 286–307.

30. Reid R, Bruce D, Allstaff K, *et al*. Validating the Readiness for Interprofessional Learning Scale (RIPLS) in the postgraduate context: are health care professionals ready for IPL? *Med Educ*. 2006; **40**: 415–22.

31. Bell FL. *Nursing in General Practice: Working on the Boundaries of Role Development* [dissertation]. Dundee: University of Dundee; 2008.

Part III

Learning for Improvement

CHAPTER 19

Safety skills

Maria Ahmed & Nick Sevdalis

INTRODUCTION

It has been more than a decade since the publication of a number of major, high-profile reports that made patient safety a political and public health priority, such as *To Err is Human*[1] in 1999 in the United States and *An Organisation with a Memory*[2] in 2000 in the United Kingdom. A wave of research studies followed, with the emerging body of evidence and concepts now recognised as forming patient safety science.[3] Following several studies that found significant care-related harm reaching patients, particularly those admitted to hospitals,[4] various approaches and interventions to improve safety have been developed and evaluated in the past 10 years – and some of them, such as checklists, have been implemented across a range of specialties aiming to improve the safety of care delivered to patients.[5–7]

Alongside such interventions, frameworks to understand patient safety, the occurrence of error, the recovery from error and ultimately the mitigation of the consequences of errors have also been developed. Among these, the 'systems approach' to errors within healthcare environments has been fairly prominent.[8,9] According to this approach, errors do not occur (solely) because of inadequacies of individual healthcare providers. Instead, the systems approach poses that numerous factors within a complex healthcare system can contribute to errors and cause harm – including the presence and adherence to protocols, the quality of team working and communication within and between clinical teams, the nature of the clinical tasks that ought to be carried out (i.e. how complex they are), and the wider organisation of clinical work (e.g. situations where junior clinicians are left to deal with very sick patients without adequate supervision), among other factors. A number of studies have found evidence for the validity of this approach in understanding error and harm and in addressing the factors that can lead to them.

Even within such systemic views of errors, however, it is widely recognised that individual healthcare providers are often the very last barrier within the complex healthcare system prior to harm reaching a patient.[10] Patient safety interventions aimed at last barriers to harm, such as double-checking medication at the point of administration or carrying out a 'time-out' prior to incision within an operating theatre, rely to a large extent on individual clinicians' own skills to ensure safety. Further, even within systems approaches the skills of individuals remain a prominent contributor to organisational performance – indeed, such skills are a key marker of clinical professionalism.

While there has been significant progress in the quest for safer healthcare, recent reports conclude that progress has been slower than hoped.[11-13] Crucially, a discussion has recently emerged within the patient safety community and literature, focused on whether 'the safety pendulum has swung too far' to create a 'no-blame' culture, with safety improvement efforts paying insufficient attention to the role of clinicians in maintaining and promoting patient safety.[11] Consistent with this overarching view, this chapter aims to highlight the role of the clinician in maintaining and promoting patient safety, to examine the qualities and attributes of the safe clinician, to explore education and training as a means of optimising the clinicians' role and discuss implications for patient safety in primary care.

QUALITIES AND ATTRIBUTES OF THE SAFE CLINICIAN

There is a growing acceptance that the qualities and attributes of the safe clinician go beyond 'simple' technical or procedural competence.[14] Analysis of patient safety incidents in healthcare,[15] and lessons from high-reliability organisations such as aviation and the nuclear power industry, has led to increasing recognition of the importance of 'non-technical skills' (NTSs) in the delivery of safe, effective healthcare.[16] NTSs are defined as 'the cognitive, social and personal resource skills that complement technical skills and contribute to safe and efficient task performance'.[16] NTSs span a broad range of skills including communication, decision-making, teamwork, leadership and situational awareness.[17,18]

BOX 19.1 Categories of 'safety skills'[1]

Anticipation and preparedness	Honesty
Awareness of the patient (including empathy)	Humility
	Leadership
Awareness of oneself	Open-mindedness
Awareness of the situation	Organisational skills and efficiency
Awareness of one's team	Responsiveness
Common sense	Team working and communication
Confidence	Technical skills
Conscientiousness	Vigilance
Crisis management	

This progress in the way researchers and healthcare practitioners think of their skills led to the broader conceptualisation of 'safety skills'. Safety skills are those skills that contribute to safe clinical practice regardless of whether they could be classified as NTSs or another type of skill. In a recent study using survey and focus group methods and samples of experienced patient safety researchers and clinicians, a list of 73 safety skills was identified and subsequently arranged into 18 broad categories listed in Box 19.1.[19] A subsequent validation survey involving 50 senior physicians and surgeons found that the majority of these skills were perceived to be important to being a safe clinician.

Interestingly, humility, honesty and empathy were uncovered as being key attributes of a safe practitioner. Indeed, these latter attributes fit well with the broader qualities that patients, the public and regulators expect the healthcare profession to espouse,[20] but which may not have previously been accepted as being of direct importance to safe clinical practice – possibly because their measurement presents difficulties. The survey respondents also believed that the majority of the identified 'safety skills' can be acquired through training. This is an important finding that may support designing educational interventions to develop these skills and so enhance the clinician's role in patient safety.

EDUCATION AND TRAINING TO IMPROVE PATIENT SAFETY

Education and training are essential means of maximising the role of the clinician in patient safety. However, while conventional health professional training equips clinicians with core technical competencies, there is little or no formal opportunity to develop many of the safety skills beyond core clinical knowledge and skills.[21] Indeed, in 2009, the House of Commons Health Committee Inquiry into Patient Safety concluded that sustainable improvements in patient safety requires major reform in medical education and recommended that patient safety should be 'fully and explicitly integrated into the education and training curricula of all healthcare workers'.[11] Broadly speaking, patient safety education may fall into two categories: (1) non-technical skills training to improve clinical practice at the front line and (2) education in the 'science' of patient safety (e.g. error theory and root cause analysis) to equip clinicians to engage in efforts to improve the wider healthcare system.[22]

In recent years there has been a huge proliferation in the number of published educational interventions in patient safety. Wong *et al.*[23] conducted a recent systematic review of courses in patient safety and quality improvement targeting medical students and trainees. They identified 41 courses published between 2000 and 2009. The courses employed a combination of didactic and experiential educational modalities to teach core concepts in quality and safety such as root cause analysis, systems thinking and quality improvement methods. Among the 27 reports that included an evaluation, the authors found that such courses were generally well received by learners and effectively improved knowledge in safety and quality improvement, with some courses leading to improvements in care processes. However, few studies were able to demonstrate changes in learners' behaviour or potential patient benefit.

Similarly, there is a growing literature of non-technical skills training in healthcare, particularly within the craft specialties of surgery and anaesthesia.[24] Training interventions to improve teamwork, communication and situational awareness have been shown to have a beneficial effect on clinical performance and safety.[17,25,26] Evidence for training in more elusive NTSs such as mental readiness and stress management has also emerged.[27,28] Interventions in NTS training employ a wide range of educational modalities from simple lecture-based teaching and video demonstrations of relevant NTSs[29] to high-fidelity, multidisciplinary team-based simulations.[30,31]

Building on published work, a number of dedicated patient safety curricula have been developed for clinicians; these include the World Health Organization's *Patient Safety Curriculum Guide for Medical Schools*[32] and more recently their multi-professional edition for students in medicine, nursing and the allied health professions.[33] Such curricula aim to guide and support educators in developing and implementing educational programmes in patient safety.

However, despite such guidance and evidence for its efficacy, the wider implementation and adoption of patient safety education have been slow.[23,34] Multiple barriers exist to the sustainable integration of patient safety education including lack of expert faculty, poor learner engagement, competing educational priorities and an unsupportive institutional culture.[35] As a result, recommendations to promote curricular integration of patient safety education aim to address these factors and include investing in faculty development,[36] promoting patient safety as a science and integrating patient safety competencies into accreditation standards and certification examinations.[23,37]

APPLICATION TO PRIMARY CARE

Just as clinicians are critical for safety in the secondary care setting, so, too, general practitioners (GPs) and the wider primary care team are critical to the safety of primary care. Comparable research into the safety skills of primary care clinicians is yet to be conducted. However, it is likely that the diverse and complex environment of primary care may require a different set of 'safety skills'. In particular, it could be argued that several of the well-recognised NTSs identified in the acute setting may actually form the core 'technical' skills of primary care – such as decision-making and teamwork. Nonetheless, such safety skills could be further developed through explicit training to ensure excellence in practice and a commitment to improving the safety and quality of care. For example, attitudes towards and engagement in key risk management interventions such as significant event analysis is known to vary widely among GPs[38,39] and members of the wider primary care team.[40] Education, and so an improved understanding of the science of safety, may help to promote uptake and engagement in subsequent safety improvement efforts.

Indeed, a recent survey of an international panel of primary care physicians and researchers as part of the European LINNEAUS collaboration showed that respondents considered education and training as one of the most important strategies to improve patient safety in primary care.[41] However, the provision of patient safety in the training of primary care health workers was considered to be severely lacking. With regard to GP specialist training, the latest iteration of the UK Royal College of General Practitioners curriculum includes a comprehensive statement on competencies in patient safety and quality of care.[42] However, there is currently little guidance or opportunity to develop these competencies in practice.

We take the view that, in order to achieve progress in the field of safety skills within the primary care context, the most effective means of delivering patient safety education in primary care ought to be considered in detail. While the use of checklists, briefings and simulation is gradually becoming commonplace within the acute care setting, the transferability of these educational modalities to primary care needs to be explored. Just like the environment and procedures of an operating theatre or an intensive care unit do not fully replicate those found in a jumbo jet cockpit,[43] the context of clinical work within primary care differs from that of a structured interventional environment. While in the latter often the diagnosis is clear and safety focuses on the execution of the relevant procedure and pre- and post-procedural care, primary care faces successive short consultations with many patients, most of whom will not be very sick but some of whom may present the GP with complex diagnostic problems, thus requiring extra attention. There are certainly many lessons to be learned from the current experience of interventions and training modules developed for secondary care environments. We believe, however, that simply 'transplanting' these into primary care may not necessarily be the most fruitful approach.

Finally, given the well-known barriers to the sustainable integration of patient safety education, there is a need to explore how best to embed such education into practice and ensure equivalent attention to traditional subjects. Capitalising on well-established levers such as the Quality and Outcomes Framework and revalidation requirements for doctors[44] may pose as potentially powerful vehicles to embed patient safety into primary care education and ensure alignment with core professional and practice standards.

SUMMARY

Safety improvement efforts have inadequately considered the role of the clinician in maintaining and promoting patient safety. A wide range of technical skills, NTSs and wider safety attributes are required to be a safe clinician. Education and training is a valuable means of developing these attributes and thereby optimising the role of clinicians in patient safety. Efforts in primary care are required to catch up with work in secondary care to verify the safety skills required of primary care clinicians and inform subsequent strategies to develop these skills. This will help ensure safe clinical practice at the front line and also promote engagement in wider safety improvement efforts across the wider healthcare system.

SUMMARY POINTS

- Clinicians have a central role in maintaining and improving patient safety.
- The key attributes of a safe clinician include safety skills (including technical and non-technical skills), humility, honesty and empathy.
- Education and training can develop these 'safety skills' to optimise the clinician's role in patient safety.
- Further research is required into safety skills in primary care to catch up with progress in secondary care specialties.

REFERENCES

1. Kohn LT, Corrigan JM, Donaldson MS. *To Err is Human: building a safer health system.* Washington, DC: National Academy Press, Institute of Medicine; 1999.
2. Department of Health. *An Organisation with a Memory.* London: HMSO; 2000.
3. Vincent C. *Patient Safety.* Chichester: Wiley-Blackwell; 2010.
4. De Vries EN, Ramrattan MA, Smorenburg SM, *et al.* The incidence and nature of in-hospital adverse events: a systematic review. *Qual Saf Health Care.* 2008; **17**(3): 216–23.
5. Pronovost P, Berenholtz S, Dorman T, *et al.* Improving communication in the ICU using daily goals. *J Crit Care.* 2003; **18**(2): 71–5.
6. Haynes AB, Weiser TG, Berry WR, *et al.* A surgical safety checklist to reduce morbidity and mortality in a global population. *N Engl J Med.* 2009; **360**(5): 491–9.
7. De Vries EN, Prins HA, Crolla RM, *et al.* Effect of a comprehensive surgical safety system on patient outcomes. *N Engl J Med.* 2010; **363**(20): 1928–37.
8. Vincent C, Taylor-Adams S, Stanhope N. Framework for analysing risk and safety in clinical medicine. *BMJ.* 1998; **316**(7138): 1154–7.
9. Vincent C, Moorthy K, Sarker SK, *et al.* Systems approaches to surgical quality and safety: from concept to measurement. *Ann Surg.* 2004; **239**(4): 475–82.
10. Taylor-Adams S. Safety skills for clinicians: an essential component of patient safety. *J Patient Saf.* 2008; **4**: 141.
11. House of Commons. *Health Committee – Sixth Report: Patient Safety.* London: The Stationery Office; 2009.
12. Shojania KG, Thomas EJ. Trends in adverse events over time: why are we not improving? *BMJ Qual Saf.* 2013; **22**(4): 273–7.
13. Wachter RM, Pronovost P, Shekelle P. Strategies to improve patient safety: the evidence base matures. *Ann Intern Med.* 2013; **158**(5 Pt. 1): 350–2.
14. Yule S, Flin R, Paterson-Brown S, *et al.* Non-technical skills for surgeons in the operating room: a review of the literature. *Surgery.* 2006; **139**(2): 140–9.
15. Gawande AA, Zinner MJ, Studdert DM, *et al.* Analysis of errors reported by surgeons at three teaching hospitals. *Surgery.* 2003; **133**(6): 614–21.
16. Flin R, O'Connor P, Crichton M. *Safety at the Sharp End: a guide to non-technical skills.* Guildford: Ashgate; 2008.

17. Sevdalis N, Hull L, Birnbach DJ. Improving patient safety in the operating theatre and perioperative care: obstacles, interventions, and priorities for accelerating progress. *Br J Anaesth*. 2012; **109**(Suppl. 1): i3–16.

18. Hull L, Arora S, Aggarwal R, *et al*. The impact of nontechnical skills on technical performance in surgery: a systematic review. *J Am Coll Surg*. 2012; **214**(2): 214–30.

19. Long S, Arora S, Moorthy K, *et al*. Qualities and attributes of a safe practitioner: identification of safety skills in healthcare. *BMJ Qual Saf*. 2011; **20**(6): 483–90.

20. General Medical Council. *Good Medical Practice*. London: GMC; 2013. Available at: www.gmc-uk.org/GMP_2013.pdf_51447599.pdf (accessed 28 March 2013).

21. Aron DC,Headrick LA. Educating physicians prepared to improve care and safety is no accident: it requires a systematic approach. *Qual Saf Health Care*. 2002; **11**(2): 168–73.

22. Ahmed M. Embedding patient safety into postgraduate medical education [PhD thesis in progress], Imperial College London; 2013.

23. Wong BM, Levinson W, Shojania KG. Quality improvement in medical education: current state and future directions. *Med Educ*. 2012; **46**(1): 107–19.

24. Flin R, Patey R. Improving patient safety through training in non-technical skills. *BMJ*. 2009; **339**: b3595.

25. McCulloch P, Mishra A, Handa A, *et al*. The effects of aviation-style non-technical skills training on technical performance and outcome in the operating theatre. *Qual Saf Health Care*. 2009; **18**(2): 109–15.

26. Neily J, Mills PD, Young-Xu Y, *et al*. Association between implementation of a medical team training program and surgical mortality. *JAMA*. 2010; **304**(15): 1693–700.

27. Arora S, Aggarwal R, Sirimanna P, *et al*. Mental practice enhances surgical technical skills: a randomized controlled study. *Ann Surg*. 2011; **253**(2): 265–70.

28. Wetzel CM, George A, Hanna GB, *et al*. Stress management training for surgeons: a randomized, controlled, intervention study. *Ann Surg*. 2011; **253**(3): 488–94.

29. Arora S, Sevdalis N, Ahmed M, *et al*. Safety skills training for surgeons: a half-day intervention improves knowledge, attitudes and awareness of patient safety. *Surgery*. 2012; **152**(1): 26–31.

30. Undre S, Koutantji M, Sevdalis N, *et al*. Multidisciplinary crisis simulations: the way forward for training surgical teams. *World J Surg*. 2007; **31**(9): 1843–53.

31. Paige JT, Kozmenko V, Yang T, *et al*. High-fidelity, simulation-based, interdisciplinary operating room team training at the point of care. *Surgery*. 2009; **145**(2): 138–46.

32. World Health Organization. *Patient Safety Curriculum Guide for Medical Schools*. Geneva: WHO; 2009. Available at: www.who.int/patientsafety/education/curriculum/EN_PSP_Education_Medical_Curriculum/en/index.html (accessed 1 February 2013).

33. World Health Organization. *Multi-professional Patient Safety Curriculum Guide*. Geneva: WHO; 2011. Available at: www.who.int/patientsafety/education/curriculum/tools-download/en/index.html (accessed 1 February 2013).

34. Woodward HI, Mytton OT, Lemer C, *et al*. What have we learned about interventions to reduce medical errors? *Annu Rev Public Health*. 2010; **31**: 479–97.

35. Wong BM, Etchells EE, Kuper A, *et al*. Teaching quality improvement and patient safety to trainees: a systematic review. *Acad Med*. 2010; **85**(9): 1425–39.

36. Ahmed M, Arora S, Baker P, *et al*. Building capacity and capability for patient safety education: a train-the-trainers programme for senior doctors. *BMJ Qual Saf*. 2013; **22**(8): 618–25.

37. Pronovost PJ, Miller MR, Wachter RM, *et al.* Perspective: physician leadership in quality. *Acad Med.* 2009; **84**(12): 1651–6.

38. Bowie P, McKay J, Dalgetty E, *et al.* A qualitative study of why general practitioners may participate in significant event analysis and educational peer assessment. *Qual Saf Health Care.* 2005; **14**(3): 185–9.

39. McKay J, Bradley N, Lough M, *et al.* A review of significant events analysed in general practice: implications for the quality and safety of patient care. *BMC Fam Pract.* 2009; **10**: 61.

40. de Wet C, Bradley N, Bowie P. Significant event analysis: a comparative study of knowledge, process and attitudes in primary care. *J Eval Clin Pract.* 2011; **17**(6): 1207–15.

41. Gaal S, Verstappen W, Wensing M. What do primary care physicians and researchers consider the most important patient safety improvement strategies? *BMC Health Serv Res.* 2011; **11**: 102.

42. Royal College of General Practitioners. *RCGP Curriculum 2012.* London: RCGP; 2012. Available at: www.rcgp.org.uk/gp-training-and-exams/gp-curriculum-overview.aspx (accessed 1 February 2013).

43. Reader TW, Cuthbertson BH. Teamwork and team training in the ICU: where do the similarities with aviation end? *Crit Care.* 2011; **15**(6): 313.

44. General Medical Council. *The Good Medical Practice Framework for Appraisal and Revalidation.* London: GMC; 2012. Available at: www.gmc-uk.org/static/documents/content/GMC_Revalidation_A4_Guidance_GMP_Framework_04.pdf (accessed 28 December 2012).

CHAPTER 20

A safety checklist for specialty training

Paul Bowie, John McKay & Moya Kelly

INTRODUCTION

The emerging evidence from a range of international sources suggests that the safety of general practice may be compromised in a significant minority of cases.[1-3] Doctors-in-training (specialty trainees) are known to be involved in a proportion of these incidents largely because of a range of systems-, knowledge-, training- and behaviour-based reasons. From an educational perspective, the World Health Organization now recognises that there is a need for patient safety training to be more explicitly integrated and prominently positioned within existing undergraduate and postgraduate curricula for all healthcare professions.[4] The UK Royal College of General Practitioners (RCGP) – which has responsibility for the content of the specialty training curriculum – has responded by developing a curriculum statement on 'patient safety'[5] and defining specific learning objectives (*see* Table 20.1). However, it is left to individual general practitioner (GP) educational supervisors to determine how the RCGP curriculum is best delivered and the related learning needs of trainees are identified and acted upon during the training period. Ensuring that all essential educational issues are identified, prioritised and satisfactorily covered during specialty training is not straightforward, given the scale and complexity of the tasks to be undertaken and the high volume of topics to be addressed.

PATIENT SAFETY AND THE TRAINING ENVIRONMENT

Within the framework of the RCGP curriculum, GP educational supervisors currently guide the activities undertaken by the trainee using a combination of locally developed induction packs, nationally promoted learning interventions and assessments, and professional experience in the workplace to match across to RCGP curriculum competencies (*see* Table 20.2). However, it is currently unclear how the patient safety-related learning needs of trainees are specifically

TABLE 20.1 Royal College of General Practitioners curriculum learning outcomes (with examples) related to patient safety

Learning outcome	Description and example of outcome
1.	**Primary Care Management** For example, contribute to the regular significant event audit meetings and observe the benefits of a multidisciplinary team
2.	**Person-Centred Care** For example, communicate openly, listen and take patients' concerns seriously. Consider patient issues when reflecting on consultation experiences
3.	**Specific Problem-Solving Skills** For example, demonstrate an awareness of the limitations of your own skills in risk management and illustrate that you understand when the skills of colleagues trained more extensively in risk management should be called upon
4.	**A Comprehensive Approach** For example, describe the risks to patient safety by considering an illness pathway or journey in which a variety of healthcare professionals have been involved
5.	**Community Orientation** For example, describe how patient groups may be put at increased risk of mishap by virtue of their particular characteristics, such as language, literacy, culture and health beliefs
6.	**A Holistic Approach** For example, describe how the lessons of patient safety can be applied prospectively to doctor–patient interactions, especially through the identification and discussion of risk
7.	**Contextual Aspects** For example, describe the impact of the working environment on the care the doctor provides and the likelihood of adverse incidents as a result of this
8.	**Attitudinal Aspects** For example, help to shape an organisational culture that prioritises safety and quality through openness, honesty, shared learning and continual incremental improvement
9.	**Scientific Aspects** For example, describe the basic principles of risk assessment

addressed when in the training environment. Given the lack of standardised guidance on how and what specific learning issues are to be covered, it is possible there is variation in GP educational supervisors' interpretation and delivery of this safety-critical element of the curriculum at the 'sharp end' of front-line educational practice.

Overall there appears to be a paucity of evidence on how postgraduate training in general practice (or lack of) may have a visible and negative impact on the safety of patients – arguably, it may be impossible to ever demonstrate clear causation. However, we know that a range of issues connected with the postgraduate training environment may act as proxy indicators of the safety of patient care being compromised unnecessarily and avoidably. For instance, medical educators may be involved in failures of, or inadequate, clinical supervision;[6] or fail to respond appropriately to trainees seeking professional guidance;[7] or conduct insufficient joint reviews of the management of complex clinical cases;[8] or provide limited feedback on drug prescribing performance;[9] and may let poorly developed attitudes and behaviour (such as lack of insight)

TABLE 20.2 A list of the 12 Royal College of General Practitioners curriculum competencies with descriptions*

Competency No.	Description of competency
1.	**Communication and consultation skills** This competency is about communication with patients, and the use of recognised consultation techniques
2.	**Practising holistically** This competency is about the ability of the doctor to operate in physical, psychological, socio-economic and cultural dimensions, taking into account feelings as well as thoughts
3.	**Data gathering and interpretation** This competency is about the gathering and use of data for clinical judgement, the choice of examination and investigations and their interpretation
4.	**Making a diagnosis/making decisions** This competency is about a conscious, structured approach to decision-making
5.	**Clinical management** This competency is about the recognition and management of common medical conditions in primary care
6.	**Managing medical complexity** This competency is about aspects of care beyond managing straightforward problems, including the management of co-morbidity, uncertainty and risk, and the approach to health rather than just illness
7.	**Primary care administration and information management & technology** This competency is about the appropriate use of primary care administration systems, effective record keeping and information technology for the benefit of patient care
8.	**Working with colleagues and in teams** This competency is working effectively with other professionals to ensure patient care, including the sharing of information with colleagues
9.	**Community orientation** This competency is about the management of the health and social care of the practice population and local community
10.	**Maintaining performance, learning and teaching** This competency is about maintaining the performance and effective continuing professional development of oneself and others
11.	**Maintaining an ethical approach to practice** This competency is about practising ethically with integrity and a respect for diversity
12.	**Fitness to practise** This competency is about the doctor's awareness of when his or her own performance, conduct or health, or that of others might put patients at risk and the action taken to protect patients

* Assessment scale: insufficient evidence; needs further development; competent; and excellent.

continue unchecked.[10] Other salient issues that are potentially safety-critical include trainees possessing different levels of clinical knowledge[11] and an inability to prioritise their clinical workloads and manage time.[8] The quality of the learning environment in which trainees are based may also affect the safety of patient care,[12] while doctors-in-training are known to be susceptible to medical errors.[13,14]

Given what is known about human error theory in the healthcare workplace,[15] and the marked differences in local safety cultures[16] and the reliability of practice systems,[1-3,14,17] it is inevitable that variation in the quality of training provision exists and that some issues will be inadequately covered or even overlooked completely. If this happens with fundamental training topics that are considered to be safety-critical then there is a likelihood that the risk of patients being harmed and other quality of care issues arising could potentially increase.

SAFETY CHECKLIST DEVELOPMENT

There is growing evidence from healthcare safety and improvement initiatives that routine adherence to the adoption and use of checklist reminders can improve the overall reliability with which care processes and tasks are undertaken, and so potentially mitigate future risks.[18-21] With this in mind, and using a range of consensus building methods with front-line educators and trainees, the most safety-critical issues to be addressed in the first 12 weeks of specialty training in the general practice environment were identified and prioritised – the training period judged to be specifically high risk and beyond which trainees are given greater clinical freedom. In doing this we aimed to help maximise early opportunities to address safety-critical issues proactively via a checklist reminder, which may lead to a reduced risk of patients being unintentionally harmed during and after the training period.

The development work identified and validated 14 safety-critical domains and 47 related items that were judged to be essential components of specialty training in general practice to be addressed by educational supervisors and trainees in the first 12-week period of training in the general practice setting. Each item was also aligned with one or more of the 12 RCGP curriculum competencies to assist and guide supervisors in delivering the curriculum and collecting supporting evidence (*see* Table 20.3). At the suggestion of supervisors, the checklist was also adapted to enable trainees to self-assess safety-related learning needs early in their specialty training and monitor future progress.

CHECKLIST IMPLEMENTATION

At a basic level, the safety domains and related items generated have the potential to be used by GP educational supervisors and general practice managers to modernise existing induction packs, or help inform the development of new induction processes. More specifically, supervisors can apply the tool as a checklist prompt or reminder to ensure that the most safety-critical educational tasks are actually carried out and are done so timeously, efficiently and without ambiguity. The potential to improve the *reliability* of educational provision in these important areas of specialty training and healthcare practice should be evident. Completion of the checklist could also be used as supporting evidence to the postgraduate training authority (e.g. during accreditation visits) that the core patient safety element of the training curriculum is being proactively considered and delivered.

TABLE 20.3 Validated safety checklist themes and related items mapped against 12 Royal College of General Practitioners (RCGP) curriculum competencies

Checklist theme and item	RCGP curriculum competency No.*
PRESCRIBING SAFELY	
1. Knowledge of high-risk medications (e.g. non-steroidal anti-inflammatory drugs, warfarin, methotrexate)	5, 6
2. Controlled drugs (e.g. knowledge of storage, dose adjustment, prescription format)	5, 12
3. Awareness of health board/formulary prescribing guidance	9
4. Knowledge of practice repeat prescribing system	7
5. Risks associated with signing repeat and special requests without consulting records	5, 6
6. Monitoring drug side effects (e.g. myalgia with statins)	5, 6
DEALING WITH MEDICAL EMERGENCY	
7. Ensuring adequate emergency treatment knowledge/confirmation of cardiopulmonary resuscitation knowledge and skills (in past 12 months)	5
8. Surgery emergency bag/tray and equipment	5
9. Contents of doctors' emergency bag or case (where appropriate)	5
10. Awareness of emergency contacts (e.g. ambulance, police, social work)	5
SPECIFIC CLINICAL MANAGEMENT	
11. Recognising and acting on red flags for serious illness (e.g. patient needs immediate admission or urgent outpatient referral)	3
DEALING EFFECTIVELY WITH RESULTS OF INVESTIGATION REQUESTS	
12. Need to follow up and act on results and hospital letters	12
13. Knowledge of practice system for results handling	7
PATIENT REFERRALS	
14. Identifying the need for referral (i.e. recognition of condition requiring further investigation and/or treatment)	3
15. Referral system (e.g. how and when to refer 'urgently' and 'routinely')	7, 9
16. Clinical appropriateness of referral (e.g. ensure correct clinical priority and correct specialty)	9
17. Quality of acute referral letter (e.g. past medical history, medication status, social circumstances)	7
EFFECTIVE AND SAFE COMMUNICATION	
18. Knowledge of internal communication processes within the practice (e.g. email, message systems, practice meetings)	7
19. How to liaise with and understand the roles of team members: who, purpose, how, where, when?	8
20. Safe communication with patients and relatives (e.g. consultations, phone calls and letters)	4

(continued)

Checklist theme and item	RCGP curriculum competency No.*
CONSULTING SAFELY	
21. How to safety net (face to face)	1
22. How to safety net (when providing telephone advice)	1
23. Awareness of guidelines for use of chaperones	11, 12
ENSURING CONFIDENTIALITY	
24. Avoiding breaches of confidentiality	11
25. Appropriate disclosure of medical and personal information	11
AWARENESS OF THE IMPLICATIONS OF POOR RECORD KEEPING	
26. Failing to keep records	12
27. Failing to keep accurate records	12
28. Failing to confirm patient identify	12
29. Failing to document all patient contacts	12
30. Knowledge of related legal issues	12
RAISING AWARENESS OF PERSONAL RESPONSIBILITY	
31. Awareness of professional accountability	12
32. Recognising the limits of own clinical competence	12
33. How and when to seek help	12
34. Personal organisation and effectiveness	12
DEALING WITH CHILD PROTECTION ISSUES	
35. Recognition of harm and the potential for harm in children	2
36. How to liaise with other agencies	8
37. Breaching confidentiality	11, 12
ENHANCING PERSONAL SAFETY	
38. How to access emergency alarms/panic button for personal safety	12
39. Dealing with aggressive and violent patients	12
40. Ensuring personal safety and security on home visits	12
EMPHASISNG THE IMPORTANCE OF THE LEARNING ENVIRONMENT	
41. Ensure rapid access to supervisory advice, feedback and support	10
42. Raise awareness of practice team contribution and support	10
43. Ensure reflective learning recorded in e-portfolio	10
44. Knowledge of clinical audit and significant event analysis	10
SAFE USE OF PRACTICE COMPUTERISED SYSTEMS	
45. Ensure proficiency in using practice computer system	7
46. How to prioritise computer system safety alerts (e.g. yellow and red traffic lights)	7
47. The need to avoid common pitfalls (e.g. leaving notes open and writing up the wrong patient)	7

* *See* Table 20.2

All of these factors are of prime importance because of the potential medico-legal implications for the GP educational supervisor if a trainee is inadequately tutored and supervised and patient safety is subsequently compromised. GP educators need to have mechanisms in place to make an early assessment of a trainee's competencies and to undertake regular performance reviews and feedback sessions as part of an overall strategy to minimise risks.

THE LEARNING ENVIRONMENT

Theory suggests that because human memory and attention are imperfect,[16] one way to mitigate errors or lapses in the execution of tasks is through the use of procedural checklists to help people perform more reliably. Compliance checklists to improve the safety or reliability of processes are standard practice in high-reliability industries,[22,23] most notably in commercial aviation and petrochemical organisations. In healthcare, checklist use is well documented, particularly in surgical,[24] obstetric[25] and intensive care[26] settings, where the implementation of checklists is associated with improved clinical outcomes, team working and productivity efficiencies.

However, despite these positive reports there is some scepticism over whether the introduction of a checklist on its own is the single greatest factor attributable to improvement success. Bosk *et al.*[27] suggest that the widespread deployment of a checklist may not be successful without a clear understanding that it is a 'technical' solution being introduced to a complex dynamic working environment where pre-existing 'sociocultural' issues may need to be contained or resolved.

Clinicians may resist or feel threatened by checklist implementation because they perceive it to impinge on their expertise, interfere with their decision-making or oversimplify the working environment. It is also known that there is variation in perceptions of local safety climate within and between general practice teams and that some may unintentionally inflate this measure because of inexperience with, or lack of knowledge of, local safety concerns.[28] Similar variation exists in the strength of team working,[29] the maturity of the learning environment[12] and commitment to quality improvement.[30] Attending to these types of psychosocial and cultural issues is, therefore, as equally important as supporting efforts into checklist development and implementation if momentum is to be gained and a successful impact made.

SELF-ASSESSMENT FOR TRAINEES

Adaptation of the checklist as a self-assessment tool for trainees was an unexpected study development. Self-assessment is a method of measuring and interpreting one's own performance and is a well-established educational intervention among all healthcare professions and as part of specialty training.[31] The use of self-assessment tools by specialty trainees to identify learning needs is routine in medicine,[32,33] but it does not appear to be well developed in terms of highlighting specific educational interventions related to patient safety. The activity takes on a greater significance when the performance focus is related to the identification of learning need associated with safety-critical education and training. Although evidence highlights the limitations of self-assessment,[31] it is still promoted as a valuable educational activity because it can be used as a baseline measure that prompts joint discussion and monitoring of performance over time by the trainee and supervisor.

CONCLUSIONS

There is clear potential for patients to be unintentionally and avoidably harmed because of what happens (or does not happen) educationally in the GP training environment. The checklist concept is but one small (albeit untested) intervention to help minimise the related risks to patients and the potential medico-legal consequences for supervisor and trainee alike.[34] The use of a checklist measure to ensure the reliable delivery of 'essential' patient safety education has potential relevance for all medical specialties and other clinical professions with similar training arrangements in the UK and internationally.

REFERENCES

1. Elder NC, Dovey SM. Classification of medical errors and preventable adverse events in primary care: a synthesis of the literature. *J Fam Pract.* 2002; **51**(11): 927–32.
2. Makeham MAB, Dovey SM, County M, *et al*. An international taxonomy for errors in general practice: a pilot study. *Med J Aust.* 2002; **177**(2): 68–72.
3. Dovey SM, Meyers DS, Phillips RL Jr, *et al*. A preliminary taxonomy of medical errors in family practice. *Qual Saf Health Care.* 2002; **11**(3): 233–8.
4. World Alliance for Patient Safety. *WHO Patient Safety Curriculum Guide for Medical Schools*. Geneva: World Health Organization; 2009. Available at: www.who.int/patientsafety/activities/technical/who_ps_curriculum.pdf (accessed 31 August 2011).
5. Royal College of General Practitioners. *GP Curriculum Statements*. London: RCGP; 2011. Available at: www.rcgp-curriculum.org.uk/rcgp_curriculum_documents.aspx (accessed 4 January 2012).
6. Kilminster SM, Jolly BC. Effective supervision in clinical practice settings: a literature review. *Med Educ.* 2000; **34**: 827–40.
7. Bruijn M, Busari JO, Wolf BHM. Quality of clinical supervision as perceived by specialist registrars in a university and district teaching hospital. *Med Educ.* 2006; **40**: 1002–8.
8. Kilminster SM, Jolly BC, Grant J, *et al*. *Good Supervision: guiding the clinical educator of the 21st century*. Sheffield: University of Sheffield; 2000.
9. Dornan T, Ashcroft DM, Heathfield H, *et al*. *FINAL Report: an in depth investigation into causes of prescribing errors by foundation trainees in relation to their medical education – EQUIP study*. London: General Medical Council; 2009.
10. Kennedy TJ, Lingard L, Baker GR, *et al*. Clinical oversight: conceptualizing the relationship between supervision and safety. *J Gen Intern Med.* 2007; **22**(8): 1080–5.

11. Van der Vleuten CP, Schuwirth LW. Assessing professional competence: from methods to programmes. *Med Educ*. 2005; **39**(3): 309–17.

12. Smith V C, Wiener-Ogilvie S. Describing the learning climate of general practice training: the learner's perspective. *Educ Prim Care*. 2009; **20**(6): 435–40.

13. Zwart DLM, Heddema WS, Vermeulen MI, *et al*. Lessons learnt from incidents reported by postgraduate trainees in Dutch general practice: a prospective cohort study. *BMJ Qual Saf*. 2011; **20**: 857–62.

14. McKay J, Bradley N, Lough M, *et al*. A review of significant events analysed in general medical practice: implications for the quality and safety of patient care. *BMC Fam Pract*. 2009: **10**: 61.

15. Singh H, Thomas EJ, Petersen LA, *et al*. Medical errors involving trainees: a study of closed malpractice claims from 5 insurers. *Arch Intern Med*. 2007; **167**: 2030–6.

16. Reason JT. Understanding adverse events: the human factor. In: Vincent CA, editor. *Clinical Risk Management: enhancing patient safety*. 2nd ed. London: Blackwell BMJ Books; 2001. pp. 9–30.

17. Sandars J, Esmail A. The frequency and nature of medical error in primary care: understanding the diversity across studies. *Fam Pract*. 2003; **20**(3): 231–6.

18. National Patient Safety Agency. *WHO Surgical Safety Checklist* London: NPSA; 2009.

19. Shillito J, Arfanis K, Smith A. Checking in healthcare safety: theoretical basis and practical application. *Int J Health Care Qual Assur*. 2010; **23**: 699–707.

20. Semel ME, Resch S, Haynes AB, *et al*. Adopting a surgical safety checklist could save money and improve the quality of care in U.S. hospitals. *Health Aff (Millwood)*. 2010; **29**: 1593–9.

21. Hales BM, Pronovost PJ. The checklist tool for error management and performance improvement. *J Crit Care*. 2006; **21**: 231–5.

22. Weick K, Kathleen M. *Managing the Unexpected: assuring high performance in an age of complexity*. San Francisco, CA: Jossey-Bass; 2001.

23. Degani A, Wiener E. *Human Factors of Flight-Deck Checklists: the normal checklist*. Moffett Field, CA: NASA; 1990.

24. Haynes AB, Weiser TG, Berry WR, *et al*. A surgical safety checklist to reduce morbidity and mortality in a global population. *N Engl J Med*. 2009; **360**: 491–9.

25. Rao K, Lucas DN, Robinson PN. Surgical safety checklists in obstetrics. *Int J Obstet Anesth*. 2010; **19**: 235–40.

26. Gawande A. The checklist: if something so simple can transform intensive care, what else can it do? *New Yorker*. 2007; **10**: 86–101.

27. Bosk CL, Dixon-Woods M, Goeschel CA, *et al*. The art of medicine: reality check for checklists. *Lancet*. 2009; **374**: 444–5.

28. de Wet C, Johnson P, Mash R, *et al*. Measuring perceptions of safety climate in primary care: a cross-sectional study. *J Eval Clin Pract*. 2010; **18**(1): 135–42.

29. Campbell SM, Hann M, Hacker J, *et al*. Identifying predictors of high quality care in English general practice: observational study. *BMJ*. 2001; **323**(7316): 784–7.

30. Apekey TA, McSorley G, Tilling M, *et al*. Room for improvement? Leadership, innovation culture and uptake of quality improvement methods in general practice. *J Eval Clin Pract*. 2011; **17**(2): 311–18.

31. Colthart I, Bagnall G, Evans A, *et al*. The effectiveness of self-assessment on the identification of learner needs, learner activity, and impact on clinical practice: BEME Guide no. 10. *Med Teach*. 2008; **30**: 124–45.

32. Davis DA, Mazmanian PE, Fordis M, *et al.* Accuracy of physician self-assessment compared with observed measures of competence: a systematic review. *JAMA.* 2006; **296**: 1094–102.
33. Overeem K, Faber M, Arah O, *et al.* Doctor performance assessment in daily practice: does it help doctors or not? A systematic review. *Med Educ.* 2007; **41**: 1039–49.
34. Mackenzie P, Anthony S. The role of the GP trainer: medico-legal aspects. *Clin Gov Int J.* 2009; **14**(1): 74–9.

CHAPTER 21

Practice-based small group learning

Ronald MacVicar

PBSGL: THE CONTEXT

A surgeon is defined by the time that he or she spends in the operating theatre; a physician, by the time he or she spends on the ward round with his or
her entourage; and a researcher, by the time spent in the laboratory. General
practitioners (GPs) are defined by the time they spend with their patient in
the consultation.

David Metcalfe[1] captured this fundamental importance of the consultation
in general practice in his William Pickles lecture entitled 'The Crucible' for the
Royal College of General Practitioners in 1986:

> If we as general practitioners are to make our unique contribution it will be as
> personal doctors whose way of listening, examining, diagnosing, advising, treat-
> ing and monitoring has as its objective not only the cure or control of disease
> but the protection or expansion of our patients' stature, autonomy and personal
> space. That is the kind of health we can deliver, even to people with disease, even
> to people who are dying. We do it in the consultation.

The importance of the consultation to general practice can be measured in the
quantity and quality of publications on the topic over the last 6 decades as general practice has matured into a distinct discipline. Michael Balint's[2] work in
the 1950s emphasising the importance of the doctor–patient relationship has
been built on by a series of influential authors, including Byrne and Long,[3] Stott
and Davis,[4] Pendleton,[5] Neighbour,[6] Stewart *et al.*[7] and Silverman *et al.*[8] Each
provided a model for the consultation by building on the insights of previous
authors, so that the learner or practitioner is offered a somewhat bewildering
menu of theoretical models, ranging from Byrne and Long's[3] six phases that
they claimed form a logical structure to the consultation, to Silverman *et al.*'s[8]
daunting list of 55 consultation skills.

While these authors focused on their theoretical models of the consultation, the precious opportunity that this time provides for both the patient and the doctor arguably transcends any model. Iona Heath[9] described this:

> The consultation brings together the human experience of suffering and the paradigms of scientific medicine, with the general practitioner acting as interpreter at the boundary between illness and disease, and a witness to suffering.

The underpinnings of what Heath described as 'the paradigms of scientific medicine' is scientific evidence gained through meta-analyses, systematic reviews and randomised controlled trials and it is on this hierarchy that the evidence-based medicine (EBM) movement is based.[10] The development of the EBM movement, which has grown since the early 1990s, poses a challenge within each and every consultation in general practice. Sweeney et al.[11] encapsulated this, with a hint of scepticism, in 1998:

> Evidence-based medicine is the new deity in clinical medicine: physicians worship it, managers demand it and policy makers aspire towards it. Clinical activity in the UK National Health Service is increasingly driven by the principles of evidence-based medicine and general practice is not immune.

From the earliest days of EBM, barriers have been described to the implementation of evidence in routine clinical practice.[12] These barriers are most apparent in general practice where applying general scientific principles to individual patients provides a particular challenge,[13-15] and where a perceived tension exists between evidence-based and patient-centred practice.[16] Furthermore, as scientific research is seldom carried out in, or directed at, general practice the results are not straightforward to apply in the primary care setting.

Given the nature of general medical practice, which exists 'at the boundary between illness and disease'[9] and where undifferentiated presentations are the norm, it is rare that clinical decisions can be made with absolute certainty. Marinker and Peckham[17] have characterised the distinctive role for GPs in dealing with this uncertainty and these undifferentiated clinical problems in comparison to the role of hospital specialists as: 'hospital doctors have to reduce uncertainty, explore possibility and marginalise error. General practitioners have to tolerate uncertainty, explore probability and marginalise danger'.

The evidence-based approach has often been contrasted with a patient centred approach, a concept that has been described with some justification as a 'fuzzy concept'.[18] However, Stewart[19] has provided a definition of patient-centred care, which encompasses five principle domains:
1. exploring the patient's concerns and need for information
2. seeking an integrated understanding of the patient's world
3. finding common ground on diagnosis and management
4. enhancing prevention and health promotion
5. enhancing the continuing relationship between the patient and the doctor.

There is little to suggest that these domains are in any way contradictory to the use of evidence in day-to-day clinical practice, and it can in fact be argued that they provide a framework to achieve this. Indeed, this is not so different from Sackett *et al.*'s[10] original description of evidence-based practice:

> The practice of evidence based medicine means integrating individual clinical expertise with the best available clinical evidence. By individual clinical expertise, we mean the proficiency and judgement that individuals acquire through clinical experience and clinical practice.

In turn, Reeve has suggested that scientific evidence be regarded as 'one of a range of knowledges' in her definition of interpretive medicine:

> IM [interpretive medicine] is the critical, thoughtful, professional use of an appro-priate range of knowledges in the dynamic shared exploration and interpretation of individual illness experience, in order to support the creative capacity of indi-viduals in maintaining their daily lives.[20]

It is clear that the EBM movement, and evidence derived from the paradigm of scientific medicine, is something that general practice neither could nor should ignore. It is therefore no coincidence that at the 'home' of EBM at McMaster University in the late 1980s, an approach to continuing professional development (CPD) for family physicians (GPs) evolved that attempted to introduce evidence-informed decision-making into day-to-day care for indi-vidual patients – practice-based small group learning (PBSGL). The rest of this chapter describes how this form of learning contributes as one way of sup-porting the role of Heath's interpreter, Sackett's individual clinical expert and Reeve's critical, thoughtful professional in the context of Metcalfe's crucible – in the consultation with the patient.

PBSGL: THE METHOD

The PBSGL programme is an innovative approach to CPD for GPs that is focused on facilitated discussions between peers. This enables a focus on the real problems that GPs encounter and the challenge of integrating evidence-based and patient-centred care for the uncertain problems with which patients present in what has been described as the 'swampy lowlands' of everyday pro-fessional practice.[21]

'Practice-based learning' is derived from problem-based learning and is based upon a peer-facilitated small group learning format where groups address topic-specific modules. The key components of this form of learning are sum-marised in Box 21.1.

The focus is on the gap between current and best practice, identification by participants of a need to change practice and a commitment to that change. To achieve this commitment to change, shared reflection on current practice

---

BOX 21.1 Key components of the PBSGL programme

Process – a peer-facilitated small group discussion focused on:
- reflection on current practice
- identification of gaps between current practice and best practice
- consideration of strategies to enhance change in practice
- commitment to change in practice

Content – evidence-based educational modules that:
- present representative cases that stimulate participants in the groups to reflect on similar cases from their own practice
- summarise best available evidence relevant to primary care practice
- promote application of scientific knowledge to the problems that participants encounter in practice, resulting in improved patient care

Trained peer facilitators who:
- are chosen by their group
- are trained in a 1-day workshop conducted by experienced trainers
- play a vital role in the enduring success of PBSGL

The development and sustenance of a community of practice that:
- is consistent with educational theory
- is borne out by the function and longevity of groups

---

is crucial, often focused on challenging cases that participants have dealt with and the small group format provides the necessary security for this to occur.

The substrate for these discussions is topic-specific evidence-based educational modules. The modules have a standard format that includes:
- an introduction that describes the gap between current and best practice
- case studies to encourage participants to reflect on similar cases from their own practices; the aim is for participants to engage with cases from their own practice rather than necessarily to solve the problems that are presented
- a summary of the best available evidence about the specific clinical topic area that is relevant to primary care at the time the module was prepared
- case commentaries that describe one way of approaching the presented cases
- a full reference list with explicit levels of evidence
- support materials such as management algorithms, decision aids or patient information leaflets.

The content (the module) and the process (peer-facilitated small group learning) are brought together at the PBSGL meeting. Groups meet at a venue, frequency and timing of their choice and a standard session discussing a single module typically lasting 90–120 minutes. There is no single preferred model for group membership; some groups consist of the team members of a single practice while others are made up from groups of friends or acquaintances. Both models have advantages, with the former providing opportunities for changes in practice to be agreed and implemented within a single practice unit, whereas the latter model stimulates cross-pollination resulting from sharing experience and perspectives between practitioners from different practices. Although the most common model is one of GPs learning together, many groups include other health professionals, most notably practice nurses and pharmacists, with growing numbers of both multi-professional groups and uni-professional pharmacy or nurse-only groups.

The cohort of trained peer-facilitators is crucial to the success of the PBSGL method. Their key task is to develop an atmosphere that encourages participants

- to identify their learning needs
- to reflect on their current practice
- to explore the application of new knowledge into their practice.

Facilitators are trained to link the discussion to participants' own practice by encouraging them to consider similarities between the cases presented in the module and those in their practices. These discussions usually serve to focus participants' attention on their own learning needs as they relate to actual practice cases or specific identified challenges. Although facilitators are not content experts, they are 'practice experts' familiar with issues common to their peers in the group. The effectiveness of the learning group depends on the willingness of participants to identify, acknowledge and share gaps between current practice and best practice, including any errors that may result from these gaps. These open and honest discussions will only occur if the facilitator develops a safe environment.

The small groups are the key component of PBSGL and they are encouraged to feed into the development of the programme by suggesting topics for future modules, contributing to module development, piloting new modules and providing feedback on the module on a 'log-sheet' after each meeting. The main function of the group log-sheet is to record group members' commitment to change. Review of these recorded commitments to change at regular intervals is encouraged.

Although new groups continually form and existing groups reconfigure, many groups have been together for many years and have developed those characteristics indicative of 'communities of practices'. A community of practice has been defined as

> a group of people who share a concern, a set of problems or a passion about a topic, and who deepen their knowledge and expertise in this area by interacting on an ongoing basis.[22]

The peer facilitator role and the honesty of members in discussing both their successes and their failures in practice are the keys to the development of a community of practice. Such an environment can only be created over time as members develop trust in and respect for the members of the group. This is facilitated by:

- a range of perspectives and experiences
- opportunities to benchmark practice with others with similar practice profiles
- enhanced opportunities for successful implementation of new knowledge into practice as participants share their strategies and successes.[23,24]

PBSGL: THE HISTORY

PBSGL originated in Canada and has grown from a single group of GPs at McMaster University in Hamilton, Ontario, in the late 1980s to now involve approximately 6000 members across Canada. A non-profit organisation, the Foundation for Medical Practice Education (FMPE), administers the programme in Canada and is aligned to McMaster University. PBSGL was introduced in Scotland in 2006 and membership has continued to grow year on year since (*see* Figure 21.1), so that approximately a third of all GPs in Scotland now participate.

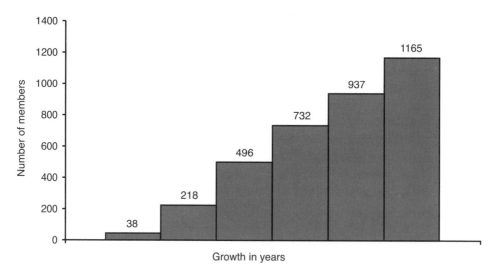

FIGURE 21.1 PBSGL Scotland membership growth 2006–11

The Scottish groups initially used modules produced by the FMPE and, while the modules were greatly valued, the cultural dissonance of Canadian case materials and Canadian norms and language were an irritant for some members. As a result, an increasingly in-depth adaptation process ('tartanisation') of Canadian modules has developed over the last few years. In addition, the PBSGL team now also produces an increasing proportion of Scottish/UK modules de novo by adopting and applying FMPE processes, so that approximately 14–16 new modules can be made available every year.

Administration of the Scottish programme is provided by NHS Education for Scotland (NES), a 'Special Health Board' with the remit as NHS Scotland's training and education body to provide educational solutions that support excellence in healthcare for the people in Scotland.

PBSGL: THE EVIDENCE

Systematic reviews suggest that a range of common educational approaches to gain new knowledge have limited impact on improving professional practice.[25-29] In contrast, interactive approaches to learning can be effective in changing practice, particularly when they involve small peer groups that foster trust, promote discussion of evidence focused on real cases, provide feedback on performance and offer opportunities to practise newly learned skills.[28,30] PBSGL describes one model of encompassing these approaches in a structure that, judging by experience in Canada and in Scotland, has proved very popular with GPs.

Evaluation of the PBSGL pilot in Scotland in 2003–04 suggested a positive change for participants, with an increase in their implementation of evidence-based practice.[31,32] The small group format and the role of the facilitator were identified as crucial factors to the success of the approach. The findings highlighted the importance of an environment conducive to learning and change and recognising the power of the group to direct their own learning without the need for invited experts. The positive evaluation supported NES's decisions to support the national roll-out of PBSGL for GPs and to commission further pilots with nurse-only and multi-professional groups.

The evaluation of the pilots with these different staff groups was also positive. Nurses reported that their habitual practices were constructively challenged in a supportive environment and participants reported that they were able to be open about gaps in their knowledge and were able to identify and address the questions that resulted.[33,34] Participants in the multi-professional groups reported that key ingredients in meeting their learning needs were increased respect and understanding of one another's different roles and perspectives and a mutual keenness to understand the perspectives of and to learn from other professions.

While self-reported increases in knowledge and improvements in practice are encouraging, they do not provide objective evidence of any change in a clinician's behaviour. The Better Prescribing Project presented an opportunity to provide this objective evidence.[35] This involved a randomised control trial of learning events for GPs that focused on PBSGL modules and/or individual prescribing portraits on treating hypertension in primary care in British Columbia. The study involved GPs caring for almost 4400 patients who were receiving treatment for hypertension. Modest but meaningful changes in prescribing were reported for the patients of GPs that used PBSGL modules and the improvements were sustained after 6 months.

A further component of the Better Prescribing Project looked at the commitment to change statements made by GPs in the study and compared them with the provincial pharmacy registry for 6 months before and after the educational intervention. In three out of four of the conditions studied, those physicians who expressed a commitment to change were significantly more likely to change their prescribing in the subsequent 6 months.[36] This is further confirmation of the correlation between GPs making commitment to change statements and subsequent change in their practice.[37-40] There is also evidence that discussing individual commitment to change statements with a group of peers may further enhance implementation.[41]

PBSGL has been widely used in North America for a number of years now as one component of family medicine residency training and it was implemented as a part of GP specialty training in Scotland in August 2009. A qualitative study of a group of trainees using PBSGL in Scotland found PBSGL was a valued and effective method of learning and that it played an important role in preparing them for independent practice and self-directed learning.[42] PBSGL has since been incorporated in the GP specialty training programmes of some deaneries in other UK home countries.

The PBSGL approach has relevance beyond general practice and primary care CPD. A group at McMaster University has adapted the format to support faculty development – for example, PBSGL education. Building on evidence of positive impact for community-based teachers in Canada,[43] this approach was used in a pilot study in the north of Scotland in 2011 that involved groups of educational supervisors from across the primary/secondary care and undergraduate/postgraduate interfaces. The aim was to investigate whether self-reported improvements in educational practice occurred and whether there was any perceived impact for participants on issues in the described interfaces. Results from this qualitative study suggested that there had been a positive impact on their educational practice and an improved understanding of one another's roles.[44]

PBSGL: PRESENT AND FUTURE
PBSGL is now established in general practice in Scotland and is being adapted and taken up by other professional groups, including nurses, pharmacists, dentists, healthcare chaplains and others. There is also growing interest in this learning method for primary care from the rest of the United Kingdom and internationally. NES and the FMPE encourage this interest and the wider implementation of PBSGL, with local adaptations, champions and a partnership approach modelled on their highly successful international collaboration over recent years.

FURTHER READING
Sample modules and a list of available modules can be viewed at:
- www.gpcpd.nes.scot.nhs.uk/pbsgl/overview.aspx
- www.gpcpd.nes.scot.nhs.uk/pbsgl/module-topics.aspx

REFERENCES
1. Metcalfe D. William Pickles lecture 1986. The crucible. *J R Coll Gen Pract.* 1986; **36**(289): 349–54.
2. Balint M. *The Doctor, his Patient and the Illness.* London: Tavistock Publications; 1957.
3. Byrne PS, Long BEL. *Doctors Talking to Patients.* London: HMSO; 1976.
4. Stott NCH, Davis RH. The exceptional potential in each primary care consultation. *J R Coll Gen Pract.* 1979; **29**(201): 201.
5. Pendleton D, Schofield T, Tate P, *et al. The Consultation: an approach to learning and teaching.* Oxford: Oxford University Press; 1984.
6. Neighbour R. *The Inner Consultation: how to develop an effective and intuitive consultation style.* Lancaster: MTP Press; 1987.
7. Stewart M, Brown J, Weston W, *et al. Patient-Centred Medicine: transforming the clinical method.* Thousand Oaks, CA: Sage Publications; 1995.
8. Silverman J, Kurtz S, Draper J. *Skills for Communicating with Patients.* Oxford: Radcliffe Medical Press; 1998.
9. Heath I. *The Mystery of General Practice.* London: Nuffield Provincial Hospitals Trust; 1995.
10. Sackett DL, Rosenberg WM, Gray JA, *et al.* Evidence based medicine: what it is and what it isn't. *BMJ.* 1996; **312**(7023): 71–2.
11. Sweeney KG, MacAuley D, Gray DP. Personal significance: the third dimension. *Lancet.* 1998; **351**(9096): 134–6.
12. Haynes RB, Sackett DL, Guyatt GH, *et al.* Transferring evidence from research into practice: 4. Overcoming barriers to application. *ACP J Club.* 1997; **126**(3): A14–15.
13. Hoey J. The one and only Mrs. Jones. *CMAJ.* 1998; **159**(3): 241–2.
14. Fox RC. Medical uncertainty revisited. In: Bendelow G, Carpenter M, Vautier C, *et al.,* editors. *Gender, Health and Healing: the public/private divide.* London: Routledge; 2012: pp. 236–53.
15. Gillies JC. Getting it right in the consultation: Hippocrates' problem; Aristotle's answer. *Occas Pap R Coll Gen Pract.* 2005; (86): 5–35.
16. McColl A, Smith H, White P, *et al.* General practitioner's perceptions of the route to evidence based medicine: a questionnaire survey. *BMJ.* 1998; **316**(7128): 361–5.
17. Marinker M, Peckham M. Clinical futures. *BMJ.* 1998; **317**: 1542.
18. Bensing J. Bridging the gap: the separate worlds of evidence-based medicine and patient-centered medicine. *Patient Educ Couns.* 2000; **39**(1): 17–25.
19. Stewart M. Towards a global definition of patient centred care: the patient should be the judge of patient centred care. *BMJ.* 2001; **322**(7284): 444.
20. Reeve J. Interpretive medicine: supporting generalism in a changing primary care world. *Occas Pap R Coll Gen Pract.* 2010; (88): 1–20.
21. Schon D. *The Reflective Practitioner.* New York, NY: Basic Books; 1983.
22. Wenger E, McDermott RA, Snyder WM. *Cultivating Communities of Practice: a guide to managing knowledge.* Boston, MA: Harvard Business Press; 2002.
23. Saint-Onge H, Wallace D. *Leveraging Communities of Practice for Strategic Advantage.* London: Routledge; 2012.
24. Wenger E. *Communities of Practice: learning, meaning, and identity.* Cambridge: Cambridge University Press; 1999.
25. Davis DA, Thomson MA, Oxman AD, *et al.* Evidence for the effectiveness of CME: a review of 50 randomized controlled trials. *JAMA.* 1992; **268**(9): 1111–17.

26. Davis DA, Thomson MA, Oxman AD, *et al.* Changing physician performance: a systematic review of the effect of continuing medical education strategies. *JAMA.* 1995; **274**(9): 700–5.

27. Oxman AD, Thomson MA, Davis DA, *et al.* No magic bullets: a systematic review of 102 trials of interventions to improve professional practice. *CMAJ.* 1995; **153**(10): 1423–31.

28. Davis D, O'Brien MA, Freemantle N, *et al.* Impact of formal continuing medical education: do conferences, workshops, rounds, and other traditional continuing education activities change physician behavior or health care outcomes? *JAMA.* 1999; **282**(9): 867–74.

29. Mazmanian PE, Davis DA. Continuing medical education and the physician as a learner: guide to the evidence. *JAMA.* 2002; **288**(9): 1057–60.

30. Marinopoulos SS, Dorman T, Ratanawongsa N, *et al.* Effectiveness of continuing medical education. *Evid Rep Technol Assess (Full Rep).* 2007; (149): 1–69.

31. MacVicar R, Cunningham D, Cassidy J, *et al.* Applying evidence in practice through small group learning: a Scottish pilot of a Canadian programme. *Educ Prim Care.* 2006; **17**(5): 465–72.

32. Kelly DR, Cunningham DE, McCalister P, *et al.* Applying evidence in practice through small-group learning: a qualitative exploration of success. *Qual Prim Care.* 2007; **15**(2): 93–8.

33. Overton GK, Kelly D, McCalister P, *et al.* The practice-based small group learning approach: making evidence-based practice come alive for learners. *Nurse Educ Today.* 2009; **29**(6): 671–5.

34. Kanisin-Overton G, McCalister P, Kelly D, *et al.* The Practice-based Small Group Learning Programme: experiences of learners in multi-professional groups. *J Interprof Care.* 2009; **23**(3): 262–72.

35. Herbert CP, Wright JM, Maclure M, *et al.* Better Prescribing Project: a randomized controlled trial of the impact of case-based educational modules and personal prescribing feedback on prescribing for hypertension in primary care. *Fam Pract.* 2004; **21**(5): 575–81.

36. Wakefield J, Herbert CP, Maclure M, *et al.* Commitment to change statements can predict actual change in practice. *J Contin Educ Health Prof.* 2003; **23**(2): 81–93.

37. Mazmanian PE, Waugh JL, Mazmanian PM. Commitment to change: ideational roots, empirical evidence, and ethical implications. *J Contin Educ Health Prof.* 1997; **17**(3): 133–40.

38. Mazmanian PE, Daffron SR, Johnson RE, *et al.* Information about barriers to planned change: a randomized controlled trial involving continuing medical education lectures and commitment to change. *Acad Med.* 1998; **73**(8): 882–6.

39. Overton GK, MacVicar R. Requesting a commitment to change: conditions that produce behavioral or attitudinal commitment. *J Contin Educ Health Prof.* 2008; **28**(2): 60–6.

40. Overton GK, McCalister P, Kelly D, *et al.* Practice-based small group learning: how health professionals view their intention to change and the process of implementing change in practice. *Med Teach.* 2009; **31**(11): e514–20.

41. Wakefield JG. Commitment to change: exploring its role in changing physician behavior through continuing education. *J Contin Educ Health Prof.* 2004; **24**(4): 197–204.

42. Hesselgreaves H, MacVicar R. Practice-based small group learning in GP specialty training. *Educ Prim Care.* 2012; **23**(1): 27–33.
43. Walsh AE, Armson H, Wakefield JG, *et al.* Using a novel small-group approach to enhance feedback skills for community-based teachers. *Teach Learn Med.* 2009; **21**(1): 45–51.
44. MacVicar R, Guthrie V, O'Rourke J, *et al.* Practice-based Small Group Learning: an evaluation of a four month programme. *Educ Prim Care.* In press.

CHAPTER 22

Protected learning time

David Cunningham

INTRODUCTION

Primary healthcare is no longer delivered solely by general practitioners (GPs) but by a team of diverse staff groups and health professionals.[1] To provide this care effectively and efficiently, teams need to coordinate their learning as well as their working, and need to develop a shared culture of quality improvement.[2,3] There is increasing pressure for primary healthcare teams to perform work that was traditionally undertaken by secondary care, and healthcare decision-makers perceive this transfer being achieved by a team-based approach to the delivery of patient care. As a consequence, primary healthcare teams will need to *learn together* how they will provide complex healthcare for their patients in the future.

A number of studies have shown that primary healthcare teams can learn with and from one another, to improve the quality of services that are delivered to patients.[4-8] To learn together takes time, and there is recognition by the government, and by academic and educational leaders, that primary healthcare teams need some time, protected from their normal service activities, in order for this shared learning to be achieved.[2,9-13]

Protected learning time (PLT) started in England in 1998 and quickly spread to many areas in the United Kingdom.[14] By using out-of-hours organisations to provide protection from service delivery, PLT can provide time for primary healthcare teams to come together and have shared learning. It is common for mid-week afternoons to be selected, as these are considered by teams to be the quietest times of their working week. Although a number of different models exist, most PLT schemes are organised by local healthcare organisations that may also provide large centrally organised events for a number of teams in the locality.[15] The majority of PLT learning events are usually practice based and are commonly planned and prepared by the primary healthcare team, and often these tasks are the responsibilities of general practice managers.[16]

Early and later reviews of PLT in the United Kingdom have shown that it is well received, that teams find it a useful resource, and that it may lead to improved services for patients.[17–24] However, not all PLT schemes are the same: the composition of learning events and of the different staff groups who attend them will vary across the country. For example, some schemes may not include non-clinicians in large, centrally organised PLT events, and some practice managers may not involve their administrative support staff or community nurses in practice-based events.[16,25,26]

Planning and preparing learning for the diverse individuals who make up the primary healthcare team, and delivering this learning as a long-term project, is not an easy task. There are barriers and obstacles that prevent some teams from using PLT effectively. A number of primary healthcare teams may exist in a nominal sense, rather than as a functioning unit.[27,28] They may be structured into a team by health authorities, but they do not work or learn from one another in the sense of a team. Studies support the concept that effective teams are small in size, with 12 members or fewer, that they involve a mix of individuals with different and complementary skills, and that team members contribute towards work that is shared. Effective teams have members who are usually committed to a common purpose, and communicate easily and readily with one another.[29–31] Additionally, effective teams need effective leadership but this *learning leader* does not necessarily have to be a GP. Individuals who have vision and the ability to communicate this to team members, and who can enthuse and inspire others, are often successful learning leaders. In addition to the attributes listed already, effective teams tend to have respect for other members, and value the roles of each other. Primary healthcare teams who do not work in these ways may find that shared learning is difficult for a variety of reasons described in this chapter.

LEARNING PROCESSES

If learning is to be useful and effective, it is important to identify the learning needs of the team, so that these needs may inform future learning activities during PLT. Primary healthcare teams may struggle with the task of identifying the learning needs of the team rather than the learning needs of a number of individuals. If this task is not achieved, or only partially achieved, then learning that is provided by healthcare organisations or practice managers will be based on the learning needs of only some members of the team, rather than all of them. Usually these team members will be the individuals with power and influence within the team, especially in relation to the practice manager, and will usually be the GPs.

As a consequence of inadequate learning needs assessment, irrelevant learning may be arranged for some staff groups during PLT. If this happens regularly, then the attendance rates of these staff groups will decline, and some individuals will disengage completely from collective learning. Administrative support staff may prefer to catch up with work during PLT, rather than participate in learning activities that are not based on their specific needs. For some teams the opportunities of PLT and the potential for team learning may be lost, and they will experience fragmented learning, rather than collective learning. Learning events may occur in the practice building, but a deeper inquiry may reveal that there are separate learning activities for each individual staff group taking place in separate rooms within the building. Some tools have been designed to enable the identification and collation of non-clinical learning needs of various staff groups within primary healthcare, so that practice managers can collate the learning needs of the team. Such tools are well received by participants.[32]

Although teams may be able to identify their learning needs, they may not be able to plan learning that meets these needs. Resources may not be readily available to organisers, or learning topics may not gain the approval of individuals with power, and as a result may not take place. Practice managers who are not given sufficient resources for learning may resort to representatives of pharmaceutical companies who will be willing to fund learning events as long as they are able to meet and influence medication prescribers.

Learning topics that are usually well received by all of the team include significant event analyses, learning about organisational systems that affect the entire team, and learning about the everyday activities of the team. Primary healthcare teams are keen to improve their performance in their everyday work, and to learn from others in their team in order to do this.[6] Other examples of effective learning topics include team communication issues, clinical and non-clinical computer software systems that the team uses, patient safety and the detection of errors, and the management and handling of prescriptions and test results for patients.

It is important to consider the impact of the learning atmosphere or learning environment at practice-based PLT, and how this impacts on which learning methods are adopted by teams. Administrative support staff may express a preference for learning events that are interactive and involve learning with the team. They may also prefer events that are fun and light-hearted, and welcome events and activities that allow the team to get to know each one another better, and this may help to reduce the hierarchy within the team. Learning events based on traditional learning methods such as lectures and presentations to large passive audiences are often poorly received by administrative staff and by other staff groups.

Some team members may spend little time working with one another, and when brought together at practice-based PLT events they may find this shared time to be uncomfortable and awkward. This is a common experience for primary healthcare teams who work from separate and different premises, or work from premises that do not have shared areas where teams can informally meet, interact, and learn from one another. As a consequence, the learning environment at practice-based PLT events may not be conducive towards shared learning, and PLT may expose the difficulties of team working for these teams.

STRUCTURAL ISSUES

Primary healthcare teams are made up of a variety of individuals. Their structural arrangements are complicated and reflect the developmental history of the National Health Service (NHS). Traditionally, GPs work in partnerships with one another and employ support staff, practice managers and practice nurses. These staff groups compose the general practice. This structure reflects the self-employed status of the GP, which predates the formation of the NHS to a time when primary care professionals often worked alone, and independently of other staff groups and professions.[33–35] The community nursing team is attached to the general practice and consists of health visitors, district nurses and their supporting teams. Local primary care organisations usually employ the community nursing team, in addition to allied health professionals, who together make up the primary healthcare team. Other employment structures exist and are becoming more prominent in the NHS.[36]

Practice managers may focus the planning and preparation for PLT events on the general practice and may not involve community nurses in these initial learning processes. Some practice managers may not consider that community nurses are part of their team, and this is often evident in teams who are not co-located or do not share work with their community nursing colleagues.

Other structural issues influence the effectiveness of PLT. Changing working practices create the need for learning events to enable teams to improve their performance in relation to patient care. An example of this is the 2004 General Medical Services contract, which is the most recent of a series of contracts for GPs and their staff, since the NHS was established in 1948. Some staff groups in the primary healthcare team who are employed by the local healthcare organisation may not be affected by these GP contracts, and therefore will feel excluded by PLT events that focus on issues arising from them.

LEARNING RELATIONSHIPS

Team members learn effectively from one another when they are known to one another and have shared work and common objectives and outcomes. Some teams have poor relationships between individuals and between staff groups. Distant relationships can persist in teams through time and can become an established method of working.[37] This is possible with support staff and GPs, and with the medical practice and attached community nursing team. Team-building events can prove useful for such teams, and are often welcomed by team members. Some icebreakers can include quizzes, practical demonstrations such as self-defence and security lessons, and physical activities such as hill-walking and cycling. At times, such events can be viewed as being illegitimate learning events from influential individuals, who are often based in central organisations, which may be distant from these teams and their work. Teams should be encouraged to undertake events that lead to shared learning and closer working patterns and arrangements.

Primary healthcare teams can be hierarchical in nature, with GPs perceived as being at the top of the hierarchy. These perceptions of hierarchy can be lessened by informality and close working arrangements. Those teams who call one another by their first names, who spend time together informally in and out of working hours, and who use humour effectively tend to experience more effective PLT events.

BOX 22.1 Some tips for effective protected learning time for primary healthcare teams

- It is important to identify what the team needs to learn and then base learning activities on these needs. The team's learning needs are different from the learning needs of individuals, or of those team members who have power or influence.
- Teams need to find diverse ways of identifying their learning needs. Some ways include formal assessments, identifying areas of weakness in the practice, or where the team feel they are underperforming in certain areas.
- If team members work in separate buildings or occupy distinctly separate areas within one building, they may need to spend time getting to know one another, and learn what others do in their jobs. This increases visibility and is a legitimate use of PLT and should be repeated until the team feels closer than before. Leaders should remember that personnel change over the years and that new team members or new staff groups need to be introduced to the team.
- Teams should be wary of 'hijackers' who seek to take over their PLT and offer learning events that suit their own agenda, rather than the team's learning needs.
- Prior to a PLT event, planning and preparation processes should involve all staff groups. These processes should be led by practice managers or any individual who has the educational skills and knowledge to do this job. These tasks may be helped by the creation of a small sub-team consisting of representatives from every staff group involved. It is important to enable those staff groups who are often overlooked (e.g. administrative staff and community nurses).
- Others in the team may want to lead on a learning topic when this is appropriate. Practice managers need to develop a strong sense of learning enablement within the team.
- Effective learning teams adopt learning methods that are well received by all in the team. Learning methods should be varied, and interactive and participatory in nature.
- Practice-based events should be planned well ahead, with a sense of competition for a time slot within the PLT afternoon. Team members feel enabled to suggest new topics and resources and their contributions are always valued and encouraged. Events should stretch the team and make the team consider learning events that are innovative and different from the past.

- Practice managers or learning leaders need to encourage evaluations of events, both formal and informal, and make changes based on the evaluations.
- Events should at times be fun, light-hearted and challenging. Events can involve team-building activities, which break down pre-existing barriers within the team.
- Team members are referred to by their first name during PLT, rather than their title or their staff group identifier. Members should be seen as individuals rather than 'doctor', 'nurse' or 'receptionist'.

SUMMARY

PLT can be a very valuable resource for primary healthcare teams, and can enable teams to develop and improve services. However, it needs to be carefully managed and requires considerable planning and preparation if it is to meet the learning needs of all those involved. Without careful maintenance, PLT can disintegrate into separate learning events and the potential wide-reaching benefits of the educational method can be lost.

REFERENCES

1. Royal College of General Practitioners. *The Primary Health Care Team RCGP Information Sheet 21*. London: Royal College of General Practitioners; 2003.
2. Calman KC. *A Review of Continuing Professional Development in General Practice*. Leeds: Department of Health; 1998.
3. Scally G, Donaldson LJ. Clinical governance and the drive for quality improvement in the New NHS in England. *BMJ*. 1998; **317**: 61–5.
4. Cross M, White P. Personal development plans: the Wessex experience. *Educ Prim Care*. 2004; **15**: 205–12.
5. Cross M, White P. Practice professional development plans: the Wessex experience. *Educ Prim Care*. 2004; **15**: 213–19.
6. McMillan R, Kelly D. A project of team involvement in development and learning (TIDAL). *Educ Prim Care*. 2005; **16**: 175–83.
7. Wilcock PM, Campion-Smith C, Head M. The Dorset Seedcorn Project: interprofessional learning and continuous quality improvement in primary care. *Br J Gen Pract*. 2002; **52**(Suppl.): S39–44.
8. Campion-Smith C, Riddoch A. One Dorset practice's experience of using a quality improvement approach to practice professional development planning. *Br J Gen Pract*. 2002; **52**(Suppl.): S33–7.
9. Rushmer R, Kelly D, Lough M, *et al*. Introducing the learning practice: II. Becoming a learning practice. *Journal of Evaluation in Clinical Practice*. 2004; **10**(3): 387–98.
10. Rushmer R, Kelly D, Lough M, *et al*. Introducing the learning practice: I. The characteristics of learning organizations in primary care. *J Eval Clin Pract*. 2004; **10**(3): 375–86.
11. Rushmer R, Kelly D, Lough M, *et al*. Introducing the learning practice: III. Leadership, empowerment, protected time and reflective practice as core contextual conditions. *J Eval Clin Pract*. 2004; **10**(3): 399–405.

12. Dean P, Farooqi A, McKinley RK. Quality improvement in general practice: the perspective of the family healthcare team. *Qual Prim Care.* 2004; **12**: 201–7.

13. Huby G, Gerry M, McKinstry B, *et al.* Morale among general practitioners: qualitative study exploring relations between partnership arrangements, personal style and workload. *BMJ.* 2002; **325**: 140–2.

14. Department of Health. *Organisational Development – National Service Frameworks.* London: Department of Health; 2002.

15. Cunningham D, Kelly D. The perceptions of educational steering committees on protected learning time in general practice. *Qual Prim Care.* 2007; **15**: 37–43.

16. Cunningham D, Stoddart C, Kelly D. Protected learning time in general practice: a questionnaire study of practice managers' perceptions of their role. *Qual Prim Care.* 2006; **14**: 225–33.

17. Cunningham D, Reid R, Cardno L, *et al.* Protected learning time: lessons from the Scottish survey. *Educ Prim Care.* 2010; **21**: 288–9.

18. Lucas B, Small N, Greasley P. Protected learning time in general practice: a question of relevance? *Educ Prim Care.* 2005; **16**: 680–7.

19. Haycock-Stuart EA, Houston NM. Evaluation study of a resource for developing education, audit and teamwork in primary care. *Prim Health Care Res Dev.* 2005; **6**: 251–68.

20. Jelphs K, Parker H. *An Evaluation of the SALT (Southern Area Learning as Teams) Protected Learning Time in Northern Ireland.* Birmingham: University of Birmingham; 2006.

21. White A, Crane S, Severs M. Evaluation of TARGET in Portsmouth: T time for A audit, R reflection, G guidelines, E education and T training. *Educ Prim Care.* 2002; **13**: 81–5.

22. Brooks N, Barr J. Evaluation of protected learning time in a primary care trust. *Qual Prim Care.* 2004; **12**: 29–35.

23. Siriwardena AN, Fairchild P, Gibson S, *et al.* Investigation of the effect of a county-wide protected learning time scheme on prescribing rates of ramipril: interrupted time series study. *Fam Pract.* 2007; **24**: 26–33.

24. Siriwardena AN, Middlemass JB, Ward K, *et al.* Drivers for change in primary care of diabetes following a protected learning time educational event; interview study of practitioners. *BMC Med Educ.* 2008; **8**(4): 1–9.

25. Cunningham D, Fitzpatrick B, Kelly D. Administration and clerical staff perceptions and experiences of protected learning time: a focus group study. *Qual Prim Care.* 2006; **14**(3): 177–84.

26. Cunningham D, Kelly D. Community nurses' perceptions and experiences of protected learning time: a focus group study. *Qual Prim Care.* 2008; **16**: 27–37.

27. Kendrick D. Role of the primary health care team in preventing accidents to children. *Br J G Pract.* 1994; **44**: 372–5.

28. Pringle M. The developing primary care partnership. *BMJ.* 1992; **305**: 624–6.

29. Katzenbach JR, Smith DK. *The Wisdom of Teams: creating the high-performance organization.* Maidenhead, UK: McGraw-Hill; 1993.

30. Wiles R, Robison J. Teamwork in primary care: the views and experiences of nurses, midwives and health visitors. *J Adv Nurs.* 1994; **20**: 324–30.

31. Mickan SM, Rodger SA. Characteristics of effective teams: a literature review. *Aust Health Rev.* 2000; **23**(3): 201–8.

32. Cunningham D, Kelly D. The evaluation of a multiprofessional learning needs assessment tool. *Education for Primary Care.* 2005; **16**: 547–55.

33. Hadfield SJ. A field survey of general practice, 1951–2. *Br Med J*. 1953; **2**(4838): 683–706.
34. Hockey L. *Feeling the Pulse: a survey of district nursing in six areas*. London: Queen's Institute of District Nursing; 1966.
35. Rivett G. *National Health Service History*. Available at: www.nhshistory.net (accessed 14 April 2011).
36. Pollock A, Price D, Viebrock E, *et al*. The market in primary care. *BMJ*. 2007; **335**: 475–7.
37. Bond J, Cartlidge A, Gregson B, *et al*. Interprofessional collaboration in primary health care. *J R Coll Gen Pract*. 1987; **37**: 158–61.

CHAPTER 23

Consultation skills

Rhona McMillan

Compared with most medicines, communication skills have undoubted palliative efficacy, a wide therapeutic index and the commonest problem in practice is suboptimal dosing![1]

INTRODUCTION

It is now widely accepted that effective doctor–patient communication enhances patient satisfaction and experience and can improve clinical outcomes.[2] In contrast, poor communication can adversely affect clinical outcomes and patient satisfaction and can increase the likelihood of litigation.[3,4] In the United Kingdom (UK), communication skills have therefore been recognised as an essential element in delivering high-quality patient care by the General Medical Council (GMC)[5] and the Royal College of General Practitioners.[6]

It is clearly established that patients' satisfaction with their care is increased if the doctor they consult with is able to acknowledge their concerns and interact effectively with them.[7,8] There is also evidence that a doctor's clinical effectiveness is enhanced by specific training in communication skills,[9,10] and a positive link between effective communication and reduced clinical risk has also been suggested.[11] More specifically, it has been found that providing established doctors and medical students with feedback about the quality of their consultation skills can lead to improvements in their subsequent attitudes and behaviour and that the changes are sustained over time.[12] Communication skills training may also help to prevent clinician 'burnout' and improve the morale of the medical workforce.[12]

Since the mid 1990s all medical students in the UK have been taught communication skills as a part of the core undergraduate curriculum.[13] General practitioner (GP) registrars, or GP specialty trainees (GPSTs) as they are now called, have received targeted consultation skills training since the early 1990s, and their consultation skills have been assessed on a summative basis since 1996.[14] There are still many UK GPs who may not have had the benefit of this training, however, including older GPs and GPs from other countries, cultures and different training programmes. It is also recognised that, after effective communication skills have been developed, they need to be practised or else they may wither.[15]

Since the introduction of communication skills training for medical students in 1993, the world has changed dramatically: medical, technical, societal and political developments have all had an impact on doctors, patients and the consultation and there have been many advances and developments in healthcare. For example, treatment regimens are increasingly complex and tailored to the individual patient, a significant amount of care formerly delivered in secondary care settings is now transferred to primary care settings and there is greater emphasis on preventive medicine. The implication of all of these factors is that GPs need to be able to discuss the issue of risk effectively with patients from many different backgrounds. Another important development is that almost every GP desk now has a computer on it, which, in many cases, can be thought of as introducing a third person into the consultation. Not least because of the requirements of the Quality and Outcomes Framework[16] within the consultation that informs the GP's agenda and which unfortunately, all too often, may be unrelated to the patient's agenda. Finally, patients of today are increasingly highly educated and much better informed about medical matters through being able to quickly and easily access the latest information in great detail about their symptoms or illnesses from a wide range of educational resources and many want to be actively involved in their care and share in the decision-making process.

In 2012 the concerns of patients about the communication skills of doctors were highlighted in two reports. The first was the GMC's annual report *The State of Medical Education and Practice in the UK*,[17] which reported a 69% rise in complaints in the preceding 12 months from patients about the standard of doctors' communication skills. Nearly half (47%) of all complaints were made against GPs, although this has to be interpreted in the context of general practice being the largest of the medical disciplines. The second report, published by the Patients Association,[18] noted that patients too often felt 'disempowered and disengaged' from their care and patronised by clinicians. In contrast, the Department of Health's 2011–12 GP patient survey described the communications skills of UK GPs more positively,[19] with the vast majority of patients (88%) reporting a good or very good overall experience of their GP surgery.

Given the importance of effective communication skills for all healthcare professionals, and recognising the desire and potential of some specialty trainees and clinicians to further improve these skills, two educational interventions were developed by the west region of NHS Education for Scotland: (1) a system of peer review of GPs' consultation skills, delivered at regular intervals, and (2) a consultation skills course for GPs.

THE CONSULTATION SKILLS COURSE

Consultation skills courses have been provided for GPs in the region since 1998. Prior to this, provision of continuing medical education in the areas of communication and consultation skills had been sparse or nonexistent, with almost all of the available educational time and training resources devoted only to the knowledge base and technical requirements deemed necessary to be a good GP.[20]

The consultation course is run using a small group format and is delivered during 2 full working days, each day 6 weeks apart. Courses are delivered by GPs who are considered experienced educationalists, and have proven facilitation skills and a passion for the consultation. Given that all younger GPs and most doctors involved in the training of GPSTs have had the opportunity to access training in communication skills, the courses are strategically aimed at established GP principals or sessional doctors such as locums or retainers.

The aims of the first day are for the participants to form a cohesive small group to enable the discussion and sharing of problems and solutions relating to consultations and practising consultation skills. The group explores models of consultation analysis and the concepts of giving and receiving effective feedback, including the pitfalls to avoid. Practicalities such as patient consent, confidentiality, recording and encrypting consultations are also covered. The first day's workshop culminates with a session where one of the facilitators demonstrates a pre-recorded consultation to the group and receives feedback from another facilitator. In this way, the group has an opportunity to see their facilitator consulting but are also able to experience the process of feedback (albeit second hand). Participants are then presented with a booklet, developed by the facilitators, expanding on the principles discussed during the first workshop.

There is then a period of 6 weeks between the first day and the second day of the course to allow the participating GPs to practise their newly acquired skills and to video record a patient consultation that they are happy to share with their group at the second workshop.

Day two begins with an icebreaker. The group is then shown a consultation conducted by the second facilitator who receives feedback from her or his colleague(s). This provides the participants with a second practical demonstration of effective consulting skills and the process of providing related formative feedback. The participants form smaller groups then revise both patient-centred consulting and feedback skills. For the duration of the day (workshop) each participant's consultation is viewed and reviewed within the safety of the small group, with focused feedback being provided with the aid of their facilitator.

The consultation course is time-consuming and requires highly skilled facilitators with the ability to lead small groups and give effective and constructive feedback, and who are able to both teach and demonstrate patient-centred consultation skills. However, the investment of time and expertise is well worth it. Evaluations of the consultation courses have been excellent overall, with evidence of:

- improved knowledge (e.g. the necessary tasks during the consultation)
- acquisition of new skills (e.g. *'I now try to identify the patient's true concerns'*)
- positive changes in attitudes (e.g. *'It was surprisingly comfortable with a group watching and giving feeding back about my video – I did not feel threatened'*)
- subsequent changes in behaviour (e.g. *'I try to clarify a patient's understanding'*).[21]

GPs deal with uncertainty on a daily basis yet rarely have the opportunity to explore and reflect on their feelings and concerns about this difficult subject. An unintentional benefit of the courses has been that the cohesive nature of the small group has offered the participating GPs an opportunity to explore areas of both clinical and non-clinical uncertainty in a safe and acceptable forum. Being able to form a cohesive group and function effectively as a group are valuable skills in their own right and potentially transferable to other situations, including managing change at the practice level. The participating GPs also identified the benefits of reduced stress and enhanced morale as a result of this educational intervention: 'I'm less stressed at the finish of my surgery' and 'I have a greater overall satisfaction if a consultation has gone well'.[21]

PEER REVIEW OF GENERAL PRACTITIONER CONSULTATION SKILLS

GPs have been able to voluntarily submit their videotaped consultations for external peer review as part of their continuing personal development since 1999 in the region. The consecutive steps of this process are outlined in Box 23.1.

BOX 23.1 The general practitioner (GP) consultation peer-review process

1. GP prepares videotape of six consultations with patients
2. GP reviews consultations
3. GP reflects on consultations using a patient-centred model
4. GP compiles a written log
5. GP submits videotape and written log
6. Videotape is reviewed by a reviewer with reference to the written log
7. Reviewer prepares written feedback, incorporating areas for development and suggestions for change
8. Feedback is sent to GP with the original videotape
9. GP further reviews and reflects upon consultations in conjunction with written feedback

---

This peer-review system was actually developed in response to regional demand from GPs for educational assessment of their consulting skills. The first stage was to establish a consultation peer-review group. The second stage was to recruit peer reviewers. The initial peer reviewers were selected from the group of GPs who had previously been trained to perform a summative assessment of the video consultations submitted by GPSTs as one of the formal requirements to complete their specialty training. However, it quickly became apparent that the consultations submitted by experienced GPs were much more complex than those submitted by GPSTs and that the summative assessment tool was not directly transferable or useful for this group.

The consultation peer-review group therefore aimed to devise and evaluate a more suitable tool for assessing the consulting skills of experienced GPs. The result was the development of a more purposeful tool based on a patient-centred model with five core components (*see* Box 23.2)[22] that can be used to assess the quality of consultations and used as a structure to provide formative feedback.

BOX 23.2 Patient-centred consultation model

1. Explore the patient's main reason for the visit, concerns and need for information
2. Seek an integrated understanding of the patient's world; that is their whole person, emotional needs and life issues
3. Find common ground on what the problem is and mutually agree on management
4. Enhance prevention and health promotion
5. Enhance consulting relationship between the patient and the doctor

---

Peer reviewers are trained to write individualised, descriptive feedback for the participating GP principals. The written feedback focuses on communication skills, partnership with patients, health enablement and development of a management plan. These areas correspond to the attributes described by the GMC in *Good Medical Practice*.[5] The video medium enables feedback not only about verbal communication but also about the often overlooked and equally important role of non-verbal communication cues in doctor–patient interactions.[23]

To date, approximately 1000 GPs have submitted video consultations for peer review. The reviewers have found a wide range in the quality of consulting skills demonstrated by these GPs, which highlighted at least three key areas for further consideration:

1. the formative versus summative nature of the peer review process
2. the nature and quality of feedback
3. recognising and dealing with GP performance that raises clinical concerns.

Formative versus summative

The purpose of the consultation peer review process is to provide constructive, structured feedback to GPs who volunteered to engage with this service to enable them to improve their consulting skills. While this aim has been achieved for the vast majority, inevitably the performance of a small number of GPs has caused the reviewers clinical concern. It has become apparent that this process, although designed to give educational feedback, can potentially serve as a filter to identify poor consultation skills in established GPs.

Nature and quality of feedback

Written feedback about consulting skills can be difficult to prepare and may not always be appropriate, especially if a large number of issues needs to be covered. When concerns have been raised about a doctor's consultation skills, feedback has been more appropriately delivered on a face-to-face basis.

Dealing with performance issues

A protocol has been developed to ensure that when a GP's clinical performance causes concern for the reviewer, the concern is highlighted and appropriate action is taken. Participants are clearly informed about this uncommon possibility in the submission guidance. According to the protocol, the first step is to invite the GP to receive feedback face to face, rather than in writing, and to further assess the potential causes for the underperformance. The most common conclusion from these meetings is that the GP whose performance caused concern was either working under significant stress or was physically and/or mentally unwell. It is typical for this not to have been apparent to the doctor or been noticed by her or his colleagues or picked up during the annual appraisal meeting. In all such cases (up to now) the doctors have been able to resubmit consultations of adequate quality after they had made a full recovery. In the unusual instances where a doctor whose performance had caused concern does not wish to engage in further education or is unwilling or unable to remedy their identified deficiencies, they are referred through local quality assurance mechanisms to be dealt with on a case-by-case basis at health authority level.

CONCLUSION

The consultation is at the heart of patient care and safety in general practice. By improving these skills doctors minimise risks, enhance patient safety and experiences, and are able to provide a higher quality of patient-centred care. However, there are limited practical and educational interventions to support GPs who wish to improve the effectiveness of their consultations with patients. This chapter described two potential methods – a consultation skills course and peer review of GP consultations – that have been particularly helpful as first steps in improving the consultation skills of GPs by providing effective feedback on their performance by colleagues trained to do so.

REFERENCES

1. Buckman R. Communications and emotions. *BMJ.* 2002; **325**(7366): 672.
2. Simpson M, Buckman R, Stewart M, *et al.* Doctor-patient communication. The Toronto Consensus Statement. *BMJ.* 1991; **303**(6814): 1385–7.

3. Health Service Ombudsman for England. *Annual Report 2004–5*. London: HMSO; 2005.

4. Levinson W, Rotor DL, Mullhooly JP, *et al*. Physician-patient communication. The relationship with malpractice claims among primary care physicians and surgeons. *JAMA*. 1997; **227**(7): 553–9.

5. General Medical Council. *Good Medical Practice*. London: GMC; 2006.

6. Royal College of General Practitioners. *GP Curriculum Statement 2012*. London: RCGP. Available at: www.rcgp.org.uk/gp-training-and-exams/gp-curriculum-overview.aspx (accessed 27 December 2013).

7. Rotor DL, Hall JA. *Doctors Talking with Patients, Patients Talking with Doctors*. Westport: Auburn House; 1992.

8. Carroll L, Sullivan FM, Colledge M. Good Health Care: patient and professional perspectives. *Br J Gen Pract*. 1998; **48**(433): 1507–8.

9. Silverman J, Kurtz S, Draper J. *Skills for Communicating with Patients*. Oxford: Radcliffe Medical Press; 1998.

10. Del Mar CB. Communicating well in general practice. *Med J Aust*. 1994; **160**(6): 367–70.

11. Vincent C, editor. *Clinical Risk Management: enhancing patient safety*. London: BMJ Books; 2001.

12. Maguire P, Fairbairn S, Fletcher C. Consultation skills of young doctors: I. Benefits of feedback training in interviewing as students persist. *Br Med J (Clin Res Ed)*. 1986; **292**(6535): 1573–6.

13. General Medical Council. *Tomorrow's Doctors*. London: GMC; 1993.

14. Campbell LM, Murray TS. Summative assessment of vocational trainees: results of a 3 year study. *Br J Gen Pract*. 1996; **46**(408): 411–14.

15. Skelton J. Everything you were afraid to ask about communication skills. *Br Gen Pract*. 2005; **55**(510): 40–5.

16. National Institute for Care Excellence. *About the Quality and Outcomes Framework (QOF)*. London: NICE; 2013. Available at: www.nice.org.uk/aboutnice/qof/ (accessed 22 November 2013).

17. General Medical Council. *The State of Medical Education and Practice in the UK Report: 2012*. London: GMC; 2012. Available at: www.gmc-uk.org/publications/somep2012.asp (accessed 22 November 2013).

18. Patients Association. *Patients Want More Involvement and Engagement from GPs on Care Decisions*. Middlesex: Patients Association; 2012. Available at: www.patients-association.com/default.aspx?tabid=80&Id=95 (accessed 22 November 2013).

19. Department of Health. *The GP Patient Survey 2011–12*. Available at: www.gp-patient.co.uk/results/ (accessed 22 November 2013).

20. Levison W, Rotor DL. The effects of two continuing medical education programs on communication skills of practising primary care physicians. *J Gen Intern Med*. 1993; **8**(6): 318–24.

21. Cameron N, McMillan R. Enhancing communication skills by peer review of consultation videos. *Educ Prim Care*. 2006; **17**(1): 40–8.

22. Stewart M, Brown JB, Weston WW, *et al*. *Patient-Centred Medicine: transforming the clinical method*. 2nd ed. Oxford: Radcliffe Medical Press; 2003.

23. Silverman J, Kinnersley P. Doctors' non-verbal behaviour in consultations: look at the patient before you look at the computer. *Br J Gen Pract*. 2010; **60**(571): 76–8.

CHAPTER 24

The power of apology

Dorothy Armstrong

We are all human – we can all make mistakes.

The quote beginning this chapter is from a man whose son died. He brought his complaint to the Scottish Public Sector Ombudsman (SPSO) to ensure that he was listened to, lessons were learned and to receive an apology. Complaints are a significant tool we can all use to improve the quality and consistency of healthcare. In my role as Professional Adviser to the SPSO, I hear first-hand from patients, relatives and carers about their experiences of healthcare. The majority of people describe their experience of healthcare as being inconsistent: exemplary care at its best coupled with failings in human interactions and communication or technical care. In general practice, the most common 'failings' that emerge from complaints are focused on poor communication, behaviours and attitudes. Issues around the standards of care and treatment provided by general practice teams are often secondary.[1]

In my work, I provide clinical advice to a team of investigators. This work involves the review of patient records, statements from staff, patients and carers and notes of meetings. In addition, I meet with staff, patients and relatives to provide an independent and impartial service. Often complaints are not upheld – that is, we do not agree with the complainant that there have been failings in the care provided. However, things can and do go wrong. Most complainants want to be listened to and want to seek reassurance that steps are in place to make sure the same mistake does not happen again. Without exception, people want to be acknowledged and receive a meaningful apology.

Within this chapter, I will first consider why people complain and highlight the emerging evidence that supports the use of apology in the prevention, escalation and management of complaints. Some useful tools will be presented that doctors, nurses and the wider healthcare team in general practice can potentially utilise. However, in order to discuss the power of apology, it is appropriate to first consider and understand why people complain and what it is they are hoping to achieve by complaining to the practice or by taking the compliant to the Ombudsman.

WHY DO PEOPLE COMPLAIN?

The most common reasons people complain are:
- to stop the problem happening again
- to learn lessons
- to be given a full explanation
- to receive feedback
- they feel humiliated, betrayed and hurt
- they want to know what happens next
- to receive a meaningful apology.

WHAT IS AN APOLOGY?

An apology is a way of communicating a message that includes a number of components: a meaningful apology requires all parts to be present. The definition of apology is 'an encounter between two parties at which one party, the offender, acknowledges responsibility for an offence or grievance and expresses regret or remorse to a second party, the aggrieved.'[2] The apology should first of all express regret as well as an acknowledgement of shortcoming or failing. Omission of one part is a partial apology and is much less powerful than a meaningful apology. Box 24.1 provides an overview of the key elements of an apology.

BOX 24.1 Elements of an apology[1]

- Accept what you have done wrong. Your apology must correctly describe the offending action or behaviour, whether or not it was intentional. It must also acknowledge the effects of the offence you have caused on the person who has made a complaint.
- Accept your responsibility for the harm done. This includes setting out who was responsible.
- Clearly explain why the offence happened. Your explanation should show that the offence was not intentional or personal. Although most people will want or need an explanation, you should understand that this is not always the case. Also, if you have no valid explanation, don't offer an explanation at all – you could just say that there is no excuse for the offending behaviour.
- Show that you are sincerely sorry. This shows that you understand the suffering of the person who has made a complaint. It can be difficult to communicate how sorry you are in writing. You should say sorry in person and then back it up by repeating it in writing.
- Assure them that you will not repeat the offence. This may include stating the steps you have taken, or will take, to deal with the complaint and the steps you will take to make sure that the harm does not happen again (where possible).
- Make amends – put things right where you can.

WHY APOLOGISE?

An apology is the superglue of life. It can repair just about anything.[3]

As children we are taught to say sorry for our mistakes, but in our working lives as adults many of us find saying sorry a real challenge. However, used well an apology can be both very powerful for the patient and empowering for staff. Many people find it difficult to apologise, though. People do not like to admit that they were wrong for a number of reasons including personal hurt, being in denial, avoiding the issue, fear of rejection and lacking the personal ability to accept responsibility. If only staff involved in a mistake or wrongdoing had been honest and open and provided an apology at the time, then the complainant may not have continued to complain and the staff concerned would have learned from the incident and avoided the potential consequences and stresses brought on by failing to apologise.[4]

FEAR OF LITIGATION

Another reason staff do not apologise readily is the fear of litigation. There is a strong sense in the National Health Service that apologising is in itself an admission of liability and should, therefore, not be performed by healthcare staff. However, this is contrary to the guidance offered by law and regulators. For example:

> An apology, an offer of treatment or other redress, shall not of itself amount to an admission of negligence or breach of statutory duty.
>
> Section 2 of the Compensation Act 2006 (an act of UK Parliament)[5]

This particular section only applies in England and Wales. When the 2006 Act was introduced the accompanying Explanatory Notes said that section 2 was intended to reflect the existing law. The SPSO understanding is that the law on this point is the same in Scotland as it is in England and Wales.

> Patients who complain about the care or treatment they have received have a right to expect a prompt, open, constructive and honest response including an explanation and, if appropriate, an apology.
>
> General Medical Council[6]

> Apologising to patients is not an admission of liability . . . The Being Open policy advises healthcare staff to apologise to patients, their families or carers if a mistake or error is made that leads to moderate or severe harm or death, explain clearly what went wrong and what will be done to stop the problem happening again.
>
> National Patient Safety Agency[7]

Overall, the evidence suggests that the offer of an apology is not linked to higher rates of legal action.[8,9] In addition, if the quality of the relationship between the doctor and patient is good and well established, and the patient feels that his or her views and values are respected, then the doctor is less likely to be sued.[10]

BOX 24.2 Example of an apology[3]

There were 11 patients given a contaminated solution that had been injected into the heart during cardiac surgery. Five of the 11 patients died following this error. One of the senior staff recalls the events:

> One of my senior colleagues called all the families together and he and I sat down with the eleven families and said, 'This is a terrible thing that has happened. It is awful. We are truly sorry that this has happened. We are not going to do another operation until we have got these patients out of the woods.' And we did not. We said, 'We are going to leave no stone unturned until we find out what the cause was.' We knew it was an infection, we knew it had occurred somewhere in the processing of that solution, which was beyond our control as individual clinicians. But we said sorry. None of those patients took legal action.

HOW SHOULD WE DELIVER AN APOLOGY?

How should an apology be delivered? The 'devil is in the detail' is an important principle here. The content and method of apologising will depend on the circumstances and what you hope to achieve. However, there are some good generic principals.

BOX 24.3 The three R's – Regret, Reason and Remedy

Regret
- Meaningful, real, acknowledge wrongdoing
- Just say 'sorry'
- Accept responsibility

Reason
- Be honest – this does not mean you will be sued
- The wrongdoing was unintentional and not personal
- Trying hard to do the right thing

Remedy
- Next steps – here is what we will do
- Investigate to find out why, such as significant events analysis
- Provide feedback

Providing a meaningful apology is part of good interpersonal and communication skills and can be taught and rehearsed as part of the pre-registration curriculum and in continuing professional development. Role play, observation, simulation and media such as film and drama can be used to encourage staff to practise their skills in offering an apology to patients. Also, by using tools such as the three R's (*see* Box 24.3), staff can practise the appropriate techniques at home as well as in the workplace.

The three R's tool can be used in everyday practice and has the power to de-escalate anger and aggression and diffuse emotion, and it can enable and empower staff to manage conflict and resolve tensions involving patients (and others).

Regret

It is important to recognise that something has gone wrong by acknowledging the wrongdoing, even if you are not at fault. Saying sorry in a meaningful and sincere manner is crucial. Often this first step is enough to de-escalate the situation.

Reason

Even if you feel criticised and hurt, it is really important to provide a reason (if there is one) for the mistake, but you must avoid being defensive when doing so. Make sure you are clear that the wrongdoing was not intentional or personal, so keep to the facts. Try to put yourself in the complainant's shoes and step back from the situation – stay objective.

BOX 24.4 Being CALM*

Composing yourself: adopt a relaxed pose, keep good eye contact with the person complaining, use open body language to stay engaged and to demonstrate your composure and readiness to respond positively. Remember that in most situations you are not being criticised personally.

Attending: give the person your undivided attention. Don't be distracted by other thoughts – this is important, so be there.

Listen: really listen to what the person is saying. Identify key emotional words 'angry', 'disappointed', 'hurt', 'disgusted' – the emotions may need to be addressed just as much as the situation that caused the reaction. Hold your response until the person has finished.

Moving on: respond positively to what the person has told you and lay the foundations for moving on. First and foremost, say you are sorry. Simply that you are sorry for whatever has happened that has made the person upset, and take the time to agree a way forwards to identify what went wrong, whether there is an explanation and what can be done to put things right.

* Adapted from Armstrong *et al.*[11]

Remedy

Try to resolve the mistake there and then, if you can. Ask the complainant what he or she would like to happen and take responsibility to investigate, if required, and to provide feedback to the complainant as soon as is practicable. Encourage colleagues to be proactive too.

When communicating verbally, the timing of the apology, the tone of voice used and the content of the message, and the body language adopted are highly important. Ensuring that both you and the complainant are as calm as possible is important to ensure the situation does not escalate. However, the very act of saying 'I'm sorry' is often enough to calm everyone down and move on towards reaching a solution to the problem that has been identified. Box 24.4 describes a useful tool to help staff respond to complaints in the moment.[11]

WHO SHOULD GIVE THE APOLOGY?

The most appropriate person should give the apology; that is, either the person who is responsible for the mistake or the person who is seen as speaking on behalf of the organisation. The most effective apology is to provide a verbal apology, followed up by a written, detailed letter. A written apology implies the seriousness of the matter and recognises the time and effort in the writing of the letter.

The apology should be natural and sincere and not defensive. Communicating shame, guilt, pain and humiliation in writing or verbally adds sincerity, as does being able to show empathy, by expressing regret, sadness, sorrow or sympathy for the harm experienced.[3]

SUMMARY

In my work at the Ombudsman, I often hear people say that they have not been listened to and they feel humiliated and powerless; that if only staff involved in a mistake or wrongdoing had been honest and open and provided an apology, they would not have continued to complain. Apologising, like people, is both simple and complex and each apology is unique. As outlined here, many factors must be considered, including the nature of the mistake in terms of differentiating the more minor issues, such as delays in being seen or unappetising food, to the more serious examples such as unprofessional behaviour or drug error. In summary, a successful apology can actually be a positive experience for all parties concerned.

FURTHER READING

For more information on the work of the Scottish Public Services Ombudsman, please visit www.spso.org.uk/.

BOX 24.5 Practical pointers

- Apologising is a key part of our lives – apology can be extremely powerful when done well.
- A meaningful apology can de-escalate a situation and can often prevent a complaint being taken forwards.
- All members of the general practice team should be empowered to say sorry, even if not directly involved.
- Use the three R's tool and the CALM tool.
- Giving an apology is a sign of strength and it can show that you are willing to learn when something has gone wrong.
- To apologise is good practice and is an important part of effectively managing complaints.
- It's not easy to apologise but it is everyone's business.

REFERENCES

1. Scottish Public Services Ombudsman. *Guidance on Apology*. Edinburgh: SPSO; 2011. Available at: www.spso.org.uk/sites/spso/files/communications_material/leaflets_buj/2011_March_SPSO%20Guidance%20on%20Apology.pdf (accessed 7 March 2014).
2. Scottish Public Services Ombudsman. *Annual Report 2012–13*. Edinburgh: SPSO; 2012. Available at: www.spso.org.uk/sites/spso/files/communications_material/annual_report/SPSO_Annual_Report_2012-13.pdf (accessed 7 March 2014).
3. New South Wales Ombudsman. *Apologies: a practical guide*. 2nd ed. Sydney: NSW Ombudsman; 2009.
4. Woods MS. What if we just said, 'I'm Sorry'? *Patient Saf Qual Healthc*. 2005 November–December. Available at: tinyurl.com/just-saying-sorry (accessed 7 March 2014).
5. Compensation Act 2006. Part 1 – Standard of Care. Available at: www.legislation.gov.uk/ukpga/2006/29/pdfs/ukpga_20060029_en.pdf (accessed 7 March 2014).
6. General Medical Council. *Good Medical Practice*. London: GMC; 2013.
7. National Patient Safety Agency. Being open: communicating patient safety incidents with patients, their families and carers. London: NPSA; 2010. Available at: www.nrls.npsa.nhs.uk/alerts/?entryid45=65077 (accessed 7 March 2014).
8. Holden J. Saying sorry is not the same as admitting legal liability [letter]. *BMJ*. 2009; **338**; b520.
9. Leape L. Understanding the power of apology: how saying 'I'm sorry' helps heal patients and caregivers. *Focus Patient Saf*. 2005; 8(4): 1–3.
10. Lazare A. *On Apology*. New York, NY: Oxford University Press; 2004.
11. Armstrong D, Sloan S, Mathieson A. *Leading Accountable and Professional Care*. Edinburgh: NHS Education for Scotland; 2011. Available at: www.nes.scot.nhs.uk/media/359458/leading_accountable_and_profressional_care_.pdf (accessed 7 March 2014).

Part IV

Managing Patient Safety

CHAPTER 25

Managing human error

Lucy Mitchell & Carl de Wet

Every 36 hours an estimated 1 million people use the National Health Service in the United Kingdom, and although the vast majority receive safe and effective care, some patients are harmed, sometimes seriously or even fatally.[1,2] Since the late 1990s numerous studies have increased our understanding of the scale of the safety problem, and the contribution of human error to avoidable patient harm.[3-8] If healthcare is, for the most part, delivered by highly skilled and motivated professionals in technologically advanced environments, why should this be the case? This is a difficult question to answer, but one that will be considered in this chapter.

This chapter's basic premise is that human error is inevitable and largely predictable because of a combination of the natural limitations of human performance and inadequate design of many healthcare systems. Different types of errors are described, before considering how they may be reduced, mitigated or prevented by considering three interlinked levels: (1) the individual (e.g. personal capabilities), (2) the task (e.g. level of complexity) and (3) the workplace environment (e.g. physical, systems and organisation). The chapter concludes by reflecting on the potential value of the science of human factors in helping to design error-resistant systems.

TO ERR IS HUMAN

Human beings are often able to perform complex mental and physical tasks simultaneously. Consider the skill involved in driving a car. Once experienced, the arm changes gears, the foot controls the pedals and, at the same time, cognitive processes monitor the changing conditions both inside and outside the vehicle as well as anticipate the behaviour of other road users.

There are at least two main reasons why *everyone* is vulnerable to making errors, despite the wide range of skills and abilities between people. The first reason is that even the most capable person has natural limitations to his or her physical and mental abilities. Consider attention span. Returning to the example of driving, it is very easy to forget parts of a journey driven before, because it may be a regular route and nothing unexpected happened. This happens because the 'long-term' or 'procedural' memory enables driving without the person having to be consciously focused on his or her actions, enabling his or her mind to wander onto other matters.

The other memory store is the 'short-term' or 'working' memory. This is very limited, in that it can only hold on to around seven 'chunks' of information at any given time. Using a telephone number as an example, a person can usually remember a 12-digit telephone number by splitting it into 'chunks'. The area code (which, if already known, will be retrieved from the long-term memory store) and the remaining digits combined together as three- or four-digit chunks, makes the number easier to remember. Writing it down or rehearsing it can maintain the memory. However, information is easily displaced from the working memory before making it into the long-term memory store, particularly by disruptions while rehearsing or writing the number down. Similarly, healthcare staff are often interrupted when carrying out a task and forget to complete it. Recognising this risk, some hospitals have changed their medication dispensing system so that nurses on drug rounds have to wear tunics that clearly state that they should not be interrupted, thereby reducing distractions.

BOX 25.1 **Adaptive mechanisms**

Pattern-matching: most people form an impression by observing the whole rather than by scrutinising every detail. An experienced clinician uses this mechanism to her advantage by rapidly reaching a diagnosis in an acutely unwell patient and the patient receives life-saving treatment in time. However, on another occasion, a rare or unusual presentation that closely mimics the familiar pattern might be mistaken, leading to a diagnostic error.

Previous success: if there are a number of options, most people will choose the option they have chosen before, or that they have some knowledge of. In practice a healthcare worker may be aware of the latest evidence and protocols, but still decide to use an unproven treatment that he has previously tried successfully.

Involuntary automaticity: most people tend to complete patterns by filling in 'blanks'. In practice, a healthcare worker may selectively choose those tests that support her diagnosis, even in the presence of other contradictory evidence.

Availability heuristic: this form of 'cognitive tunnel vision' means that undue weight is given to facts that come readily to mind, while other options are 'ignored'. One practical implication is that the differential diagnoses list (a list of possible causes) is prematurely limited by the clinician excluding some test results that do not 'fit'.

Confirmation bias: people tend to select cues and information from the available evidence to support their choice rather than attend to other information that would result in altering the course of action.

The second reason is that most people naturally posses a range of adaptive mechanisms or 'short cuts' that they learn and develop as result of interactions with their environment and through work-related tasks.[9-11] These mechanisms normally enable them to deal with new or complex problems in an effective and efficient manner. However, at other times the *same* mechanisms may lead them to err unconsciously. A selection of adaptive mechanisms and their clinical implications are shown in Box 25.1.

ERROR AND ERROR TYPES

The term 'error' is colloquially understood and ubiquitous, yet a standard definition still eludes the research community.[12] For the purposes of this chapter, error can be defined as the result of choosing the wrong plan to achieve an aim, or not initiating or completing the right plan as intended.[4] Errors are unintentional and should not be confused with violations, which are deliberate actions that are inconsistent with the rules or recommended practices that should be familiar to a healthcare professional.

Errors can be divided into two main groups: active and latent. Active errors are committed by front-line staff and tend to have direct patient consequences. Latent (or system) errors create the conditions, context and potential for active errors. They seldom have immediate consequences, but they can potentially affect many more patients. Examples would be understaffed wards or inadequate equipment. Error traps or 'resident pathogens' are the latent errors that contribute to patient safety incidents and are unfortunately often overlooked or underappreciated during analysis of incidents.

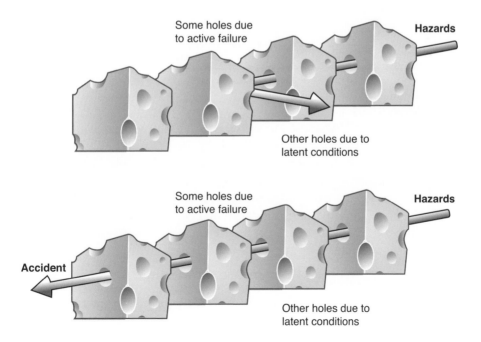

FIGURE 25.1 Reason's Swiss cheese model[4]

Thankfully, not all errors result in harm. In fact, it usually requires a string of errors to result in harm to patients. On a different day, the same contributing factors would be caught and an adverse event would instead be classed as a 'near miss'. It is not uncommon for a healthcare professional to think 'that was close' at the end of a patient case when the outcome is perhaps not ideal but could have been worse.

Professor James Reason illustrated this concept through his well-known 'Swiss cheese model' (*see* Figure 25.1).[4] In this model, the slices of cheese represent the various system defences between hazards and adverse events and the holes represent active and latent errors. The slices of cheese are in constant motion. The holes generally do not form a straight line, with at least one slice blocking hazards from reaching patients. Most incidents of harm occur when the holes in the slices of cheese (the active and latent errors) temporarily align, allowing hazards to reach patients. The model's key principles and their implications are shown in Table 25.1.

TABLE 25.1 Key principles and implications of the Swiss cheese model of error

Principle	Implication
1. Serious patient safety incidents are usually caused by multiple systems failures – only rarely are they caused solely by front-line staff error.	A systems-approach to patient safety improvement is essential.
2. Errors may occur many times without any obvious consequence, making them seem trivial and unimportant. However, the holes in the cheese only have to align once to cause a disaster.	Front-line staff should not become complacent.
3. Many errors do not result in harm.	Errors provide organisations and front-line staff with potential learning opportunities to prevent harm before it occurs.

MANAGING ERROR

One of the most effective ways of improving the quality and safety of healthcare is through detecting, mitigating and preventing errors – in other words, through managing error. Error management can be conceptualised on three interlinked levels: (1) the individual level, (2) the level of tasks (jobs) and (3) the systems level. The three systems exert a combined positive or negative influence on the safety-related behaviour of all healthcare workers. Negative influences may lead to adverse incidents in some instances. Ideally, error management strategies should include interventions at every level.

The individual level

Examples of different factors that may protect or dispose to error at this level include the technical skills (clinical examination), non-technical attributes (interpersonal skills, team working), physical abilities (fatigue levels, eyesight, hearing) and mental characteristics (attitudes, resilience, stress management) of healthcare professionals. Some of these factors, including suggestions for effective error management, are described in other chapters: safety skills (*see* Chapter 19), professional appraisal (*see* Chapter 15), enhanced significant event analysis (*see* Chapter 31) and practice-based small group learning (*see* Chapter 21).

The level of tasks (jobs)

Examples of different factors that may protect or dispose to error at this level include task complexity, job design, workload, equipment design, distractions and the physical environment. There are many possible error management strategies and tools, including task analysis (*see* Chapter 7), consultation skills (*see* Chapter 23) and the out-of-hours environment (*see* Chapter 37).

The systems level

Examples of different factors that may protect or predispose to error at this level include the safety culture of the organisation and team, degree of senior leadership support, quality of communication, effective team working and access to training and educational resources. There are many possible error management strategies and tools for this level, including considering safety culture (*see* Chapter 3), process mapping (*see* Chapter 8), enhanced significant event analysis (*see* Chapter 31), policies, protocols and procedures (*see* Chapter 9) and systems thinking (*see* Chapter 6).

MANAGING ERROR AT THE INDIVIDUAL LEVEL

Non-technical skills are the cognitive, social and personal resource skills that complement a professional's technical skills. This term was originally used in civil aviation to describe all the skills that were not technical but which were equally necessary for safe and effective performance.[13] Social skills are used in communication, teamwork and leadership, while cognitive skills underpin situation awareness and decision-making, and personal resource skills include coping with pressure and managing stress and fatigue.

In primary care, as in other areas of healthcare, different methods of communication are used to share information including verbal, non-verbal and written forms of communication via computer, informal Post-it notes and by directly entering information into patient notes. Because of the dynamic nature of the work, it is difficult to standardise methods (i.e. the system) to communicate or share information; however, consequently, it is easy to see how information gets lost or misplaced, misinterpreted or not conveyed to everyone who needs to know. Taking verbal communication as an example, it is not enough for the person giving the message to assume that the information has been received and understood, unless the receiver acknowledges receipt. When the receiver does acknowledge receipt of the message, this 'closed loop' communication can help provide the 'sender' with the comfort that the information has reached the intended recipient, particularly if action is required. Equally, the recipient is afforded the opportunity of furnishing further details or relaying information straight back to the originator, via the person delivering the message. This is one method that can be invoked to minimise confusion surrounding content and to safeguard the delivery of the information.

Leadership is a factor at the individual and system levels. At the individual level it is a non-technical skill that is required for any team leader. Team leadership involves directing and coordinating the activities of team members. Skills in this regard include encouraging team members to work together, delegating tasks, developing knowledge, skills and abilities as well as motivating, planning, organising and fostering a positive team atmosphere. However, leadership is not just a skill for the overall team leader, since other team members are often required to develop leadership skills, particularly when team members have different expertise and training backgrounds, as in healthcare.

The cognitive skill of situation awareness put simply is: 'knowing what is going on around you', specifically in ever-changing, dynamic or even volatile situations. Components of situation awareness include using one's senses by listening, watching, touching and understanding 'cues' in the environment, understanding what those different elements mean, anticipating what might happen next and acting accordingly. Healthcare professionals are able to function safely by absorbing these cues and processing them relative to their performance. Good decision-makers constantly gather information, process the information and anticipate what might happen next as a result of their actions.

Pressure, stress and fatigue are also aspects of human function that have to be managed.[14] It is known that some people 'thrive' on pressure and that manageable levels of stress can enhance performance – for example, by using an 'adrenaline rush' in a positive way. However, individuals are different in how they manage situations and what is stressful to one may be manageable or even exciting to another. At one end of the spectrum, if the demands of a task outweigh the personal resources or capabilities of that individual for coping then stressful symptoms will impact negatively on performance. At the opposite end of the spectrum, boredom or rust-out can be experienced if an individual's resources far exceed the demands of the task. A balance is where the individual judges his or her available resources to be equal to the demands of the situation. The 'three bucket' model is a tool that may help to facilitate this.

Professor Reason proposed the 'three bucket' model to help healthcare professionals evaluate their relative risk to err in a given situation and time.[3] Using the model, healthcare professionals rate their perceived risk as low, medium or high in each of the following three 'buckets' (components).

1. *Self*: this bucket concerns the state of the individual healthcare professional. For example, is he or she fatigued and does he or she have the necessary experience and knowledge to deal with the demands at that time?
2. *Context*: this bucket represents all contextual factors, including environmental factors (distractions, interruptions and handovers), equipment failures, and available resources and time.

3. *Task*: this bucket contains all factors related to the task at hand and includes factors such as task complexity, duration and its physical demands on the healthcare professional.

The likelihood of error is represented by a combination of the entire contents of all the buckets. Each bucket can contain positive and negative factors. For example, the healthcare worker may be well rested and in a supportive environment but faced with a very complex task. The buckets can never be completely empty, given that healthcare professionals are constantly performing tasks within a context. In other words, there is always risk – only the degree of risk changes. However, full buckets do not always lead to error, just as nearly empty buckets are no guarantee of safety. The buckets simply provide an estimation of the probability of error. As the probability of error increases, healthcare workers should first acknowledge this fact, increase their vigilance and consider whether they should request support.

Investigations of serious incidents too often conclude by warning staff to 'be more careful' or with the recommendation to 're-educate' staff. This type of recommendation may be valid, but it completely misses the opportunities to identify and improve the underlying predisposing system factors.

ERROR MANAGEMENT AT THE SYSTEMS LEVEL

> *We cannot change the human condition, but we can change the conditions under which humans work.*[4]

If human fallibility is a given, error management and improvement initiatives have to rely on well-designed systems to support healthcare professionals in their workplaces. Recently, there has been considerable interest in the science of human factors and the potential value it has to improve the quality and safety of healthcare, especially through improved systems design and reliability.

The science of human factors (or ergonomics) is 'the practice of learning about human characteristics, and using that understanding to improve people's interaction with the things they use and with the environments in which they use them'.[15] Human factors is concerned with work-related behaviour, performance and well-being as a result of the interactions and interfaces between professionals, equipment and technology, tasks and systems, and the wider organisational environment. A selection of practical examples of specific systems designs to help reduce human error is shown in Box 25.2.

However, the reality is that the physical, cognitive and organisational issues in the workplace routinely interact to contribute to human error, low productivity, suboptimal care and health and safety problems. Often, issues such as inadequate workplace systems, poor task and equipment design, the physical environment, high workloads and weak management results in low staff motivation, distractions, irritations, job dissatisfaction, stress and fatigue, which can then impact on personal and organisational performance and well-being. These issues *cannot* be considered in isolation because of their interconnectedness.

BOX 25.2 A selection of system designs to help reduce human error

- *Automate* systems where possible and appropriate
- *'Forcing functions'* should be added where possible – for example, adding reminders and 'double-clicks' to confirm doses, dosing intervals and durations of high-risk medications
- *Standardise* systems to reduce reliance on memory
- Devise and use *checklists* – increasingly being used in Scottish hospitals, in pre-operative settings, for example
- Minimise staff *interruptions and distractions*
- Reduce the *number of steps and handover* (i.e. transferring a task or patient to another team member) in a given procedure or intervention to minimise the risks of information being lost, missed out or misinterpreted
- Add 'redundancies' (double-checks) for high-risk processes, such as having two nurses check intravenous medication

---

SUMMARY POINTS

- People are vulnerable to errors in a predictable manner in all aspects of their life, due to a number of natural human limitations.
- Error management strategies should consider three interlinked levels: the individual, task and systems levels.
- At the individual level, the 'three bucket' model is one method for health-care professionals to self-assess their susceptibility to err in a given situation and time.
- The science of human factors has potential value to improve the design of systems so they become reliable 'error traps'.

REFERENCES

1. Vincent C. *Patient Safety*. Edinburgh: Elsevier Churchill Livingstone; 2006.
2. Brennan TA, Leape LL, Laird NM, *et al.* Incidence of adverse events and negligence in hospitalised patients. Results of the Harvard Medical practice study I. *N Engl J Med.* 1991; **324**(6): 370–6.
3. Reason J. Beyond the organisational accident: the need for 'error wisdom' on the front line. *Qual Saf Health Care.* 2004; **13**(Suppl. 2): ii28–33.
4. Reason J. Human error: models and management. *BMJ.* 2000; **320**(7237): 768–70.
5. House of Commons Health Committee. *Patient Safety, Sixth Report of Session 2008–09.* Volume 1. London: The Stationery Office; 2009.
6. Kohn KT, Corrigan JM, Donaldson MS. *To Err is Human: building a safer health system.* Washington, DC: National Academy Press; 1999.

7. Vincent C, Aylin P, Franklin BD, *et al*. Is health care getting safer? *BMJ*. 2008; **337**: a2426.

8. Walshe K. International comparisons of the quality of health care: what do they tell us? *Qual Saf Health Care*. 2003; **12**(1): 4–5.

9. Alvarado CJ. The physical environment in health care. In: Carayon P, editor. *Handbook of Human Factors and Ergonomics in Health Care and Patient Safety*. Mahwah, NJ: Lawrence Erlbaum Associates; 2007. pp. 287–321.

10. Carthey J, Clarke J. *Patient Safety First: implementing human factors in healthcare – 'how to' guide*. London: Clinical Human Factors Group; 2009.

11. Flynn R, Winter J, Sarak C, *et al*. *Human Factors in Patient Safety: review of topics and tools*. Geneva: World Health Organization; 2009.

12. Yu KH, Nation RL, Dooley MJ. Multiplicity of medication safety terms, definitions and functional meanings: when is enough enough? *Qual Saf Health Care*. 2005; **14**(5): 358–63.

13. Amalberti R, Woland L. Human error in aviation. In: Soekha H, editor. *Aviation Safety*. Utrecht: VSP Publishers; 1997. pp. 91–108.

14. Cox T. *Stress Research and Stress Management: putting theory to work*. Sudbury: HSE Books; 1993.

15. Wilson JR. A framework and a context for ergonomics methodology. In: Wilson JR, Corlett EN, editors. *Evaluation of Human Work: a practical ergonomics methodology*. 2nd and revised ed. London: Taylor & Francis; 1995. pp. 1–39.

CHAPTER 26

Diagnostic error

Brian Robson

CHAPTER OVERVIEW

The three aims of this chapter are to (1) describe the incidence and importance of diagnostic errors in general medical practice; (2) explore important contributory and causative factors; and (3) suggest potential strategies to reduce such errors.

THE INCIDENCE AND IMPORTANCE OF DIAGNOSTIC ERROR

Timely diagnosis and accurate diagnosis are essential prerequisites for cost-effective and high-quality medical care. Unfortunately, diagnostic errors are a common and major safety threat worldwide.[1,2] Their prevalence is estimated to be as high as 21% of all consultations in general practice,[2,3] while the overall diagnostic error rate in patients admitted to hospital from primary care ranges from 2% to 4%.[2] When we consider that there are more than a million consultations every day in the United Kingdom (UK) in this setting, the potential scale of the problem becomes apparent. Diagnostic errors are also the most common reason for medico-legal claims against general practitioners (GPs).[4,5] However, despite their relative frequency and potentially devastating impact on patients and healthcare providers, diagnostic errors are rarely reported through incident reporting systems and they remain understudied and poorly understood when compared with, for example, medication errors.[1]

In primary care systems where GPs have a 'gatekeeping' function, diagnostic errors are especially important. For example, the healthcare systems in the UK, Australia and Canada depend on GPs to assess, diagnose and 'triage' an undifferentiated patient population. One of the key requirements to successfully fulfil this 'gatekeeping' role in an appropriate, efficient and effective manner is the clinical ability to accurately assess risk and to strike the right balance between 'over-' and 'under-' investigation, treatment or referral. In other words, an important task for GPs is 'sifting out the serious from the self-limiting'.[6]

It is a daunting task to correctly diagnose a single patient with serious disease out of the many who present with minor or self-limiting conditions. The following examples and accompanying statistics illustrate the diagnostic difficulty for the GP:

- 200 patients with cough – one new diagnosis of lung cancer
- 350 patients with back pain – one serious underlying condition
- 20 patients with chest pain – one serious underlying cause.[6]

Even in patients presenting with life-threatening conditions, diagnostic error remains common for certain conditions. For example, the diagnosis of meningococcal disease is missed in approximately half of all children during their first presentation.[7]

The responsibility of making a timely and accurate diagnosis is complicated by the plethora of possible variations on clinical presentations and situations that provide ample opportunity for diagnostic error.[8] It is true that some symptoms and clinical conditions have been shown to be associated with an increased risk of diagnostic error, including abdominal pain, fever, fatigue, malignancy, pulmonary embolus and coronary artery disease.[3] However, diagnostic error is not condition specific, even though it may appear that way because certain conditions, such as malignancy, myocardial infarction and infective diseases such as meningitis, are more memorable or may lead to litigation more often.

WHY DO DIAGNOSTIC ERRORS OCCUR?

Diagnostic error often has multiple causes. A recent review of diagnostic error in UK healthcare settings found five distinct factors or 'features' that increased diagnostic difficulty (and therefore error):

1. patients presenting with *atypical symptoms* or signs
2. patients presenting with *non-specific symptoms*
3. conditions that have a *very low prevalence*
4. the presence of *co-morbidity*
5. *perceptual* features.[1]

On a more practical level, it is worth noting that the majority of errors are caused by incomplete history taking and clinical examination.[2] It is also important to recognise the human element inherent in diagnostic error, as our natural limitations and cognitive processes predictably predispose us to err. Examples of cognitive processes include diagnostic overshadowing, hypothesis generation and satisficing (pattern matching).[9,10] 'Satisficing' is much faster than hypothesis-generation processes and therefore generally decreases the time required to make a diagnosis, but it increases the risk of missing rare conditions. In other words, satisficing is *normally* a useful approach that allows experienced clinicians to deal with the vast majority of patients in an efficient manner. Unfortunately, the very strength of this method is also its metaphorical Achilles heel. Cognitive processes are neither 'good' nor 'bad' but context and operator dependent, with the implication that diagnostic error may be very difficult to eliminate.

However, it is possible to identify specific types of cognitive failures that more commonly contribute to diagnostic error. Four types of cognitive failures are shown in Box 26.1.[5]

BOX 26.1 Types of cognitive failures that may contribute to or cause diagnostic error

- *Faulty knowledge*: knowledge deficits resulting in failure to recognise a diagnostic condition or order the correct diagnostic investigation.
- *Data gathering failure*: incomplete history or physical examination resulting in failure to have sufficient information to inform an accurate diagnosis.
- *Data synthesis failure*: failure to interpret the physical findings or laboratory results correctly resulting in failure to reach accurate diagnosis.
- *Cognitive bias*: 'premature closure' where clinicians decide on a specific diagnosis too early and fail to consider other diagnoses or carry out further inquiry to challenge their initial diagnosis.

If we understand why each of these cognitive failures occurs, it may provide opportunities to design and implement specific, targeted interventions to address their root causes. However, it is recognised that attitude also contributes to cognitive failure.[11] For example, a clinician's unrealistic or unfounded confidence in her own ability may be a greater factor in her failure to appropriately process all the available information than insufficient clinical knowledge or information.[12]

The 'dual processing' model describes two different cognitive mechanisms – 'analytical' and 'non-analytical' mechanisms.[13,14] Analytical processing typically involves a slow, structured and considered approach to making a diagnosis. Non-analytical procession typically involves intuitive processing of information through pattern recognition, considering the frequency of symptoms or signs and the clinician's previous experience and knowledge of the clinical problem. The non-analytical approach increases efficiency but it potentially restricts the differential diagnoses through premature closure of all possibilities. While the old adage that 'common things occur commonly' may be true, it could lead clinicians to fail to consider less-common possibilities.

HOW CAN DIAGNOSTIC ERROR BE REDUCED?

Given the multifactorial aetiology of diagnostic error, there is unfortunately no single intervention or 'silver bullet' to prevent every one. However, there are some recommendations and emerging evidence of interventions that may help to reduce these types of error.

Diagnostic errors still remain unrecognised in many instances. One of the first steps would therefore be to raise clinical staff's awareness of the nature, impact and causes of this important problem. Singh and Graber[14] describe a systems-based approach to address diagnostic error using 'Five Rights', which are summarised in Box 26.2.

BOX 26.2 The 'Five Rights'*

1. *Right teamwork*. Teams deliver primary care. This is essential to coordinate the many different care processes and activities effectively – review of laboratory results, timely referrals, diagnosing and arranging clinical follow-up. These tasks need to be delegated clearly and appropriately to the responsible team members while developing and monitoring their knowledge, competency and skills.

2. *Right data and information management*. General practices in the UK typically have access to information communication technologies (ICT). However, practice protocols for care processes such as results and referral management have to be developed and agreed by each team. ICT diagnostic support tools are being developed that offer point-of-care prompts that may serve to alert clinicians to consider possible diagnoses. ICT systems may be especially important to help manage and summarise the large volumes of patient data generated through referrals and investigations so that it can be accessed quickly.

3. *Right measurement and clinical governance*. The practice team members regularly review their critical processes, including laboratory results handling and the quality of their referral letters and participate in regular significant event analysis team meetings, involving colleagues from other agencies when relevant, to learn from patient safety incidents resulting from diagnostic error.

4. *Right patient 'activation'/empowerment*. Patients and their carers and relatives can have an important role to help mitigate diagnostic error. Clinicians should actively encourage patients to raise any concerns about their diagnosis through clear communication channels.

5. *Right safety culture*. Measuring the safety culture or 'safety climate' of teams and organisations is increasingly being promoted as part of initiatives to improve the safety of care. It may be helpful to identify specific culture issues or error risks that may then be addressed.

* Adapted from Singh and Graber[14]

A number of strategies are suggested to help clinicians deal more effectively with diagnostic uncertainty.[6]

- Recognise and acknowledge your intuition. Many clinicians report a 'gut feeling' when they 'know something just isn't right' which develops over time and with experience.

- Make judicious use of the available investigations and measures at your disposal.
- Develop a reliable system of 'safety-netting'[15,16] with advice for the patient or carer of what to expect and when and how to access further care.
- A 'watchful wait' approach with regular, scheduled opportunities allowing clinical review to confirm resolution of the problem or to gather additional information.
- Adopt diagnostic algorithms and consider decision-making support software.

However, these strategies are highly dependent on adequate and appropriate training and clinical experience and may therefore be less effective for younger or less experienced clinicians.

Decision-making support software is one possible way to reduce diagnostic error, as it temporarily prompts the clinician to switch from a 'non-analytical' to an 'analytical' cognitive mechanism.[14] These so-called 'cognitive forcing functions' may therefore reduce a potential over-dependency on simplistic pattern recognition and 'convenience' diagnoses.

General practice currently faces a number of important challenges. How do we care for an increasingly elderly population with multiple co-morbidities? What is the role of the GP within the multidisciplinary team, especially as other healthcare professionals such as nurses and pharmacists adopt new and expanding roles in diagnosing and prescribing for patients? How can we best utilise the 'activated' patients and their carers in mitigating against error, given their increasing access to a wealth of online knowledge?

To meet these challenges, the ability to successfully recognise and deal with diagnostic uncertainty will remain a key requirement in general practice. Amid much uncertainty, timely and accurate diagnoses will remain the cornerstone of safe, quality care.

SUMMARY POINTS
- Diagnostic error is common, yet seldom reported; it remains the most common reason for malpractice claims in general practice.
- The aetiology of diagnostic error is usually multifactorial, with systems and human factor components. We discussed different types of cognitive processes and failures as practical examples of this.
- The risk of diagnostic error may be reduced by considering a 'Five Rights' systems-based approach: (1) effective teamwork; (2) supportive information technologies (including decision support software); (3) feedback and clinical governance systems; (4) involving patients; and (5) measuring and improving the safety culture of the practice.

REFERENCES

1. Kostopoulou O, Delaney BC, Munro CW. Diagnostic difficulty and error in primary care: a systematic review. *Fam Pract.* 2008; **25**(6): 400–13.
2. Singh H, Thomas EJ, Khan MM, *et al.* Identifying diagnostic errors in primary care using an electronic screening algorithm. *Arch Intern Med.* 2007; **167**(3): 302–8.
3. Ely JW, Kaldjian LC, D'Alessandro DM. Diagnostic errors in primary care: lessons learned. *J Am Board Fam Med.* 2012; **25**(1): 87–97.
4. Phillips RL Jr, Bartholomew LA, Dovey SM, *et al.* Learning from malpractice claims about negligent, adverse events in primary care in the United States. *Qual Saf Health Care.* 2004; **13**(2): 121–6.
5. Graber M. Diagnostic errors in medicine: a case of neglect. *Jt Comm J Qual Patient Saf.* 2005; **31**(2): 106–13.
6. Buntinx F, Mant D, Van den Bruel A, *et al.* Dealing with low-incidence serious diseases in general practice. *Br J Gen Pract.* 2011; **61**(582): 43–6.
7. Thompson MJ, Ninis N, Perera R, *et al.* Clinical recognition of meningococcal disease in children and adolescents. *Lancet.* 2006: **367**(9508): 397–403.
8. Allen J, Gray B, Crebolder H, *et al.* WONCA Europe. *The European Definitions of General Practice/Family Medicine.* Barcelona: Europe; 2005.
9. Elstein AS, Shulman LS, Sprafka SA. *Medical Problem Solving: an analysis of clinical reasoning.* Cambridge, MA: Harvard University Press; 1978.
10. Schmidt HG, Norman GR, Boshuizen HPA. A cognitive perspective on medical expertise: theory and implications. *Acad Med.* 1990; **65**(10): 611–21.
11. Norman GR. Diagnostic error and clinical reasoning. *Med Educ.* 2010; **44**(1): 94–100.
12. Berner ES, Graber ML. Overconfidence as a cause of diagnostic error in medicine. *Am J Med.* 2008; **121**(Suppl.): S2–33.
13. Croskerry P. The cognitive imperative: thinking about how we think. *Acad Emerg Med.* 2000; **7**(11): 1223–31.
14. Singh H, Graber M. Reducing diagnostic error through medical home-based primary care reform. *JAMA.* 2010; **304**(4): 463–4.
15. Almond S, Mant D, Thompson M. Diagnostic safety-netting. *Br J Gen Pract.* 2009; **59**(568): 873–4.
16. Croskerry P. Clinical cognition and diagnostic error: applications of a dual process model of reasoning. *Adv Health Sci Educ Theory Pract.* 2009; **14**(Suppl. 1): S27–35.

CHAPTER 27

Medication error[*]

Rachel Spencer

INTRODUCTION

Medication error is an important area of clinical risk in primary care and constitutes a significant proportion of all healthcare-related harm. Adverse drug events (ADEs) affect up to 20% of patients irrespective of country or specific clinical setting,[1-3] of which up to two-thirds may be preventable.[4,5] The majority of ADEs in general practice are of minor or moderate severity, but a substantial minority is serious, with as many as 7.6% associated with a hospital admission.[2,6] In addition to the harm patients suffer, there is also the additional costs incurred in treating patients harmed by these adverse events and the cost of litigation.

Medication use processes are often simplified into four stages: (1) prescribing, (2) dispensing, (3) administration and (4) monitoring. Garfield *et al.*[7] were the first to map out the whole UK primary care medicines management system and to systemically review the evidence of cumulative medication errors in it. They found errors in every stage, with error rates in excess of 50% for repeat prescribing reviews, interface prescribing, communication and patient adherence. As a result, the minority of patients (4%–21%) achieved optimum benefit from their medication. They recommend routine monitoring of adherence, clinical effectiveness and related hospital admissions as initial steps to improve the quality of the medication system.

ADEs are usually caused by 'complex and multifaceted' errors that occur in all stages of the medication use system.[4,7] Examples include drug–drug interactions, discrepancies between prescribed and administered drugs, communication failures and knowledge gaps. A handful of medications – cardiovascular drugs, non-steroidal anti-inflammatory drugs (NSAIDs) and anticoagulants – are associated with the majority of ADEs.[5,8] Other drug categories frequently associated with ADEs are anti-infective agents, diabetogenic

---

[*] This chapter is adapted from the following published article: Spencer R, Avery A, Serumaga B, *et al.* Prescribing errors in general practice and how to avoid them. *Clin Risk.* 2011; **17**(2): 39–42.

medication and analgesia.[9,10] Conversely, some drugs may cause preventable hospital admissions if they are not prescribed – for example, anti-anginals and asthma preventers.[11]

Current evidence indicates that some patient groups are more at risk of harm from medication errors than others. Older, frail patients are especially at increased risk of suffering ADEs. Barber *et al.*[4] studied UK nursing homes and found one or more errors in 69.5% of patient records, and 1.9 mean errors per resident. Other factors that may increase ADE risk include female gender, very young age (<4 years), multiple prescription items, number of daily doses, multiple co-morbidities and high consultation rates.[2,10,12,13] Also of concern are patients who are ambivalent about taking medication or have difficulty understanding and remembering instructions. Errors are most commonly associated with the prescribing and monitoring stages.[5]

This chapter describes common causes of primary care medication errors, and prescribing error in particular, from the perspective of the actors (prescribers, pharmacists and patients) and processes (communication between primary and secondary care, monitoring of medication and repeat prescribing). Eight patient case studies are provided to help illustrate the main learning points through real-life patient safety incidents. A number of potential interventions to help reduce or prevent medication error are also discussed, with a focus on practical solutions that can be adapted for use in general practitioner (GP) surgeries.

PRESCRIBERS AND PHARMACISTS

Slips and lapses are two common types of human error that can lead to patient harm. Slips are incorrectly executed plans, and usually the result of attention failures. They are unconscious and unintentional. Two examples: while selecting a medication from a drop-down list of options, the prescriber selects penicillamine rather than penicillin, and methotrexate is inadvertently prescribed for daily rather than weekly use, despite the prescriber's knowledge to the contrary. Lapses occur when a plan (or part of plan) is not executed and are normally the result of memory failures. Case 1 is an example of a 'lapse', with the prescriber forgetting to complete an action.

> **Case 1.** A 96-year-old patient was admitted to hospital because of a life-threateningly high potassium blood level. The admission occurred because clinicians at her practice were not aware that she was already taking co-amilofruse (a combination diuretic) and additionally prescribed further antihypertensive therapy. This happened because a paper prescription for co-amilofruse was previously issued during a home visit, but the GP did not record the prescription in the electronic medical record on his return to the practice (a lapse).
>
> When interviewed after the incident, the GP admitted: '*and it should have been, that's not actually on here, is it? What one hopes one does is then add that to the medication as an outside prescription. So it's one I clearly didn't.*'[6,14]

One 'error-trapping' method that prescribers can use is to perform a final analytical check before signing a prescription. Briefly pause and actively consider: *'Did I choose the correct medication for this patient in these circumstances and is the dose, form and quantity correct?'*

Community pharmacists provide a potential safety net for 'catching' prescribing errors. Good working relationships and effective communication can improve their role of mitigation. Unfortunately, some pharmacists feel unable to question doctors about prescriptions, resulting in avoidable harm.[15] A community pharmacist reflecting on this problem said: *'They might not take too kindly to, you know, you interfering if you've not got all the details'.*[6] Promoting and developing better relationships and effective communication between prescribers and pharmacists are therefore desirable. One way to achieve this may be through shared educational events. In response, NHS Education for Scotland is evaluating the experiences and perceptions of pharmacists and GPs of sharing practice-based small group learning (*see* Chapter 21).

Information technology (IT) can also be used to reduce or prevent prescribing error through well-designed computer warning systems.[16] Current software packages in most practices are able to automatically identify and alert to potential drug interactions. In the future, prescribing could be linked to investigation results, so that abnormal results with implications for choices of drug type and dosage would automatically be 'flagged up' to the prescriber.[17] IT systems need to be robust, reliable (*see* Case 2) and designed to reduce the nuisance element and information overload effect of frequent alerts about clinically insignificant interactions. One way to achieve this may be by involving clinicians in the initial and ongoing design of software. GPs could also play an advisory role in determining the severity grading of different alerts.[18] For example, co-prescribing a nitrate and a phosphodiesterase inhibitor could potentially lead to more severe harm than co-prescribing an antibiotic and a phosphodiesterase inhibitor.

> **Case 2**. An 82-year-old patient was admitted to hospital after collapsing from hypoglycaemia. This was precipitated by a reduced requirement for insulin as a result of acute on chronic renal failure, which in turn was attributed to the prescription of rofecoxib (a NSAID that has now been withdrawn).
>
> The patient's GP reflected on the role of computer alerts in relation to this incident: *'The computer does warn us at times, but clearly, not that time.'*[6]

One might assume that clinicians' familiarity with the drugs they prescribe would help to reduce error, but this is not always the case. Clinicians may overestimate their knowledge of even commonly prescribed drugs, and it has been found that clinicians' prescriptions have fewer errors if they look drugs up in the *British National Formulary*, as opposed to prescribing from memory.[19] Case 3 illustrates a patient safety incident resulting from a clinician being unfamiliar with a drug she prescribed.

Case 3. A GP prescribed the anti-malarial mefloquine for a couple before their holiday abroad. She incorrectly specified a dose of 250 mg per day, rather than the correct dosing interval of once a week, for the duration of the holiday and for one month on their return. The couple suffered significant side effects, including abdominal pain, diarrhoea, vomiting, dizziness, ataxia and headaches. They both also had acute anxiety and depression, which are known side effects of the medication. The couple's subsequent claim for lost earnings was successful.[20]

Medication errors can be reduced or prevented if GPs regularly update their knowledge of drugs and therapeutics, thereby becoming aware of and avoiding unnecessary risks to patients. This is facilitated by easy access to reliable, independent and useful information, and particularly so for the many new products launched in the market. A recent example of the changing fortunes of a drug is rofecoxib (a NSAID) – initially greeted as a panacea, it fell out of favour after a few years when evidence came to light of the potentially serious risks associated with its use. Case 4 is a preventable patient safety incident that was caused by failure to address a well-known risk associated with anticoagulants – a class of drugs commonly prescribed. In this case, the risk was further magnified because of two different anticoagulants that were co-prescribed.

Case 4. A 73-year-old patient was prescribed aspirin and warfarin as prophylaxis against suffering another stroke or myocardial infarction on his discharge from hospital. When the patient questioned this combination, the cardiology registrar allegedly told him that it was *'OK, it was the decision of the consultant.'* The GP also queried the prescription but was likewise reassured and there was no computer alert warning about the potential interaction between aspirin and warfarin. Neither the hospital nor the GP considered offering the patient gastric protection. The patient was subsequently admitted to hospital as an emergency with profuse rectal bleeding from a gastric ulcer.[20]

THE PATIENT

Patients' attitudes and knowledge about medication have been shown to be partially responsible for a number of medication-related adverse events.[6] Ideally, prescribing involves a joint decision between the doctor and patient and should include a discussion of significant and common side effects. Prescribers need to respect patients' autonomy with respect to their prescribing. Problems arise, however, when patients are ambivalent about their medication or have communication difficulties with their doctor, as illustrated through Case 5.

Case 5. A 56-year-old man was admitted to hospital as an emergency after he was discovered, unconscious, with profuse gastrointestinal haemorrhage attributed to his prescribed NSAID. Previously, the patient was consuming >20 units of alcohol per day, but had told his GP he was consuming 'only' 10 units per day. At the time of the prescription the GP had advised him to halve his consumption. If the patient had provided more accurate information, his GP may not have issued the prescription.[14]

The onus rests with clinicians in the first instance to provide patients with clear information. With chronic conditions such as diabetes mellitus, asthma and coronary heart disease this can usually be done over the course of a number of consultations. Other professionals such as practice nurses and pharmacists can play a valuable part in this process, as can directing patients to online educational resources.

Patients' myriad disabilities, such as poor hearing, poor eyesight or impaired manual dexterity, can result in them being unable to take their medication correctly. For example, prescribing a metered-dose inhaler for a patient with deforming rheumatoid arthritis increases the risks of non-adherence. This type of error is preventable if patients' individual contexts are known and taken into account. Carers and community pharmacists also have a role to play. Clinicians should familiarise themselves with the packaging and devices of commonly prescribed drugs. Pharmaceutical companies may be able to provide placebo products and devices that can be used to demonstrate to patients and carers how to administer the drug and to check that they are able to.

COMMUNICATION BETWEEN PRIMARY AND SECONDARY CARE

Effective and timely communication between primary and secondary care is critical to ensure the continuity and safety of care delivered to patients. According to the Care Quality Commission report on the management of medications at the time of hospital admission, up to 24% of patients are referred without information about their co-morbidities,[13] although 98% of referring clinicians did provide information about the patients' prescribed medication. However, approximately 80% of practices reported that the information they received from secondary care regarding medications on discharge was often wrong or incomplete. About half of practices reported that the discharge summaries were routinely received so late that they were no longer useful.[21] Further risk factors identified by the report include that in 17% of practices, non-clinical staff were tasked with the responsibility of reconciling discharge medication with the medication record of the practice. This is potentially a complex task and one that is recommended clinicians perform (*see* Chapter 28).

The expectation is that an IT approach that integrates primary and secondary care systems may improve communication, but it is unlikely that it will remove all risk for error. Case 6 illustrates the risk of ineffective interface communication.

> **Case 6**. A 68-year-old patient with chronic renal failure was discharged with a summary document to his GP advising to 'monitor U&Es [urea and electrolytes] closely' and on metolazone (a potent diuretic). The GP interpreted this instruction to mean weekly monitoring, while the hospital had intended daily monitoring.

The patient lost considerable weight, became dehydrated and was readmitted with acute chronic renal failure.[14]

Communication from primary to secondary care could be improved by introducing a standardised referral form for all admissions. Such a form could be generated automatically from the practice records and would contain extracted data about medication and co-morbidities. Out-of-hours referrals remain problematic, but strategies such as 'green bag' and 'patient's own medication' schemes may help in this regard and improve patients' understanding of and participation in their own care. In some areas hospital clinicians now have access to a Summary Care Record, which includes information about patients' medication. Medication reconciliation should become a routine function at the time of discharge. Ideally, a pharmacist or GP should perform the medication reconciliation, as they have the clinical knowledge and professional skills to perform what can be very complex tasks. Unfortunately this is a time-critical and often laborious process and clarification often has to be sought from the hospital.

MEDICATION MONITORING

Errors in medication monitoring processes may account for as much as a quarter of preventable medication-related hospital admissions, and even more so for elderly patients with renal impairment.[6] There is currently insufficient evidence of the optimum intervals for monitoring different medications and, as such, recommendations from different sources may vary considerably. This suggests the need for national guidance for GPs to standardise the monitoring of hazardous medications. Case 7 illustrates why any practice needs a robust and reliable medication monitoring system.

> Case 7. A 40-year-old patient was discharged from a psychiatric ward after her mood was stabilised with lithium. The expectation was that her practice would take over her management. She was reviewed in the practice on several occasions and repeat prescriptions for lithium were issued, but no lithium blood level was requested for 4 years. Shortly after being prescribed co-amilozide (an antihypertensive) she started complaining of 'shakes' and constipation; she became progressively more confused and was admitted to hospital as an emergency. During the admission she was found to be lithium toxic. She subsequently filed a case against her practice, alleging failure to have a system in place for monitoring, and failure to supervise repeat prescribing. The case was settled in her favour for £28 000.[20]

REPEAT PRESCRIBING

Repeat prescriptions improve efficiency in busy surgeries, but also pose potentially significant risks, as demonstrated by Case 8.

Case 8. A patient was started on steroid eye drops by an ophthalmologist, and her GP was asked to issue repeat prescriptions. The ophthalmologist subsequently decided to wean and stop the steroid drops, but this decision was never communicated to the practice and the patient continued to receive the medication. She unfortunately developed bilateral steroid-induced glaucoma, required surgery and subsequently lost the vision in one eye. A successful case was brought against the GP and a body of experts concluded that *ongoing repeat prescriptions* should not have been given without ophthalmology advice. They also highlighted failings in communication between secondary and primary care and the lack of a computer fail-safe mechanism.[20]

Medication reviews have the potential to reduce the frequency of errors in repeat medication prescribing. More complex reviews should ideally be done during a dedicated consultation slot with either a GP or a pharmacist. The National Service Framework for older people recommends that patients over the age of 75 and who are prescribed four or more medications should have a dedicated medication review every 6 months.[22] Despite the national rate of compliance with the Quality and Outcomes Framework target on medication review being 95%, there is also evidence to suggest that only half of recorded medication reviews are performed with the patient present.[21] Repeat prescriptions should be subject to review by a suitably qualified medical practitioner when they have reached their issue limit and this review should cross-reference the medical record. Patients need to be educated as to how the repeats system works at their practice. They should be encouraged to use the printed repeat slip (or another reliable method) in order to avoid errors in the selection of repeats and to help the practice process their request in a timely fashion.

CONCLUSION

This chapter described common causes of primary care medication errors from the perspective of the actors and processes involved. Strategies for avoiding medication errors include clinician and patient education; ensuring clinicians have access to all the information they need when making prescribing decisions; effective communication; checking of procedures; and increased adoption of well-designed IT solutions. The standardisation of timely and accurate information transfer across healthcare interfaces is also a priority. There is emerging evidence that pharmacists, patients and GPs may effectively mitigate some medication errors.[3,23] However, reducing medication error will likely require multiple interventions as well as improved understanding of the causes.[9]

REFERENCES

1. Tache SV, Sonnichsen A, Ashcroft DM. Prevalence of adverse drug events in ambulatory care: a systematic review. *Ann Pharmacother.* 2011; **45**(7–8): 977–89.
2. Miller GC, Britth HC, Valenti L. Adverse drug events in general practice patients in Australia. *Med J Aust.* 2006; **184**(7): 321–4.
3. Kuo GM, Phillips RL, Graham D, *et al.* Medication errors reported by US family physicians and their office staff. *Qual Saf Health Care.* 2008; **17**(4): 286–90.
4. Barber ND, Alldred DP, Raynor DK, *et al.* Care homes' use of medicines study: prevalence, causes and potential harm of medication errors in care homes for older people. *Qual Saf Health Care.* 2009; **18**(5): 341–6.
5. Gurwitz JH, Field TS, Harrold LR, *et al.* Incidence and preventability of adverse drug events among older persons in the ambulatory setting. *JAMA.* 2003; **289**(9): 1107–16.
6. Howard R, Avery A, Bissell P. Causes of preventable drug-related hospital admissions: a qualitative study. *Qual Saf Health Care.* 2008; **17**(2): 109–16.
7. Garfield S, Barber N, Walley P, *et al.* Quality of medication use in primary care: mapping the problem, working to a solution: a systematic review of the literature. *BMC Med.* 2009; **7**: 50.
8. Howard RL, Avery AJ, Slavenburg S, *et al.* Which drugs cause preventable admissions to hospital? A systematic review. *Br J Clin Pharmacol.* 2007; **63**(2): 136–47.
9. Morris CJ, Rodgers S, Hammersley VS, *et al.* Indicators for preventable drug related morbidity: application in primary care. *Qual Saf Health Care.* 2004; **13**(3): 181–5.
10. Tam KW, Kwok KH, Fan YM, *et al.* Detection and prevention of medication misadventures in general practice. *Int J Qual Health Care.* 2008; **20**(3): 192–9.
11. Howard RL, Avery AJ, Howard PD, *et al.* Investigation into the reasons for preventable drug related admissions to a medical admissions unit: observational study. *Qual Saf Health Care.* 2003; **12**(4): 280–5.
12. Doubova Dubova SV, Reyes-Morales H, Torres-Arreola Ldel P, *et al.* Potential drug-drug and drug-disease interactions in prescriptions for ambulatory patients over 50 years of age in family medicine clinics in Mexico City. *BMC Health Serv Res.* 2007; **7**: 147.
13. McCarthy L, Dolovich L, Haq M, *et al.* Frequency of risk factors that potentially increase harm from medications in older adults receiving primary care. *Can J Clin Pharmacol.* 2007; **14**(3): 283–90.
14. Howard R. *A Qualitative Exploration of the Underlying Causes of Preventable Drug-Related Morbidity in Primary Care, Resulting in Hospitalisation.* Nottingham: University of Nottingham; 2007.
15. Chen Y, Avery A, Neil K, *et al.* Incidence and possible causes of prescribing potentially hazardous/contraindicated drug combinations in general practice. *Drug Saf.* 2005; **28**: 67–80.
16. Schedlbauer A, Prasad V, Mulvaney C, *et al.* What evidence supports the use of computerised alerts and prompts to improve clinicians' prescribing behaviour? *J Am Med Inform Assoc.* 2009; **16**(4): 531–8.
17. Fernando B, Savelyich B, Avery A, *et al.* Prescribing safety features of general practice-computer systems: evaluation using simulated test cases. *BMJ.* 2004; **328**: 1171–2.
18. Kuperman G, Bobb A, Payne T, *et al.* Medication-related decision support in computerised provider order entry systems: a review. *J Am Med Inform Assoc.* 2007; **14**(1): 29–40.

19. Dornan T, Ashcroft D, Heathfield H, *et al.* An indepth investigation into causes of pre-scribing errors by foundation trainees in relation to their medical education: EQUIP study. London: GMC; 2009.

20. Medical Protection Society. *Casebook series*. London: MPS; 2010. Available at: www.medicalprotection.org/default.aspx?dn=f0c10d67-a680-44a7-a599-ba1b3c7384e0 (accessed 7 March 2014).

21. Care Quality Commission. *Care Quality Commission National Report: managing patients' medicines after discharge from hospital*. London: CQC; 2009.

22. Department of Health. *National Service Framework for Older People*. London: Department of Health; 2001.

23. Swinglehurst D, Greenhalgh T, Russell J, *et al.* Receptionist input to quality and safety in repeat prescribing in UK general practice: ethnographic case study. *BMJ*. 2011; **343**: 6788.

CHAPTER 28

Medicines reconciliation: a case study

Rachel Bruce

INTRODUCTION

Taking a medicine is the most common intervention patients use to improve their health. Older people and those with long-term conditions often take multiple medicines (polypharmacy) to treat and manage their illnesses. Evidence shows that there is a greater risk of error and potential harm from medicines when patients move between care settings, resulting in 30%–70% of patients experiencing an error or unintentional change in their medication when their care is transferred.[1]

Incidents of avoidable harm to patients can result in unnecessary hospital readmissions, with an estimated 72% of adverse events after discharge due to medications[2] and 38% of readmissions considered to be medicines related (61% of these are judged to be preventable).[3] Apart from the clear patient safety risks there are also implications for professionals, with 19.3% of general practitioner (GP) negligence claims relating to prescribing and medication (3.8% of which were due to supplying incorrect or inappropriate medication).[4]

Medicines reconciliation is an essential component of patient safety, in promoting the safer use of medicines with effective communication when patients move between care settings. The Scottish Government defines it for patients as:

> The process that the healthcare team undertakes to ensure that the list of medication, both prescribed and over the counter, that I am taking is exactly the same as the list that I or my carers, GP, Community Pharmacist and hospital team have. This is achieved in partnership with me through obtaining an up-to-date and accurate medication list that has been compared with the most recently available information and has documented any discrepancies, changes, deletions or additions resulting in a complete list of medicines accurately communicated.[5]

Medicines reconciliation is an issue at all interfaces of care but it is particularly important when patients are admitted and discharged from hospital. A schematic detailing the key transitions of care where medicines reconciliation should be done is shown in Figure 28.1. There is evidence that this process does not happen reliably,[6,7] with local audits conducted in a single health authority reporting just over half of patients admitted to one of its hospitals had one or more of their usual medicines unintentionally omitted from their prescription chart.[8] In total, 60% of patients had medication discrepancies on discharge – specifically, relating to medicines that had been started and/or stopped during the admission.[9,10]

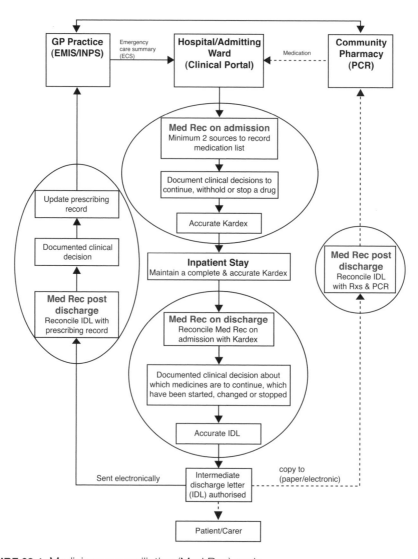

FIGURE 28.1 Medicines reconciliation (Med Rec) cycle

Much of the work on medicines reconciliation has been focused in secondary care. However, the principles are equally important in, and transferable to, primary care. Poor or unreliable processes in general practice in carrying out medicines reconciliation can potentially lead to medication errors, patient harm and hospital readmissions.

Improvement in the reliability of reconciliation processes in primary and secondary care will have potential benefits at the patient, practice and the system-wide levels. A robust and reliable process for carrying out timely medicines reconciliation in general practice post hospital discharge ensures the GP prescribing record is current and accurate. This in turn improves the accuracy of the Emergency Care Summary (ECS). The ECS is a summary of basic but clinically important information about a patient including a list of current medication being prescribed, which is extracted from the GP systems twice a day. The ECS is often used as a source of information to carry out medicines reconciliation when a patient is admitted to hospital. Inaccurate or incomplete medicines reconciliation in the primary care setting will result in an inaccurate GP prescribing record and therefore a flawed ECS for any medicines reconciliation on admission.

IMPROVING MEDICINES RECONCILIATION: A CASE STUDY

The improvement intervention described in this case study was centred on GP practices having a robust process when actioning immediate discharge letters and prescriptions. A primary care medicines reconciliation 'care bundle' was tested as part of the Scottish Patient Safety Programme in Primary Care. Care bundles (as described in more detail in Chapter 33) are a quality improvement tool that can help care teams to drive improvement and ensure safe and reliable care. It is a structured way of improving processes to deliver optimum care at every patient contact, with the aim of enhancing safety and achieving better clinical outcomes. The reliable implementation of this care bundle (*see* Table 28.1) is a means to ensure that patients' discharge information is processed in a timely manner; that they are prescribed the correct medicines and in the correct doses appropriate to their current clinical presentation; and that the risk of avoidable harm from medicines is reduced.

A key feature of this specific care bundle is the focus on patient involvement and communication – ensuring the patient is made aware of any changes to their medication post hospital discharge. The care bundle is also designed to help improve practice team working. Different members of the practice team from the reception staff to the GPs have a responsibility for different components of the bundle. Overall compliance with the care bundle requires reliable delivery of all the components by the responsible practice staff members.

Five general practices within the health authority tested the medicines reconciliation care bundle. Measurement of care bundle compliance for a random sample of 10 patients from the defined cohort was gathered on a monthly basis. For those practices with very large numbers of discharges, priority was given to 'high-risk' patients such as elderly patients with polypharmacy and those on high-risk medicines. The aim was that all practices would achieve the minimum

TABLE 28.1 Medicines reconciliation (med rec) care bundle for general practice

Bundle component	Measure	Definition of terms
1. Handling of IDLs	Has the IDL been 'workflowed' on the day of receipt?	The IDL should be sent to the appropriate GP on the day of receipt. The definition of 'workflow' will depend on the process used in the practice (i.e. electronically via a software package like 'Docman' or passing on a paper copy). Prompt initial processing of the IDL ensures timely initiation of the med rec process.
2. Med rec	Has medicines reconciliation occurred within 2 working days of the IDL being 'workflowed' to the GP?	Med rec in practical terms means the staff member responsible (usually a clinician) compares the IDL medication list with the current practice prescribing record. Clinical decisions require to be made at this point regarding appropriate ongoing therapy.
3. Documentation	Is it documented that any changes to the medication have been acted upon?	This step is required to fulfil the definition of med rec given here. Any changes must be accurately documented in the patient record. Prescribing decisions made during the med rec process should be clearly documented.
4. Communication and patient involvement	Is it documented that any changes to the medication have been discussed with the patient or their representative within 7 days of receiving the IDL?	Internal audit suggests that <30% of patients know what medicines they are taking when discharged from hospital. Patient education and communication of any changes are necessary to increase their understanding and reduce risk. Practices should choose the most effective and reliable method to achieve this as part of the med rec process and implement it.
5. Overall compliance with bundle	Have all four components been delivered?	This is a process measure with an agreed standard of minimum overall compliance of 90% for all practices.

IDL = immediate discharge letters; GP = general practitioner

target of 90% overall compliance with the care bundle by March 2013. Practices used the Plan-Do-Study-Act method (*see* Chapter 34) to make improvements to their reconciliation processes on an iterative basis.

The run chart in Figure 28.2 shows the collated care bundle compliance over the time period of the pilot.

When compliance was first measured in 2011, shortly after implementing the care bundle, the baseline overall compliance with all bundle components for all practices was approximately 40%. Over the subsequent months compliance increased gradually, as practice teams identified areas they were not meeting the set standards and consequently made system improvements using the Plan-Do-Study-Act method. Then, in September 2012 there was a significant drop in care bundle compliance. This coincided with the introduction of TrakCare, a new patient management system used in secondary care in the health authority, which fundamentally altered the way discharge letters were produced. This had an unintended consequence on primary care, as it essentially changed the processes by which GP practices managed discharge communication. However, once practices affected by this change reviewed and adapted their processes to account for this new way of working, care bundle compliance again increased steadily and the target of 90% overall compliance by all practices was achieved in January 2013.

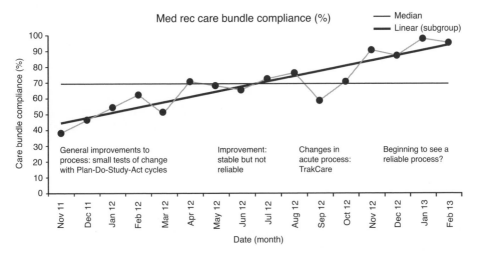

FIGURE 28.2 Run chart of the overall bundle compliance of all participating practices

DISCUSSION

Towards the end of the testing phase, practices completed a reflection sheet giving them the opportunity to highlight the benefits and challenges of implementing the care bundle. Prior to the care bundle work, all practices felt they had robust processes in place for medicines reconciliation. However, on testing they realised improvements could be made. The individual compliance measure that practices found most challenging was informing the patient (or representative) of changes to his or her medication. This is arguably one of the most important elements of the care bundle from a safety perspective, and one that patients find of great value.

> 'Although the extra work is time consuming our practice team feel that this is worthwhile and beneficial for patients.' (GP, Practice 1)

> 'We are now happy with our system for checking discharge medication. We previously often assumed a patient was aware of changes. Now we always check.' (GP, Practice 3)

> 'Initially I thought this was not my job but now that I have started contacting patients after discharge I can see that there is a need for this to happen.' (GP, Practice 4)

Audit is not a new concept for GP practices, but monthly data collection to determine overall compliance with a small number of components as part of a care bundle was a novel concept for all of the practices involved. The benefit of measuring compliance on a monthly basis was that it provided practices with real-time data with which to make improvements within their practice, and helped to quickly identify new issues that could affect their care processes – such as, in this case, the TrakCare roll-out. Measuring in real time provided the evidence quickly to practices to enable them to intervene more efficiently. In turn, this afforded them the opportunity to feed back a number of recommendations to TrakCare providers to improve the interim discharge letter, which enhanced this aspect of patient safety in primary care overall.

The initial proposed outcome measure for this improvement pilot was to achieve a measureable reduction in hospital admissions. However, with only five of 261 practices across a very large health board participating in this improvement pilot, it was not possible to assess this reliably. Therefore, the improvement pilot's outcome measure was changed to process reliability. The overall care bundle compliance was set at a minimum of 90%, with improvement in compliance observed over the time of the pilot work. Data from January and February 2013 showed practices continued to achieve the target, but more data are required before one could conclude that the improvements are sustainable. As part of the evaluation of this pilot, patient views were sought on the benefits of the care bundle approach using a questionnaire.[11] Thirty patients completed the questionnaire and all rated the communication by the GP practice on their discharge as being either 'useful' or 'very useful' in terms of understanding any changes to their medicines.

The benefits observed through practice reflection include improved and standardised processes for medicines reconciliation including standard documentation of any changes and applying consistent clinical codes of the performed actions in patients' electronic records. Practices reported more and improved communication with patients and community pharmacy because of bundle component 4 (see Table 28.1), although they acknowledged that it is one of the more challenging and time-consuming components to deliver. However, it is warmly received by patients and there are many patient stories demonstrating that if the medicines reconciliation (and care bundle) had not been applied, it would most likely have resulted in readmission to hospital.

Using the care bundle as a means to implement a robust and reliable procedure should ultimately reduce care variations and the associated clinical risks. This approach potentially also has workload benefits from the reduction in patient harm. Where appropriate, patients should be much more involved and informed in the discussion around changes to their medication on discharge and this additional contact by the practice allows greater opportunity for patients to ask questions. Having a robust process in primary care for medicines reconciliation also has a positive impact on the accuracy of the GP prescribing record, which, in turn, improves the quality of the ECS and facilitates any medicines reconciliation processes in hospital.

PRACTICAL POINTERS

- Be open-minded – don't assume your practice process is reliable.
- Involve your whole practice team for best results, including locums.
- Be innovative in your approach, particularly when communicating changes with patients.
- Inform the community pharmacy of changes, especially if your patient is on a compliance aid.
- Using a standardised practice template can improve documentation of interventions and subsequent measurement of compliance.
- Use the compliance measures to improve your processes and not as a performance management tool.

REFERENCES

1. National institute for Health and Care Excellence; National Patient Safety Agency. *Technical Patient Safety Solutions for Medicines Reconciliation on Admission of Adults to Hospital: NICE patient safety guidance 1*. London: NICE; 2007. Available at: http://guidance.nice.org.uk/PSG001 (accessed 7 March 2014).
2. Forster AJ, Clark HD, Menard A, *et al.* Adverse events affecting medical patients following discharge from hospital. *CMAJ*. 2004: **170**(3): 345–9.
3. Witherington EMA, Pirzada OM, Avery AJ. Communication gaps and readmissions to hospital for patients over 75 years and older: observational study. *Qual Saf Health Care*. 2008; **17**(1): 71–5.
4. Silk N. *An Analysis of 1,000 Consecutive General Practice Negligence Claims*. Unpublished report from the Medical Protection Society. 2000. Leeds, Medical Protection Society.
5. Scottish Government Health and Social Care Directorates. *Safer Use of Medicines: medicines reconciliation – revised definition, goals and measures and recommended practice statements for the Scottish Patient Safety Programme. Ref: CMO(2013)18*. Edinburgh: Scottish Government; 2013. Available at: www.sehd.scot.nhs.uk/index.asp?name=&org=%25&keyword=&category=9&number=10&sort=tDate&order=DESC&Submit=Go (accessed 7 March 2014).
6. Collins DJ, Nickless GD, Green CF. Medication histories: does anyone know what medicines a patient should be taking? *Int J Pharm Pract*. 2004; **12**(4): 73–178.
7. Dodds LJ. Unintended discrepancies between pre-admission and admission prescriptions: results of a collaborative service evaluation across east and SE England. *Int J Pharm Pract*. 2011; **18**(Suppl. 2): 9–10.
8. McInally J, Bissett C. Safe as houses? Are inpatients receiving the medications that they would normally take at home? GG&C Audit (Unpublished), 2009 July.
9. O'Gorman N, Lawson P. Bridging the gap: an audit of medicines reconciliation at the primary/secondary care interface in medicine for the elderly admissions. GG&C Audit (Unpublished), 2011 February.
10. West Dunbartonshire CHP. Audit of discharge medication information and communication issues. GG&C Audit (Unpublished), 2008 July.
11. Varkey P, Cunningham J, O'Meara J, *et al.* Multidisciplinary approach to inpatient medication reconciliation in an academic setting. *Am J Health Syst Pharm*. 2007; **64**(8): 850–4.

CHAPTER 29

Safe results handling

Paul Bowie, Julie Price & John McKay

INTRODUCTION

The reliability of tracking systems to oversee the management of laboratory test ordering and results handling is problematic and a significant source of error in primary care settings worldwide.[1-4] For patients and their relatives this may have multiple consequences in terms of contributing to avoidable harm and unnecessary distress; suboptimal clinical management of illness and delayed treatments; poor experience of, and dissatisfaction with, care; miscommunication of test results by healthcare staff; and the inconvenience of return appointments, repeating blood tests or making formal complaints.[5-7]

For general practitioners (GPs), a range of professional, legal and accountability issues make the safe handling of laboratory test results a high-level priority because of the patient safety evidence outlined. Poor laboratory test follow-up, missed results and delays in communication are likely to have a greater impact on patients whose investigation outcomes point to the need for timely medical treatment or intervention. Lack of, or inadequate, results handling systems can therefore lead to clinical judgements on diagnostic and treatment decisions being delayed based on the availability of incomplete information, which limits therapeutic options, thereby potentially affecting the safety of patient care.[5,6,8-10]

The implications for the GP of this type of unsafe practice may also include having to cope with formal complaints by patients or relatives, litigation claims for financial compensation in the event of proven clinical negligence or upheld complaints, and possible licensure sanctions by medical regulators. A further consequence may be a difficulty in repairing and maintaining the bond of trust in the doctor–patient relationship.[5,7,11,12]

At the system level, the published evidence suggests that general practices do not always have adequate processes to track requests for investigations, to record the results of clinically significant abnormal investigations that are returned from laboratories, or to confirm whether follow-up action has taken place before results reports are filed in patients' records.[6,8-10] Furthermore, the majority of general practices do not have effective systems in place to reliably notify patients of normal results either, thereby shifting a level of responsibility onto the patient to contact the practice to obtain the results.[5,9] The impact of poor results handling is evident in the associated financial costs incurred and use of human resources to problem-solve system failures and repeat related work tasks.[8] Additionally, the experience of poor healthcare service by patients may also have wider local community effects, in terms of creating bad publicity or a poor professional reputation.[5,13]

BOX 29.1 Example of a laboratory results handling patient safety incident

A 68-year-old patient attended the family doctor complaining of non-specific tiredness. The doctor ordered a thyroid check to exclude hypothyroidism, a glucose level to exclude diabetes and a full blood count (FBC) to exclude anaemia. The patient's blood sample was taken 2 days later by the phlebotomist. The patient phoned 1 week later for the results. The administrator informed the patient that the doctor said the results were 'normal'. The administrator did not realise that although the thyroid and sugar test were normal, the FBC had not been returned to the practice. When the patient attended a further appointment 3 months later it was noticed that the FBC had not been returned to the practice. The original result had been sent to the wrong practice. It demonstrated a possible iron-deficiency anaemia. Follow-up investigations confirmed the iron deficiency, with secondary care investigation finding the cause was a colonic cancer.

In the absence of specific evidence-based guidance on this important topic, this chapter describes a rigorous project approach by the NHS Education for Scotland primary care team to building consensus on 'good practice' guidance statements to inform the front-line implementation of safe systems for ordering laboratory tests and managing results in primary care settings internationally.

PROJECT CONTEXT

The safety and reliability of two-way systems for communicating the ordering of laboratory tests and returned test results at the interface between primary and secondary care is a topic of concern in most healthcare systems.[14,15] However, the focus here is specifically on what happens in primary care. The justification is that in most modern healthcare systems, clinical laboratory settings operate at a high level of reliability and these performance standards are periodically verified as part of external quality accreditation processes.[16]

Internationally there is variation in primary healthcare design, information technology decision support and practice systems for coordination of laboratory test ordering and result handling in and across most countries. A key focus was to ensure that the 'good practice' guidance generated was largely relevant in principle to all countries, regardless of the primary care systems in operation.

Also, given the scope, range and complexity of clinical investigations that can be ordered by primary care clinicians, the project team agreed at the outset to narrow the focus to include only common, high-volume biochemistry and haematology blood test requests – although it was recognised that the principles underpinning any developed guidance would apply more widely.

PROJECT DESIGN

Mixed methods were used in the United Kingdom and Ireland contexts, and then consensus was sought on these findings at the wider European level (*see* Figure 29.1). As a first step a steering group was formed to coordinate project networking and development activities, and then analyse, interpret, integrate and triangulate[17-19] result data as they were generated. The group was made up of highly experienced front-line primary care staff representatives including GPs, practice nurses and practice managers, as well as patient safety researchers, clinical educators, and human factors and medical indemnity specialists. The main output was a draft document divided into 10 safety domains, with a total of 93 related statements of 'good practice' identified and agreed.

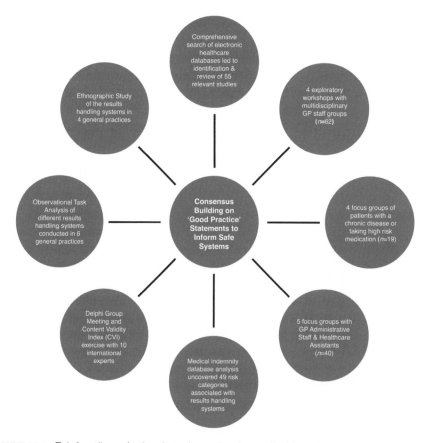

FIGURE 29.1 Brief outline of mixed study methods applied to achieve consensus

FINAL CONSENSUS BUILDING

A total of 10 international experts representing 11 discrete national healthcare systems for handling laboratory results then attended a Delphi meeting. The purpose was to critically appraise and ultimately agree on a final set of high-level safety domains and related 'good practice' statements of relevance in international settings (irrespective of whether some or many elements of this guidance were currently desirable or achievable within the differing political, economic or healthcare policy contexts with regard to improving patient safety in primary care). Experts were also asked to identify any missing issues of high relevance that they deemed important for guidance inclusion.

CONSENSUS FINDINGS

The final international meeting led to consensus on 10 generic safety domains and the inclusion of 77 evidence-based 'good practice' statements that were judged to be relevant to creating patient safety and minimising risks in laboratory test ordering and subsequent results handling systems in European primary care settings. There was much discussion on the possibility of developing other safety domains or new statements of 'good practice', but after consideration no new additions were appended.

The 10 safety domains and a small number of examples of related 'good practice' statements are outlined in Table 29.1. The first two safety domains are concerned with the requirements needed to engender and maintain a commitment to improving local safety culture among team members, and the necessity for training and development of staff in relation to results handling. Both domains recommend taking a whole-system approach as one way to improve primary care team knowledge and understanding of the different human interfaces, interactions, responsibilities and actions that are necessary to build and maintain system reliability.[6,12,20,21]

The remaining eight domains focus directly on outlining the guiding principles identified as creating safety at each discrete stage of the laboratory test ordering and results handling system. Specifically, much of the detail in these statements underpins the need for practice teams to ensure that they have a recognised high-reliability process for tracking clinical investigations ordered by clinicians, reconciling these ordered tests with results received from the laboratory, ensuring that the results are then clinically reviewed and actioned or filed, and ensuring the outcome is safely communicated to the patient with follow-up arranged, where clinically appropriate.[6–13,20,21]

TABLE 29.1 High-level safety domains and examples of 'good practice' statements*

	High-level safety domain	Subcategory	Examples of 'good practice' statements
A	Commitment to a systems approach and improving safety culture	System issue	The prevailing practice culture 'permits' or 'allows' clinical and administrative staff to freely raise potential safety risks and other quality-of-care issues, viewing these as valuable opportunities for collective learning and improvement
B	Commitment to staff training and raising awareness of roles and responsibilities	System issue	Clinical and administrative staff are knowledgeable of the risks associated with laboratory test ordering, results tracking and communication and the potential consequences for patient safety
C	Ordering laboratory tests	Process issue	The practice should have a formal process for identifying patients who do not make appointments for tests or who do not attend for a related appointment
D	Obtaining a sample	Communication issue	Ensure up-to-date patient contact details are confirmed
E	Administration of samples	Process issue	Ensure all relevant staff are trained in handling samples appropriately (e.g. develop and use protocols for spinning)
F	Transport sample to laboratory	Process issue	A process exists for tracking all samples sent to the laboratory and reconciling the results that are returned
G	Managing results returned to the practice	Process issue	Assign responsibility to an individual staff member to conduct small-scale 4-weekly tracking audits of random samples to reconcile tests ordered with results returned and appropriately actioned
H	Clinical review of laboratory results	Communication issue	Every action should contain clear information and specific free-text words (avoiding medical jargon) to be fed back to patients by a telephone call, letter or face to face
I	Results actioned or filed	Communication issue	The practice protocol should detail patient choice on leaving results-related information on answerphones or voicemail devices (e.g. what level of information should be communicated, and how and when this should be done and by whom)
J	Patient monitored through follow-up	Communication issue	The practice protocol should outline what is agreed to be a sufficient number of direct attempts made by staff to get the patient to follow up an action (e.g. return to the practice for further tests)

* A full copy of the guidance statements can be downloaded from www.linneaus-pc.eu/Tools_Resources. html

---

BOX 29.2 Key messages

- Laboratory test ordering and results handling processes are a significant source of error and avoidable patient harm in international primary care.
- Lack of or inadequate safety systems to guide 'good practice' and mitigate errors are common, creating risks for patients and GPs.
- Safety is created and risks minimised by introducing and standardising processes to improve the reliability of results management systems.
- However, the practice culture must embrace a systems approach to this issue and a commitment to staff training and development.
- The outputs of this development work are of direct interest to front-line clinicians, managers and staff, educators, patient safety advisors, health service researchers, professional bodies and policymakers.

DISCUSSION

A whole range of safety-critical issues judged to be relevant to 'good practice' in the systems-based management of laboratory results were identified and prioritised by front-line primary care team members, international experts and safety specialists. In achieving this, two methods where particularly innovative and of value in studying the topic: (1) undertaking observational task analyses[22] of results management systems in a range of practices and (2) interrogating a national medical indemnity database containing information on a plethora of risks associated with results management systems – enabling the project team to tap into arguably the largest known source of empirical data on the subject. There was a high level of concordance with the United Kingdom and Ireland issues raised in both the published literature[6,8–12,20,21] and when developing consensus with the international experts, who strongly agreed that the safety principles underpinning the great majority of 'good practice' statements translated to their national contexts.

At a fundamental level, primary care teams can immediately adapt elements of this guidance to help them develop new systems, or augment existing systems, to minimise the risk of error and avoidable harm to patients. Similarly, it may also be used to improve existing induction packs for new GPs, temporary doctors, GP trainees and other staff groups to educate them about the associated safety implications and professional accountability expectations, as well as describing how the internal system is designed and the related roles and responsibilities of relevant team members. In particular, for individual GPs, the guidance reinforces the fact that the ultimate responsibility for following up blood test results lies with the clinician who ordered the test, therefore relying (as many do) on the patient to contact the practice is a potential clinical and medico-legal risk.[7,11]

Unlike other health sectors (e.g. acute hospital care), primary care teams in many countries inhabit comparatively small, non-bureaucratic organisations that have the power and resources to develop and redesign their own internal systems for managing patient care, including laboratory results handling. The GP, and to a lesser extent the practice manager and the administrative support staff, is pivotal to the decision-making and problem-solving governing this aspect of care. However, a key issue for GPs in considering the safety improvement merits of this guidance is to appreciate more explicitly the psychosocial factors (e.g. low levels of work autonomy, poor working relationships, heavy workloads and high job stress among individual staff members) and sociocultural and organisational issues (e.g. staffing levels, strength of team working, commitment to staff training and professional development and quality improvement, and dominant power hierarchies) that will influence the effective implementation of guidance.[23,24] Therefore, where existing psychosocial and practice culture issues militate against this purely 'technical solution', it is quite likely that problems will arise when guidance implementation is attempted.[25]

For primary care educators the implications of this work may include the need for short, targeted training interventions for GPs and other front-line staff. For example, on how GPs could communicate test results in more specific, precise and less-ambiguous terms to reception staff to enable them in turn to inform patients in a safe, effective manner and with greater clarity. Similar interventions are also needed for key staff on improving knowledge of whole-system thinking in the workplace,[26] and perhaps even on interpreting and implementing aspects of the guidance itself.

It is likely that much work is required to raise awareness of both the safety-critical nature of the results handling issue and the developed guidance among policymakers, senior healthcare management, clinical leaders and professional bodies across most European primary care systems. Potential indicators of success in this regard would be inclusion of the topic in national patient safety programmes or through pay-for-performance or quality accreditation schemes, while allocation of funding for related quality improvement or research initiatives may also be a favourable outcome.

REFERENCES

1. McKay J, Bradley N, Lough M, *et al*. A review of significant events analysed in general medical practice: implications for the quality and safety of patient care. *BMC Fam Pract*. 2009; **10**: 61.
2. Elder NC, Dovey SM. Classification of medical errors and preventable adverse events in primary care: a synthesis of the literature. *J Fam Pract*. 2002, **51**(11): 927–32.
3. Jacobs S, O'Beirne M, Derflingher LP, *et al*. Errors and adverse events in family medicine: developing and validating a Canadian taxonomy of errors. *Can Fam Physician*. 2007; **53**(2): 271–6, 270.
4. Health Foundation. *Evidence Scan: levels of harm in primary care*. London: Health Foundation; 2011. Available at: www.health.org.uk/publications/levels-of-harm-in-primary-care/ (accessed 10 May 2013).
5. Makeham MA, Kidd MR, Saltman DC, *et al*. The Threats to Australian Patient Safety

(TAPs) study: incidence of reported errors in general practice. *Med J Aust.* 2006; **185**(2): 95–8.

6. Elder NC, Graham D, Brandt E, *et al.* The testing process in family medicine: problems, solutions and barriers as seen by physicians and their staff. A study of the American Academy of Family Physicians' National Research Network. *J Patient Saf.* 2006; **2**(1): 25–32.

7. Bird S. Missing test results and failure to diagnose. *Aust Fam Physician.* 2004; **33**(5): 360–1.

8. Poon EG, Gandhi TK, Sequist TD, *et al.* 'I wish I had seen this test result earlier!' Dissatisfaction with test result management systems in primary care. *Arch Intern Med.* 2004; **164**(20): 2223–8.

9. Elder NC, McEwen TR, Flach JM, *et al.* Management of test results in family medicine offices. *Ann Fam Med.* 2009; **7**(4): 343–51.

10. Mold JW. Management of laboratory test results in family practice: an OKPRN study. *J Fam Pract.* 2000; **49**(8): 709–15.

11. Bird S. A GP's duty to follow up test results. *Aust Fam Physician.* 2003; **32**(1–2): 45–6.

12. Hickner JM, Fernald DH, Harris DM, *et al.* Issues and initiatives in the testing process in primary care physician offices. *Jt Comm J Qual Patient Saf.* 2005; **31**(2): 81–9.

13. Kljakovic M. Patients and tests: a study into understanding of blood tests ordered by their doctor. *Aust Fam Physician.* 2012; **41**(4): 241–3.

14. National Patient Safety Agency. *Seven Steps to Patient Safety for Primary Care.* London: NPSA; 2005.

15. Health Foundation. *Evidence Scan: improving safety in primary care.* London: Health Foundation; 2011. Available at: www.health.org.uk/publications/improving-safety-in-primary-care/ (accessed 10 May 2013).

16. Clinical Pathology Accreditation (UK). *Standards for EQA Schemes in Laboratory Medicine.* Sheffield: CPA; 2004. Available at: www.cpa-uk.co.uk/files/PD-EQA-Standards_4.02_Dec_2004.pdf (accessed 10 May 2013).

17. Golafshani N. Understanding reliability and validity in qualitative research. *Qualitative Report.* 2003; **8**(4): 597–607.

18. Jones J, Hunter D. Qualitative research: consensus methods for medical and health services research. *BMJ.* 1995; **311**(7001): 376–80.

19. Yaghmaei F. Content validity and its estimation. *J Med Educ.* 2003; **3**(1): 23–5.

20. Elder NC, McEwen TR, Flach JM, *et al. Creating Safety in the Testing Process in Primary Care Offices.* Rockville, MD: Agency for Healthcare Research and Quality; 2007. Available at: www.ahrq.gov/professionals/quality-patient-safety/patient-safety-resources/resources/advances-in-patient-safety-2/vol2/Advances-Elder_18.pdf (accessed 10 May 2013).

21. Hickner J. Reducing test management errors in primary care office practice. *J Patient Saf.* 2005; **1**(1): 70–1.

22. Reason J. Combating omission errors through task analysis and good reminders. *Qual Saf Health Care.* 2002; **11**(1): 40–4.

23. de Wet C, Johnson P, Mash R, *et al.* Measuring perceptions of safety climate in primary care: a cross-sectional study. *J Eval Clin Pract.* 2010, **18**(1): 135–42.

24. Apekey TA, McSorley G, Tilling M, *et al.* Room for improvement? Leadership, innovation culture and uptake of quality improvement methods in general practice. *J Eval Clin Pract.* 2011; **17**(2): 311–18.

25. Bosk CL, Dixon-Woods M, Goeschel CA, *et al.* The art of medicine: reality check for checklists. *Lancet.* 2009, **374**(9688): 444–5.
26. De Savigny D, Adam T, editors. *Systems Thinking for Health Systems Strengthening.* Geneva: Alliance for Health Policy and Systems Research, WHO; 2009.

CHAPTER 30

Never Events

Carl de Wet, Catherine O'Donnell & Paul Bowie

This chapter defines the term 'Never Event' and summarises the origins and potential usefulness of this new approach to improve safety in primary care. Specific criteria to help select appropriate Never Events for the general practice setting are proposed. A validated preliminary list of Never Events recently developed for this setting through a range of consensus building methods is then reported. Finally, specific challenges associated with the Never Event concept are considered and its potential application for managing risk in general practice is explored.

WHAT IS A NEVER EVENT?

The current definition of a Never Event is 'a serious, largely preventable patient safety incident that should not occur if the available preventable measures were implemented by healthcare workers'.[1] An unambiguous example of a Never Event in the acute hospital context is performing a surgical procedure on the wrong limb. Therefore, the rationale for devising and implementing lists of Never Events in healthcare is to mitigate or eliminate the risks associated with these types of serious but preventable occurrences.

Never Events were conceived in the United States following legislation in 2006 that constrained hospitals' ability to financially charge a medical insurer or patient for eight selected 'higher-paid diagnosis-related' groups if certain clinical complications were to occur.[2] These clinical groups were selected from the list of 'serious reportable events' and became known as Never Events – a phrase coined because of its 'extra psychological charge'.[3]

Evidence is now emerging that the Never Event approach is associated with improved patient care safety in selected clinical settings.[4–8] More specifically, the Never Events approach is thought to confer at least four benefits.

1. Awareness of highly important patient safety issues is increased among the healthcare workforce.
2. Front-line organisations and teams can implement preventive measures, thereby proactively improving healthcare safety.
3. Local healthcare organisations can alert front-line care workers and teams

of Never Event policies and work with them to put in place preventive strategies – for example, by the promotion and introduction of surgical 'time outs' and checklists to help prevent wrong-site surgery.
4. It demonstrates accountability to patients and the public through acknowledging and dealing with potentially serious patient safety incidents.

THE NEVER EVENT APPROACH IN SECONDARY CARE

Patient safety in healthcare is now a global concern because of mounting evidence, particularly in acute hospital settings, that patients are unintentionally but frequently harmed in situations often judged to have been preventable. Such events are difficult, sometimes harrowing, and when extreme they can result in political responses, organisational change and widespread media reporting, such as observed during and after the recent Francis Inquiry into the deaths at the Mid Staffordshire Hospitals NHS Trust.[7] In response, many countries, including the United Kingdom (UK), have devised and implemented national improvement strategies to reduce avoidable harm,[8,9] including the introduction of policies to help prevent Never Event occurrences.[10]

Most Never Event policies have four main requirements:
1. mandatory reporting of a specified incident (Never Event) when it occurs
2. a rigorous, organisational-level investigation to determine why the incident occurred and to identify associated risk factors
3. a responsibility to act on the findings and initiate changes to prevent a recurrence
4. an apology to the patient concerned, where appropriate.

Never Event lists and policies have now been developed and implemented for acute hospital settings in many national healthcare systems, including the NHS in England and Wales,[10] and increasingly for specific settings and clinical disciplines.[11–14] Never Event policies are also in place for some community-based settings, such as home care agencies[15] and community nursing.[16]

NEVER EVENTS AND GENERAL PRACTICE

Given the reported benefits of Never Event policies in acute hospital care, and the growing recognition of the need for patient safety to be at the forefront of care delivery in general practice,[17] NHS Education for Scotland recently identified the need to pilot the Never Event approach in the general practice setting. The initial aims were informed by the design and implementation strategy applied in acute care:
● to define criteria to identify suitable Never Events for general practice
● to develop and validate a preliminary list of Never Events for this setting.

To achieve these aims, a range of consensus building methods was used with front-line general practice staff (345 general practice team members, made up of 243 general practitioners, 23 practice nurses and 79 practice managers), a group of 'informed' staff (n = 15) and a UK-wide panel of patient safety experts (n = 17). The methods included qualitative generation of potential Never Events; a consensus-building workshop; a modified Delphi exercise; and a content validation exercise.[18]

Never Event criteria

The criteria to identify general practice Never Events are shown in Box 30.1. The National Patient Safety Agency's five criteria for defining Never Events in acute hospital and mental health settings[19] were used to inform the development process, which involved participation by a multidisciplinary group of clinical, managerial and administrative primary care staff with leadership roles in patient safety initiatives across Scotland.

BOX 30.1 Criteria to identify general practice Never Events[18]

A Never Event:
1. is known to cause severe harm to a patient, or has the potential to do so
2. is preventable by the healthcare professional, team or organisation
3. can be clearly and precisely defined
4. can be detected
5. is not the result of an unlawful act.

Criterion 5 refers to 'unlawful acts', which may include, for example, accessing medical records without a clinical reason, misappropriating controlled drugs, ignoring a patient's living will or working while intoxicated. While these incidents are clearly undesirable and should ideally 'never' happen, they are excluded from a list of *preventable* Never Events. If we consider the example of 'working while intoxicated', exclusion from the list is justified for the following three specific reasons.
1. Unlawful incidents, such as this one, are violations (*deliberate* actions that are inconsistent with rules or recommended practice that should be familiar to a healthcare worker) rather than human error (the *unintentional* result of choosing the wrong plan to achieve an aim, or not initiating or completing the right plan as intended).
2. Never Events should, by definition, be preventable in every single instance by every organisation. While organisations may do much to detect and support healthcare workers with substance abuse problems, they cannot influence every individual's decision.
3. The main benefits of a Never Event policy are reporting, analysing and learning from an incident, to safeguard against its future occurrence. There are already existing organisational policies to deal appropriately with this type of incident.

Preliminary Never Event list

Given the inherent subjectivity and emotive potential of the Never Event concept, the final list (*see* Box 30.2) was refined and validated through consensus-building methods, by two different groups of experts and in two stages. Prescribing issues are a major contributor to the list, which is not surprising, as medication-related errors are a known major threat to patient safety in general practice.[20]

BOX 30.2 Preliminary list of Never Events for UK general practice[18]

1. Prescribing a drug to a patient that is recorded in the practice system as having previously caused him or her a severe adverse reaction
2. A planned referral of a patient, prompted by clinical suspicion of cancer, is not sent
3. Prescribing a teratogenic drug to a patient known to be pregnant (unless initiated by a clinical specialist)
4. Emergency transport is not discussed or arranged when admitting a patient as an emergency
5. An abnormal investigation result is received by a practice but is not reviewed by a clinician
6. Prescribing aspirin for a patient ≤12 years old (unless recommended by a specialist for specific clinical conditions, e.g. Kawasaki's disease)
7. Prescribing systemic oestrogen-only hormone replacement therapy for a patient with an intact uterus
8. Prescribing methotrexate daily rather than weekly (unless initiated by a specialist for a specific clinical condition, e.g. leukaemia)
9. A needle-stick injury due to a failure to dispose of 'sharps' in compliance with national guidance and regulations
10. Adrenaline (or equivalent) is *not* available when clinically indicated for a medical emergency in the practice or GP home visit.

This list is considered 'preliminary' for the following three reasons.
1. It is likely that there are other Never Events than those in Box 30.2 that were not considered.
2. The final selected Never Events may not be acceptable to everyone.
3. It is the first known list of Never Events for this setting.

However, while the list may be preliminary, and the incidence of these specific Never Events and their likelihood of occurrence are currently unknown, all of them have the potential for catastrophic consequences for some patients and any systematic approach to reducing their occurrence must therefore be valuable. In addition, even though they were generated in the UK, the identified items are generic and have international relevance. Finally, another potential benefit of having this preliminary list is that it makes it possible to proceed to the next stages of testing the Never Event approach in general practice. Research is currently under way to determine the incidence of Never Events, develop feasible and universally applicable preventive strategies and determine the overall utility of this approach as a safety improvement intervention.

PRACTICAL APPLICATION AND POTENTIAL CHALLENGES

At least three main concerns about secondary care Never Event policies remain unresolved. It is worth considering these concerns in more detail, as they may be equally valid in general practice. The first concern is that some Never Events included on current lists may not be preventable in every instance, despite the best efforts, intentions and adherence to clinical guidelines of the healthcare workforce and organisations.[4,21,22] For example, specific patient characteristics such as obesity, age, diabetes mellitus and other co-morbidities have been found to be independent risk factors that increase the chance of Never Events occurring. It is also known that patients in teaching hospitals and those undergoing certain high-risk surgical procedures are at greater risk of experiencing a Never Event. The implication is that those healthcare providers who care for more vulnerable patients and perform more high-risk procedures, or have better systems of error detection and reporting, may paradoxically be penalised disproportionately and unfairly.

One of the definitional criteria (*see* Box 30.1) is that a Never Event in general practice is preventable through implementation of existing interventions available to all at-risk clinicians and teams. There is emerging evidence of mitigation or reduction of patient safety incidents in some of the safety-critical areas of healthcare where Never Events were selected – for example, prescribing issues[23] and management of investigation results.[24] However, it is currently unclear whether all of the Never Events in the preliminary list (*see* Box 30.2) are truly preventable, or which of the available interventions will be most acceptable, feasible and useful to front-line staff.

A second concern pertains to the proliferation and 'broadening' of the Never Events concept.[25] The Centers for Medicare and Medicaid Services have expanded their original list in the United States, as has the Department of Health in England. For example, the number of Never Events in the England policy has increased from eight to 25 over a 3-year period from 2009. The potential risk is that the core essence of the Never Event concept as a means of focusing attention on relatively rare but serious patient safety incidents may be diluted in this process. This seeming tension between 'worthy goals' and 'overzealous application' requires careful consideration to agree an acceptable compromise,[25,26] and it should also be considered in relation to the primary care setting.

A third concern is that Never Event policies may have unintended and unwanted consequences. The following points are some examples.

- 'Overzealous' application of the Never Event approach may reduce tertiary centres' incentive to treat high-risk patients.

- 'Punitive' policies reduce the quality and frequency of incident reporting and may lead to organisations providing incomplete data or adopting alternative metrics favouring positive outcomes.
- Patient safety incidents are only considered Never Events if patients develop them during their healthcare journey. Therefore, there is an imperative to indiscriminately screen for venous thromboembolism, or organisms associated with healthcare-acquired infections, or any other potential 'Never Event' at first presentation, irrespective of clinical presentation.
- Efforts to prevent Never Events may divert resources, lead to 'improvement fatigue' among the healthcare workforce and have high opportunity costs, given the relative rarity of some incidents.
- Never Event lists may become synonymous with medical negligence.[26-30]

In addition to these concerns, there are a number of important challenges to be overcome if the Never Event approach is to be successfully implemented in general practice. For example, how do you enforce mandatory reporting in general practice settings where engagement in voluntary incident reporting systems is minimal and inconsistent?[31] A second challenge is whether the specified Never Events can be detected reliably by every general practice. Recent research on the effort required to identify adverse events shows, unsurprisingly, that the rarer the event, the greater the number of patient records to be reviewed to identify such events.[32] Other challenges include determining who should be responsible for implementation of such a policy and how this would be resourced, promoted and prioritised.

SUMMARY POINTS
- 'Never Event' lists are used in many secondary care settings in the UK and internationally as part of efforts to improve patient safety.
- A Never Event list provides a potential new approach to engage front-line staff in explicitly considering and acting on a range of safety-critical issues that may cause avoidable harm to patients in general practice.
- Criteria have been developed to define Never Events in general practice, and this has helped to generate a validated preliminary list.
- This preliminary list is an important first step in determining the potential value of the Never Event approach as a safety improvement intervention in general practice.

REFERENCES
1. Department of Health. *The 'Never Events' List for 2011/12*. London: Department of Health; 2011.
2. Milstein A. Ending extra payment for 'Never Events': stronger incentives for patients' safety. *N Engl J Med*. 2009; **360**(23): 2388-90.
3. National Quality Forum. *Serious Reportable Events*. Washington, DC: NQF; 2013.

Available at: www.qualityforum.org/Topics/SREs/Serious_Reportable_Events.aspx (accessed 5 April 2013).

4. Lohse GR, Leopold SS, Theiler S, *et al.* Systems-based safety intervention: reducing falls with injury and total falls on an orthopaedic ward. *J Bone Joint Surg Am.* 2012; **94**(13): 1217–22.

5. Rosenthal K. Targeting 'Never Events'. *Nurs Manage.* 2008; **39**(12): 35–8.

6. Gillen S. Procedures and training review aims to bring an end to 'Never Event'. *Nurs Stand.* 2012; **26**(52): 12–13.

7. Francis R. *Independent Inquiry into Care Provided by Mid Staffordshire NHS Foundation Trust January 2005 – March 2009.* Volume 1. London: The Stationery Office; 2010.

8. www.scottishpatientsafetyprogramme.scot.nhs.uk/programme

9. Health Foundation. *Learning Report: safer patients initiative.* London: Health Foundation; 2011.

10. Keogh SB, Beasley DC. Policy update: Never Events. *Nurs Times.* 2011; **107**(23): 12–13.

11. Kwong LM. Never events and related quality measures following total hip and total knee replacement. *Orthopedics.* 2010; **33**(11): 838.

12. Murphy RX Jr, Peterson EA, Adkinson JM, *et al.* Plastic surgeon compliance with national safety initiatives: clinical outcomes and 'Never Events'. *Plast Reconstr Surg.* 2010; **126**(2): 653–6.

13. Jaryszak EM, Shah RK, Amling J, *et al.* Pediatric tracheotomy wound complications. *Arch Otolaryngol Head Neck Surg.* 2011; **137**(4): 363–6.

14. Simpson KR. Obstetrical 'Never Events'. *MCN Am J Matern Child Nurs.* 2006; **31**(2): 136.

15. Suter P. Home care agencies take note: the herald of CMS 'Never Events'. *Home Healthc Nurse.* 2008; **26**(10): 647–8.

16. Lomas C. PCT leads by example on community 'Never Events'. *Nurs Times.* 2010; **106**(23): 1.

17. Healthcare Improvement Scotland. *Scottish Patient Safety Programme in Primary Care.* Edinburgh: Healthcare Improvement Scotland; 2012. Available at: www.healthcare improvementscotland.org/programmes/patient_safety/patient_safety_in_primary_ care.aspx (accessed 28 September 2012).

18. de Wet C, O'Donnell C, Bowie P. Development of a preliminary 'Never Event' list for general practice using consensus-building methods. *Br J Gen Pract.* In press.

19. National Patient Safety Agency. *Never Events Framework 2009/10.* London: NPSA; 2009.

20. Garfield S, Barber N, Walley P, *et al.* Quality of medication use in primary care: mapping the problem, working to a solution: a systematic review of the literature. *BMC Med.* 2009; **7**: 50.

21. Murphy RX Jr, Peterson EA, Adkinson JM, *et al.* Plastic surgeon compliance with national safety initiatives: clinical outcomes and 'Never Events'. *Plast Reconstr Surg.* 2010; **126**(2): 653–6.

22. Brown J, Doloresco F 3rd, Mylotte JM. 'Never Events': not every hospital-acquired infection is preventable. *Clin Infect Dis.* 2009; **49**(5): 743–6.

23. Schedlbauer A, Prasad V, Mulvaney C, *et al.* What evidence supports the use of computerized alerts and prompts to improve clinicians' prescribing behavior? *J Am Med Inform Assoc.* 2009; **16**(4): 531–8.

24. Elder NC, McEwen TR, Flach J, *et al.* The management of test results in primary care: does an electronic medical record make a difference? *Fam Med.* 2010; **42**(5): 327–33.

25. MacLeod JB. Broadening never events: is it a plausible road to improved patient safety? *Arch Surg.* 2010; **145**(2): 151–2.

26. Adetayo OA, Salcedo SE, Biskup NI, *et al.* The battle of words and the reality of never events in breast reconstruction: incidence, risk factors predictive of occurrence, and economic cost analysis. *Plast Reconstr Surg.* 2012; **130**(1): 23–9.

27. Teufack SG, Campbell P, Jabbour P, *et al.* Potential financial impact of restriction in 'Never Event' and periprocedural hospital-acquired condition reimbursement at a tertiary neurosurgical center: a single-institution prospective study. *J Neurosurg.* 2010; **112**(2): 249–56.

28. Piazza G, Goldhaber SZ. Medicare's new regulations for deep vein thrombosis as a 'Never Event': wise or worrisome? *Am J Med.* 2009; **122**(11): 975–6.

29. Thomas BW, Maxwell RA, Dart BW, *et al.* Errors in administrative-reported ventilator-associated pneumonia rates: are Never Events really so? *Am Surg.* 2011; **77**(8): 998–1002.

30. Pronovost PJ, Goeschel CA, Wachter RM. The wisdom and justice of not paying for 'preventable complications'. *JAMA.* 2008; **299**(18): 2197–9.

31. National Patient Safety Agency. *Patient Safety Incident Reports in the NHS: reporting and learning system quarterly data summary.* Issue 13. London: NPSA; 2009.

32. de Wet C, Johnson P, O'Donnell C, *et al.* Can we quantify harm in general practice records? An assessment of precision and power using computer simulation. *BMC Med Res Methodol.* 2013; **13**(39): 1–14.

Part V

Improvement Methods

CHAPTER 31

Enhanced significant event analysis

Paul Bowie, Elaine McNaughton,
Christopher Williams & David Bruce

INTRODUCTION

Significant event analysis (SEA) is well established as a safety improvement intervention in primary care in the United Kingdom (UK), particularly in general medical practice.[1] Clinicians and care teams apply the method to investigate and learn from suboptimal care or other issues of 'significance' that are highlighted for attention. The term 'significant event' is routinely used in UK primary care but its broad-based definition can denote a positive incident (e.g. a successful cardiopulmonary resuscitation attempt) or a negative incident (e.g. a prescribing error leading to avoidable harm) of 'significance' to the health-care team.[1,2]

However, the great majority of significant events (*see* Box 31.1) highlighted in general medical practice involve patient safety incidents[3,4] – circumstances where a patient was harmed (also known as an adverse event), whether physically or psychologically and regardless of severity, or could have been harmed (also known as a 'near miss'). Most practitioners also choose to forgo the opportunities to learn from 'positive' events in favour of problem-solving where things have gone wrong.[5,6]

The importance of SEA to the patient safety agenda cannot be overstated. Documentary evidence of participation is now a key element of the general practitioner (GP) specialty training curriculum and it also forms part of professional appraisal in support of medical revalidation.[2] More recently, SEA is being encouraged in the vocational training and professional development environments of general dental practice, general practice management and nursing, and community pharmacy.[7]

BOX 31.1 Examples of significant events (errors and system failures)

- Disease diagnosis and disease management (e.g. missed or delayed diagnosis of cancer, terminal care pain management)
- Prescribing, dispensing and other drug issues (e.g. wrong or inappropriate drug prescribed or administered, warfarin issue)
- Patient and relatives (e.g. patient behaviour, anger or upset)
- Investigations and results (e.g. incorrect results given to patient, results not acted upon)
- Communication (e.g. lack of communication, unsuccessful communication, inadequate communication)
- Administration (e.g. complaint, breach of protocol)
- Medical records and confidentiality (e.g. breach of confidentiality, wrong records accessed)
- Home visits and external care (e.g. delay in arrival, visit request not done)
- Equipment (e.g. computer search facility ineffective, difficulty accessing cupboard containing medical supplies)

Taking part in SEA prompts the care team to hold regular structured meetings to prioritise and reflect on events that are recognised as being opportunities for improvement and helps them to identify learning needs and plan effective action. Importantly, when undertaken constructively, it provides a forum for meaningful reflection, discussion and analysis in what should be a non-threatening and empathic environment. If done well, SEA can enhance team working and morale, and improve communication and understanding between team members, all of which helps to build a more positive safety culture in GP surgeries.[2,5,6]

However, there is strong evidence to suggest that many investigations into safety incidents in primary care are poorly conducted.[2,3,6] At least two key issues contribute to this problem. First, for clinicians and others, being involved in a significant event is similar to receiving a form of negative feedback. The subsequent emotional reaction to this type of feedback can interfere with the personal ability to assimilate and process the information beyond the 'self' level,[8,9] thereby potentially impeding an objective and constructive approach to significant events and their analyses.

Further complications are that the health and emotional well-being of clinicians involved in these types of events can suffer (the so-called 'second victim' syndrome) leading to increased stress and anxiety levels and feelings of guilt, helplessness, frustration and anger.[10,11] Additionally, a prevailing 'blame culture' is widely perceived within healthcare, which impacts on the preparedness of clinicians to highlight patient safety issues because of concerns about punitive action and professional embarrassment.[12] The implications are that many are highly selective in the types of safety incidents they raise for team-based discussion and analysis, potentially ignoring those of a complex, serious or highly sensitive nature and opting instead for less-controversial examples, or even for non-engagement in this learning activity overall.[5]

Second, a structured analytical framework that can be used as a guiding prompt by primary care teams when reviewing significant events is lacking. Although there is strong engagement with SEA in primary care, the evidence for its impact on improving the quality and safety of patient care is mixed.[2] The standard of reflection and critical analyses of such events is poor in a substantial proportion of SEAs undertaken by primary healthcare teams, with most lacking a necessary understanding of the systems and organisational factors contributing to these incidents. Indeed, a recent review of SEA reports shows that most clinicians tend to view the causes of incidents as being mainly attributable to their own actions,[3] which can be contrary to human error theory.[13]

Consequently there are multiple implications associated with what is highly likely to be a routine everyday occurrence in UK and international primary care settings, including numerous missed opportunities for individual, team-based and wider organisational learning from patient safety incidents to minimise the risks of recurrence; wasted time, efforts and financial resources associated with participating in (frequently predictable) suboptimal learning and improvement efforts; and the impact on stress and sickness levels among the primary care workforce, not least of which is the longer-term impact on the psychological well-being of healthcare professionals.[14]

There is a pressing need, therefore, to consider the emotional barriers faced by the individual when raising a significant event, and to apply an integrated team-based human factors approach to the analysis of errors.[13,15] Reflecting on and incorporating these concepts offers the practice team a means to differentiate between the personal and systems-levels factors at play, while this deeper understanding of why significant events can often happen should also go some way to deflecting the potential to 'blame' individuals. Building on over a decade's experience in this area, this chapter describes the recent development work of the NHS Education for Scotland primary care team (in partnership with the UK Health Foundation) in designing an *enhanced* SEA method based on human factors systems principles.

ADDRESSING THE PERSONAL IMPACT OF THE SIGNIFICANT EVENT (INDIVIDUAL LEVEL)

Being involved in a significant event is often an opportunity for healthcare professionals to learn and enhance patient safety. The research evidence suggests that the application of 'human factors systems' knowledge enhances performance in the workplace and improves understanding of the complex interactions that contribute to significant events.[13,15] A simple way to view the discipline of 'human factors' is to think about the interactions between three work-related factors – people, activity and the environment – and how they combine to impact on people's health and safety-related behaviour (*see* Figure 31.1).

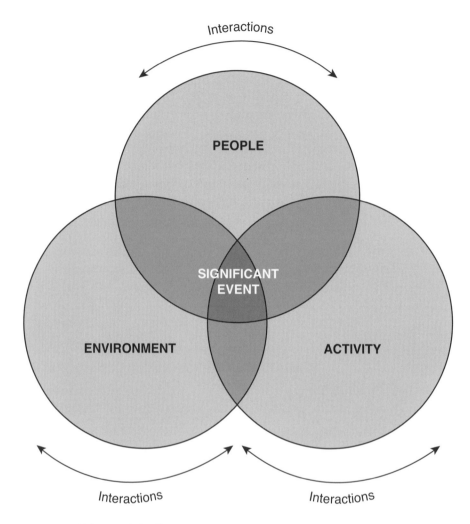

FIGURE 31.1 Enhanced significant event analysis human factors systems framework

It is important for healthcare professionals to think through how they feel about their involvement in a significant event, which may make effective analysis of the event potentially difficult. Responses such as feeling anxious, stressed, angered or indifferent are all known to affect those individuals directly involved in safety incidents.[10–12] However, by reflecting on these responses using a systems-based human factors approach, individuals can achieve a better readiness to analyse and learn from the significant event more effectively.

How an individual healthcare professional feels about a significant event influences how they think and what they do. They may feel upset, lacking in confidence, 'strangely neutral', or think this is an important opportunity to improve patient care. It is perfectly normal for individuals to feel some degree of personal responsibility for a significant event. However, human error theory suggests that significant events are rarely fully related to the actions of a single healthcare professional. Research on SEAs in primary care shows that there are often wider work-based 'contributory factors' that combine to cause the incident (*see* Table 31.1).[3]

TABLE 31.1 Examples of contributory factors that often combine to cause significant events

People	Activity	Environment
Individual, e.g. physical, psychological, personality or social issues; cognitive factors, competence, skills, attitudes, risk perception, training issues	**Complexity of work process or task, guidelines, policies and procedures**, e.g. not up to date, not available, unclear or unusable, not followed	**Work setting**, e.g. staffing, environmental conditions, workload or hours of work, design of physical environment, administrative and/or time factors
Team, e.g. roles, support, communication, leadership	**Design or organisation of work process or system**, e.g. level of complexity, workload, poor design	**Organisational**, e.g. safety culture, priorities, external risks, organisational structure
Patient, e.g. clinical condition, physical, social, psychological, relationship factors	**Equipment**, e.g. positioning, not available, not working, not calibrated, usability issues	**Communication**, e.g. verbal, written, non-verbal systems, poor communication, failure to communicate
Others, e.g. other health and social services		**Education and training**, e.g. supervision, competence, availability/accessibility, appropriateness
		Societal, cultural and regulatory influences

APPLYING A HUMAN FACTORS SYSTEMS FRAMEWORK (TEAM LEVEL)

Human factors science helps explain workplace interactions that contribute to significant events. Focusing SEA meetings on the three contributory factors outlined may identify work tasks, practice systems and organisational issues that need to be (re)designed and improved, thereby reducing future risks. The personal impact of an event on the individual healthcare professional may impede its analysis; therefore, it is very important that everyone considers their feelings about the event and is sensitive to, and supportive of, all colleagues. Prior to the SEA meeting, a decision should be made on who should lead the analysis (normally the person who raised the issue) and who should take notes of the meeting, the conclusions reached and the actions agreed. The draft SEA report (*see* Box 31.2) should be distributed for comment and final agreement among those present. The case study outlined here is a worked example of how a significant event can be analysed using the human factors systems framework.

The significant event[16]

A GP surgery decided to have their health visitor trained to administer childhood immunisations to ease their practice nurse's workload. The health visitor started working under the supervision of another qualified health visitor after

---

BOX 31.2 Recommended enhanced SEA report format (headings and subheadings)

1. About the significant event
- Describe what happened
- What the impact or potential impact of the event was

2. Contributory human and systems factors
- Outline the different People, Activity and Environment factors involved and how these combined to contribute to *why* the event happened

3. Lessons learned
- Describe the lessons learned from the event analysis
- Describe the learning needs identified at the individual, care team and organisational levels

4. Action plan for improvement
- Describe how the chances of the event happening again are now minimised
- Describe who is responsible for ensuring agreed actions are implemented and how these will be monitored and sustained

---

completing her training. A 3-month-old girl attended one of the 'new' immunisation clinics to receive her second booster. The clinic was very busy. The MMR and DTP/Hib vaccinations were placed on the same table. The health visitor picked up the 'wrong' vial while attempting to answer some of the mother's general questions and accidentally administered the MMR rather than the required DTP/Hib vaccine. She realised her error when performing the 'double-check' of the vial *after* administering the vaccine. The health visitor immediately informed the GP and the parents and apologised for '*my accident*'. The GP and the health visitor contacted the local hospital paediatric department to check for likely complications and reassessed the child on several further occasions. The child did not suffer any harm and received the appropriate vaccinations a few days later.

The actual and potential impacts

The event resulted in distressed parents and staff and the potential (low) risk of harm to the baby. There was a need to access expert advice on risks and there was the potential for a complaint to be made as well as adverse media publicity and a breakdown in the doctor–family relationship. Additionally, there was a need to apologise verbally and in writing to the parents and to offer reassurance. There was also the inconvenience for the family of having to return to the practice for the appropriate vaccination on another day.

People factors

- The health visitor had just finished her training. She had adequate knowledge but she required additional experience and supervision.
- She was distracted during the process by questions asked by the parents.
- The second health visitor had assumed the correct vaccine would be administered.
- Staff felt under pressure because of the busy workload.
- Staff can go into an 'automatic pilot' mode of working (a cognitive mechanism known as involuntary automaticity), whereby the problem is not making errors but missing them.[17]

Activity factors

- There was only one table for all vaccines and the room was too small to accommodate healthcare workers, the patient and several family members.
- The different vaccines were placed in close proximity.
- The different vaccines looked very similar.
- High volume of patients and vaccines.

Environment factors

- Increased workload resulted in the decision to create new roles and duties.
- Efficiency savings resulted in different age groups attending a combined

Learning issues (individual and practice level)	Action plan (system improvements)
- The existing immunisation system failed to properly protect the safety of a child – no formal, reliable system was in place. - Because of this system flaw, human error was inevitable. - Staff administering vaccinations should be empowered to develop, implement and follow a systems based protocol. - There was a lack of communication between staff and between staff and parents. - The combined clinics and volume of associated workload contributed to the error. - An assumption was made that the immunisation training body would have developed a protocol and would be responsible for this. - Responsibility and liability is a practice issue.	- The practice sent a written apology to the family and informed them that an investigation led to a new immunisation system being introduced. - A system protocol was developed, laminated and placed in the room used for immunisations. It was added to the practice protocols folder and the new staff induction pack. - In the fridge, one designated and clearly marked shelf would hold all the childhood vaccinations. - A wall-mounted sign was introduced to remind staff to keep work surfaces uncluttered to provide a good overview of different vaccines, which should be clearly separated. - Separate designated immunisation clinics were introduced to allow more time for vaccination and recording. - The issue will be monitored at SEA meetings until the new system is embedded in routine practice.

clinic for different types of vaccination, rather than vaccination-specific clinics.

- Lack of a formal protocol outlining the system for the safe management of the whole vaccination process, including double-checking with a colleague and the patient or carer.
- The practice wrongly assumed that the local primary care organisation would have trained both health visitors to develop and follow a relevant protocol.

BARRIERS IMPEDING SUCCESS

A recent review of the SEA evidence[2] suggests that the following issues may hinder potential success and need to be borne in mind by care teams:

- sensitive events may provoke a barrier of defensiveness and be too uncomfortable, threatening and emotionally demanding
- the focus is often on the role of individuals rather than the weak, inadequate or missing processes and systems within the practice to minimise risks
- employed staff may feel low in the hierarchy, find it difficult to act confidently as equals and feel vulnerable in speaking out
- medical domination of meetings is possible without strong leadership and facilitation
- the process may be destructive for poorly established teams – the team dynamic may militate against the critical appraisal of care delivered
- inadequate leadership can hinder the non-threatening environment, the appropriateness of topics and the uncovering of hidden agendas
- prioritisation may focus on 'safe' events rather than on complex or serious ones to minimise embarrassment, conflict or concerns about confidentiality and litigation
- 'positive' events are rarely chosen because care teams perceive a greater challenge in resolving 'negative' events, which are more likely to initiate change and improvement.

CONCLUSION

At its core, SEA is based on sound educational principles. It is one key element among others in a 'learning organisation' that promotes an effective safety culture within the practice team and facilitates change for improvement.[18] Importantly, SEA encourages a culture of honesty in the team as well as both individual and team-based reflection. However, to make SEA a much more meaningful experience a deeper consideration of the emotional demands involved in highlighting an event (at the individual level) and the most professionally appropriate and effective way to analyse the event (at the team level) is required. Guiding the analysis using a basic human factors framework can depersonalise the incident and focus attention on the 'true' contributory factors – that is, how the complexity of tasks, processes, systems and wider organisational issues can interact with the human element in the practice to increase the risk of healthcare error.

FURTHER READING

To learn more about enhanced SEA please visit: www.nes.scot.nhs.uk/shine/.

REFERENCES

1. Pringle M, Bradley C, Carmichael C, *et al. Significant Event Auditing: a study of the feasibility and potential of case-based auditing in primary medical care.* Occasional Paper No. 70. London: Royal College of General Practitioners; 1995.
2. Bowie P, Pope L, Lough M. A review of the current evidence base for significant event analysis. *J Eval Clin Pract.* 2008; **14**(4): 520–36.
3. McKay J, Bradley N, Lough M, *et al.* A review of significant events analysed in general medical practice: implications for the quality and safety of patient care. *BMC Fam Pract.* 2009; **10**: 61.
4. Cox SJ, Holden JD. A retrospective review of significant events reported in one district in 2004–2005. *Br J Gen Pract.* 2007; **57**(542): 732–6.
5. Bowie P, McKay J, Dalgetty E, *et al.* A qualitative study of why general practitioners may participate in significant event analysis and educational peer review. *Qual Saf Health Care.* 2005; **14**(3): 185–9.
6. Bowie P, McCoy S, McKay J, *et al.* Learning issues raised by the educational peer review of significant event analyses in general practice. *Qual Prim Care.* 2005; **13**: 75–84.
7. Bradley N, Power A, Hesselgreaves H, *et al.* Safer pharmacy practice: a preliminary study of significant event analysis and peer feedback. *Int J Pharm Pract.* 2009; **17**(5): 283–91.
8. Sargeant J, Mann K, Sinclair D, *et al.* Understanding the influence of emotions and reflection upon multi-source feedback acceptance and use. *Adv Health Sci Educ.* 2008; **13**(3): 275–88.
9. Kluger AN, DeNisi A. Effects of feedback intervention on performance: a historical review, a meta-analysis, and a preliminary feedback intervention theory. *Psychol Bull.* 1996; **119**(2): 254–84.
10. Scott SD, Hirschinger LE, Cox KR, *et al.* The natural history of recovery for the healthcare provider 'second victim' after adverse patient events. *Qual Saf Health Care.* 2009; **18**(5): 325–30.
11. Wu AW, Steckelberg RC. Medical error, incident investigation and the second victim: doing better but feeling worse? *BMJ Qual Saf.* 2012; **21**(4): 267–70.
12. O'Beirne M, Sterlin P, Palacios-Derflingher L, *et al.* Emotional impact of patient safety incidents on family physicians and their office staff. *J Am Board Fam Med.* 2012; **25**(2): 177–83.
13. Reason J. *Human Error.* New York, NY: Cambridge University Press; 1990.
14. Sirriyeh R, Lawton R, Gardner P, *et al.* Coping with medical error: a systematic review of papers to assess the effects of involvement in medical errors on healthcare professionals' psychological well-being. *Qual Saf Health Care.* 2010; **19**(6): e43.
15. Carthey J, Clarke J. *Patient Safety First: implementing human factors in healthcare – 'how to'*

guide. London: Clinical Human Factors Group; 2010. Available at: www.patientsafety first.nhs.uk/ashx/Asset.ashx?path=/Intervention-support/Human%20Factors%20 How-to%20Guide%20v1.2.pdf (accessed 12 May 2013).

16. Bowie P, Pringle M. *Significant Event Audit: guidance for primary care teams.* London: National Patient Safety Agency; 2008. Available at: www.nrls.npsa.nhs.uk/ resources/?entryid45=61500 (accessed 10 November 2013).

17. Toft B, Mascie-Taylor H. Involuntary automaticity: a work-system induced risk to safe health care. *Health Serv Manage Res.* 2005; **18**(4): 211–16.

18. Health Foundation. *Research Scan: improving safety in primary care.* London: Health Foundation; 2011.

CHAPTER 32

Criterion audit

Paul Bowie, Carl de Wet & John McKay

INTRODUCTION

Over the past two decades, clinical audit has arguably been the foremost policy instrument for monitoring and improving the quality of clinical care and services in the National Health Service (NHS) in the United Kingdom (UK). Levels of participation in audit by clinicians, the cost-benefits of the activity and its actual impact on improving professional practices and patient care have been subject to much scrutiny and critical debate since its formal introduction to the NHS.[1-4]

From the outset, audit has attracted criticism because the theoretical method outlined was ill-defined and untested, contributing to confusion among participants on how it should be implemented and practised.[5-9] Inevitably, this has led to differences in approach being adopted by healthcare teams resulting in variations in the rigour and validity of the methods applied and the subsequent findings from a proportion of these audit studies.[10,11]

However, a Cochrane systematic review of 140 studies of audit and feedback use to influence health professional behaviour and patient health concluded that the overall strength of evidence for this type of approach was moderate – ranging from no or limited effect to substantial effect.[12] In terms of 'success' as a quality improvement intervention (*see* Box 32.1), this ranked highly as an effective strategy (>10% increase in appropriate care or equivalent measure) compared with many other approaches.[13]

In general practice, there is good evidence (via external review by trained peer colleagues) that many general practitioners (GPs) (qualified and in training) can implement a defined method of criterion-based audit and successfully demonstrate potentially sustainable improvements in patient care, although a significant proportion can struggle with this approach.[10,11]

BOX 32.1 Factors associated with effective audit and feedback[12]

- The health professionals are not performing well to start out with
- The person responsible for the audit and feedback is a supervisor or colleague
- It is provided more than once
- It is given both verbally and in writing
- It includes clear targets and an action plan

CRITERION-BASED AUDIT

Criterion-based clinical audit is a widely accepted method for monitoring, assessing and improving care quality,[14] particularly in UK general practice, where a defined method was developed and successfully implemented by Lough and colleagues.[15] The method is strongly influenced by Donabedian's[16,17] theoretical approach to improving the quality of healthcare, which advocates focusing on measuring and evaluating aspects of healthcare in one or more of three areas: (1) structure (e.g. number of practice nurses or daily appointment capacity); (2) process (e.g. compliance with the different recommendations of a clinical guideline or Quality and Outcomes Framework target); and (3) outcomes (e.g. improved health status or patient satisfaction).

Demonstrating the ability to improve patient care by applying audit method is a lifelong expectation for all GPs and other clinicians. Audit is a mainstay of *Good Medical Practice* and a key part of quality improvement in support of GP appraisal and medical revalidation.[18] In general practice audit is known to be an effective improvement tool when it is applied robustly and with a strong mix of leadership and team involvement. Research strongly suggests that small, highly focused audits often lead to a much better chance of meaningful improvements in patient care being implemented and sustained.[10,12]

THE AUDIT CYCLE

The audit cycle or loop is the traditional theory behind the method that is followed when carrying out an audit project (*see* Figure 32.1). There are a number of different stages to the audit cycle and all of them must be closely followed to enable a successful audit outcome. Failure to do so invariably leads to an audit project being left incomplete or abandoned altogether.

CHOOSING AN AUDIT TOPIC

This is a very important first step. The aim is to achieve consensus within the practice that the chosen topic for audit is a worthwhile area to study – that is, you are unsure of current practice in that area or there is agreement that this is an area where practice could be greatly improved. Choosing a topic in an area where you know that performance is 'strong' may result in you being unable

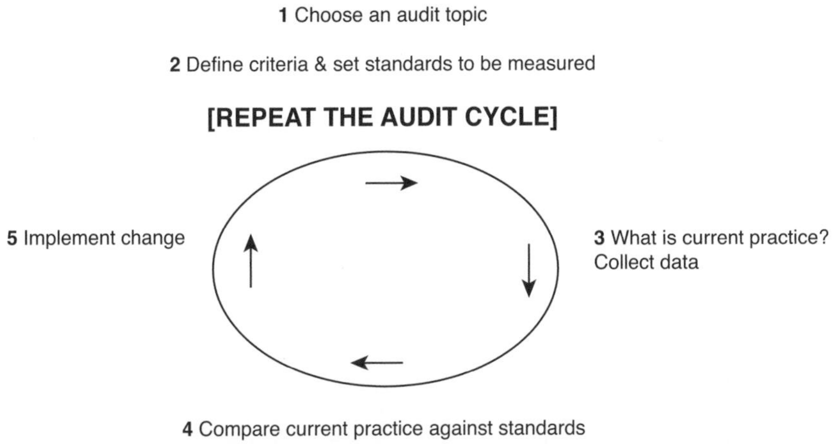

1 Choose an audit topic

2 Define criteria & set standards to be measured

[REPEAT THE AUDIT CYCLE]

5 Implement change

3 What is current practice?
Collect data

4 Compare current practice against standards

FIGURE 32.1 The audit cycle

to identify opportunities for change or further cycles of data collection, leading to an incomplete project.

Undertaking an audit project in isolation from colleagues will potentially lead to a number of difficulties and should be avoided at all costs – for example, staff or colleagues may not be as keen to help with data collection if they feel uninvolved or suspect that the audit has been imposed on them. Difficulties, or even hostility, can be experienced in getting others to change practice in light of your audit findings, if they have not been informed or involved since the start. It is extremely important, therefore, that all relevant staff are aware of what you intend to do, how you intend to do it, and are agreed at the outset that it is a worthwhile exercise and are willing to support you.

It cannot be stressed highly enough that keeping your audit projects short, simple and easily manageable is critical to success.

Sampling issues

Ideally, a practice would look at all the cases concerned with their chosen audit topic. This is not always feasible because of time and resource constraints. For some topics the quality of your data will not be improved by studying all the cases. If this is the case you should sample from the audit population. The sample should be small enough to allow rapid data collection and analysis, yet large enough to be representative of the population under study. Samples can be time or number driven.

- *Case number audits*: the number of cases should reflect the prevalence of the condition or therapy and be large enough to generalise from the findings to the population group being studied.
- *Time-based audits*: 1–3 months should be adequate for the majority of audits. Consider whether there may be a seasonal impact on your audit (e.g. attendance rates for flu-like symptoms are higher in winter).

EFFECTIVE AUDIT PRACTICE

We recommend following the eight-stage process outlined in this chapter when undertaking and reporting a completed audit cycle, for the following very specific reasons.

● It naturally follows the aforementioned audit cycle.
● It is validated as a 'best practice' method[10,15] to not only conduct an audit in general practice but also to assess the standard of the audit project undertaken (under the previous UK GP training system).
● Each stage becomes one of eight very obvious headings to be included in a full written report of a completed audit cycle, which allows for consistent and coherent reporting of audit findings for appraisal and other purposes.

UNDERTAKING AND REPORTING AN AUDIT PROJECT

In this section we outline how a completed audit project can be written up using the validated template provided. A description of what should happen at each stage of the audit cycle is illustrated with practical examples. The audit report should be structured according to eight recognised stages with the following headings.

1. Reason for the audit
2. Criterion or criteria to be measured
3. Setting standards
4. Preparation and planning
5. Data collection (cycle 1)
6. Change(s) to be evaluated
7. Data collection (cycle 2)
8. Conclusion

The report format can be easily adapted for audits in their third, fourth or later cycles that are still demonstrating improvement, although some may not fit the template exactly as they have successfully achieved their improvement goals after a number of short cycles and the implementation of change has successfully embedded in routine practice. Each of the stages is described in more detail here.

1. Reason for the audit

The opening section of the report should clearly explain why the audit topic was chosen and that, as a result of this choice, there is the potential for improvement to be introduced which is relevant to patients, the practice or you as an individual practitioner. Suitable topics should have some or all of the following characteristics:

● potential for healthcare improvement
● high-volume activity
● high-cost activity
● reflects national guidance, standards or audit topic criteria

- identified as a result of a patient safety incident or patient complaint or via the trigger review method of auditing the clinical records of high-risk patient groups.

POINTS TO CONSIDER WHEN WRITING UP YOUR COMPLETED AUDIT CYCLE REPORT

- Clearly indicate why and how this specific audit topic was chosen.
- Describe the perceived potential for relevant improvement and benefit to you, your practice and patients.

---

2. Criterion or criteria to be measured

Criteria are very precise, logical statements that are used to describe a definable and measurable item of healthcare, which describes quality and can be used to assess it. Confusion between the meaning and role of audit criteria and standards is often cited as problematic. Both can cause doctors and others great difficulty in understanding and putting into practice. It is of key importance to understand and differentiate between an audit 'criterion' and a 'standard', and demonstrating this clearly indicates having a basic grasp of criterion audit method.

EXAMPLES OF AUDIT CRITERIA

- Patients with a previous myocardial infarction (MI) should be prescribed aspirin (or equivalent), unless contraindicated.
- Patients with chronic asthma should be assessed at least every 52 weeks.
- Patients should wait no longer than 20 minutes in the surgery before consultation.
- The GP's medicine bag should contain a supply of in-date adrenaline.
- Surgeries should start within 5 minutes of their allotted time.
- The blood pressure of known hypertensive patients should be <140/85.

It is best to restrict the number of criteria to be measured for any given audit. Focusing on a criterion or two criteria makes data collection much more manageable and the introduction of small changes to practice much less challenging. Overall, it offers a better chance of the audit being completed successfully within a reasonable time span.

It is important that audit criteria should be backed up with quoted evidence (e.g. from a clinical guideline or a review of the relevant literature). However, depending on the topic, suitable evidence is not always readily available. In this case simply explain this, but also stress that there is agreement among your colleagues on the importance of the topic and the chosen criteria.

POINTS TO CONSIDER WHEN WRITING UP YOUR AUDIT

- Focus on a small number of criteria only
- Define each criterion as a short, precise logical statement (as in the examples given earlier)
- Justify the choice of each criterion by citing supporting evidence or the consensus agreement of professionals or colleagues

---

3. Setting standards

An audit standard quite simply describes the measurable level of care to be achieved for any particular criterion. It is unlikely that you will find actual percentage standards quoted in the literature or in clinical guidelines. You should arrive at the desired level of care (standard) by discussing and agreeing the appropriate figure(s) with colleagues. There is no hard rule about standard setting – the agreed level is based on professional judgement and this will obviously vary between practices for a variety of medical and social reasons.

EXAMPLES OF AUDIT STANDARDS

- **90%** of patients with a previous MI should be prescribed aspirin (or equivalent), unless contraindicated.
- **80%** of patients with chronic asthma should be assessed at least every 52 weeks.
- **75%** of patients should wait no longer then 20 minutes after their allotted appointment time.
- **100%** of GPs' medicine bags should contain a supply of in-date adrenaline.
- **95%** of surgeries should start within their allotted times.
- **70%** of blood pressure measurements of known hypertensive patients should be <140/85.

Agree on a standard that your practice believes to be an ideal or desired level of care and briefly explain why each standard was chosen (remember that different standards can be applied to each criterion). The standard(s) set should be outlined together with a timescale of when you expect it to be achieved (e.g. within 3 months, if that is how long you envisage to complete the audit project). In some cases you might require to set realistic targets and a timescale towards the desired standard over a longer period of time (e.g. 50% of asthmatic patients should have a management plan within 16 weeks, rising to 70% in 52 weeks, and surpassing 80% within 104 weeks). Consider the use of Plan-Do-Study-Act (PDSA) cycles to drive small systems-based improvements in the reliability of care processes in order to meet your chosen standards (*see* Chapter 34).

> **POINTS TO CONSIDER WHEN WRITING UP YOUR AUDIT**
> - Agree a desired percentage standard for each criterion.
> - Add a realistic timescale to achieve each standard.
> - Briefly explain why each standard level was agreed upon.

4. Preparation and planning

This is an important section that is often overlooked when compiling an audit report. As explained previously, audit should not be undertaken in isolation. Teamwork, leadership, communication, motivating and delegating are essential audit skills and these should be demonstrated in the project and the report. Quite simply, explain who was involved in discussing and planning the audit; how the data were identified, collected, analysed and disseminated; and who gave you assistance at any stage of the project (e.g. with a literature review or with collecting or analysing data) if this was required.

> **POINTS TO CONSIDER WHEN WRITING UP YOUR AUDIT**
> - Describe the preparation and planning involved in undertaking the audit.
> - Demonstrate evidence of teamwork, leadership and communication in the preparation and planning of the audit.

5. Data collection (cycle 1)

The initial (or baseline) data collected should be presented using simple descriptive statistics in table format or using graphs (bar charts, pie charts, run charts, and so forth). Remember to quote actual numbers (n) as well as the percentage (%). Do not quote irrelevant data (e.g. on age, gender or past medical history) if it bears no relation to your chosen audit criteria.

Example of presentation: data collection (cycle 1)				
Criterion	*Number of MI patients (n)*	*Number contraindicated (n)*	*Number of patients on aspirin*		*Standard (%)*
Patients with a previous MI should be prescribed aspirin (or equivalent), unless contraindicated	53	3	30/50	**60%**	80%

In the example provided here the initial audit shows that current practice is below the set standard. It is important to comment on the difference between the first collection of data (current practice in this area) and the standard previously set (the desired level of care).

> **POINTS TO CONSIDER WHEN WRITING UP YOUR AUDIT**
> - Summarise the relevant data and present it in a logical manner
> - Show numbers and percentages
> - Compare the initial findings against the standard and comment on the observed variation

6. Change(s) to be evaluated

The essence of audit is to change practice in order to improve the reliability of patient care and services. This section should adequately describe any changes that were discussed, agreed and introduced to practice by the team and how you believe this will lead to improved care. The role of others involved in this process should also be described. An explicit example of the change(s) – ideally systems based to ensure more effective implementation – that was introduced should be attached in evidence as an appendix to the report, where this is possible. Examples could include a new or amended protocol, guideline or flow chart that is introduced to practice, or a letter that is sent to a group of patients inviting them in for a medical review.

There are different ways in which change can be implemented. Often it is through a meaningful action plan that is agreed by the team and led by a designated individual. Another method is the aforementioned use of PDSA cycles, which requires clinicians to make a number of small, sequential changes and then evaluate their effectiveness before gradually spreading any improvements in practice to other areas.

It is also important to agree and indicate the specific review date when implemented changes are to be evaluated. This 'evaluation' involves further data collection (cycle 2) and is described here.

> **POINTS TO CONSIDER WHEN WRITING UP YOUR AUDIT**
> - Adequately describe considered change(s), when and how it was implemented and the role of involved staff.
> - Attach a practical example or evidence to illustrate the change that was introduced, where possible.

7. Data collection (cycle 2)

After change is agreed and implemented and a reasonable period of time has elapsed to allow any new practices or systems to take effect (remember to monitor progress with colleagues), then you must complete the audit cycle. The failure to complete the second audit cycle is arguably the single most common reason why many audit projects are doomed to fail. As well as being a waste of time and resources, this leads to frustration for those involved, as well as many missed opportunities to improve patient care.

Completion of the audit cycle is achieved by carrying out a second data collection in order to measure and evaluate what impact the newly introduced change has had on improving practice in the area being audited. If no change has been introduced or it has not been given enough time to take effect then there is no point in undertaking a second data collection – the findings are unlikely to show any improvement in the time that has elapsed because there has been no effective intervention.

Data from the second data collection should be presented in a similar way to the first round of data, but also include the results from data collection cycle 1 alongside your desired standard as well so that comparisons can be easily made. Remember to comment on the comparison between data collection cycles 1 and 2, and the desired standard to be achieved. If the standard is not attained, explain why you think this is the case and how you would propose to reach it in future.

Example of presentation: data collection (cycle 2)					
Criterion: patients with a previous MI should be prescribed aspirin, unless contraindicated					
Audit	Number of MI patients (n)	Number contraindicated (n)	Number of patients on aspirin(n)		Standard (%)
Data collection (cycle 1) March 2011	53	3	30/50	**60%**	80%
Data collection (cycle 2) June 2012	56	3	48/53	**94%**	80%

In this example, the second cycle of collected data shows that the practice's performance exceeded the agreed standard after the implemented changes. If the standard had not been attained, it may have been necessary for the individual or team to reflect on the reasons and consider further action, including implementation of other changes and re-evaluating performance (through a third or fourth cycle).

Once standards have been met, the practice needs to seriously consider how this improvement can be sustained and monitored. Monitoring systems usually measure performance in a small sample at regular intervals. A full audit is only undertaken if performance deteriorates.

POINTS TO CONSIDER WHEN WRITING UP YOUR AUDIT

- Compare the findings of the first and second cycle with each other and with the standards set – comment on the observed variations.
- Depending on the result, you may wish to either implement further change or implement a monitoring system.
- Comment on the potential for sustaining the improvement(s) and who will be responsible for leading on this.

8. Conclusion

The final section of the audit report should conclude by briefly summarising what the audit achieved in terms of improvement and learning. In doing this, the benefits achieved through the audit should be discussed, along with any problems encountered with the process or findings. Consideration should also be given as to how improvements in care will be sustained and whether the audit will be repeated in future and if so, when and by whom.

PEER REVIEW OF COMPLETED AUDIT CYCLE REPORTS

The method described above is routinely used in UK general practice. It is worth noting that a review of the standard of 336 criterion audit reports using this approach found a number of *'application of method'* issues which impacted on the potential for effective change and care improvement.[10,19] For example during the initial design stages of the audit, 95 projects (72%) had difficulty in adequately defining appropriate criteria to be measured against. A similar proportion (96 projects, 73%) had an issue in clearly setting defined and measurable standards of care that were linked to the relevant criteria, while 76 projects (76%) failed to document full and clear evidence of adequate preparation and planning. In total, 118 projects (89%) were judged to have an initial project design issue that effectively invalidated the remainder of the audit study.

Similarly, with regard to the adequate analysis of first audit cycle data, a methodological issue such as a failure to present any data or link data to criteria being measured was raised for 93 projects (71%). In terms of the change management associated with the audits, a total of 83 projects (63%) were judged to have failed in successfully negotiating, agreeing or implementing change that would lead to improvement. A methodological issue with the presentation of data for the second audit cycle, such as reporting data that is inconsistent with audit criteria or data presented in the first cycle, was highlighted for 100 projects (76%). In total, 119 projects (90%) were judged to have at least one methodological deficiency in the data analysis and change management stages of the audit.

SUMMARY

The evidence is clear that when criterion audit is applied by adhering to its defined methodological principles in combination with good leadership, planning and change management, then meaningful and sustainable improvements in the quality of patient care can be achieved. Clinicians in primary care now have a similar array of methods (e.g. trigger review, clinical care bundles and PDSA cycles) to choose from in the pursuit of quality improvement. All are a variation on a cyclical audit theme. None is superior, and all have limitations. The challenge is to match your improvement goals to the most feasible method for the task in hand, while ensuring that the prevailing practice culture is amenable and supportive of your care quality ambitions.

REFERENCES

1. Miles A, Bentley P, Polychronis A, *et al*. Clinical audit in the National Health Service: fact or fiction? *J Eval Clin Pract*. 1996; **2**: 29–35.

2. Lord J, Littlejohns P. Evaluating healthcare policies: the case of clinical audit. *BMJ*. 1997; **315**: 668–71.

3. Bowie P, Bradley N, Rushmer RK. Clinical audit and quality improvement: time for a rethink? *J Eval Clin Pract*. 2012; **18**(1): 42–8.

4. Hopkins A. Clinical audit: time for a reappraisal? *J R Coll Physician*. 1996; **30**: 415–25.

5. Johnston G, Crombie IK, Davies HTO, *et al*. Reviewing audit: barriers and facilitating factors for effective clinical audit. *Qual Health Care*. 2000; **9**: 23–36.

6. Nolan M, Scott G. Audit: an exploration of some tensions and paradoxical expectations. *J Adv Nurs*. 1993; **18**: 759–66.

7. Fulton R. Goals and methods of audit should be re-appraised. *BMJ*. 1996; **312**: 1103.

8. Buttery Y, Walshe K, Rumsey M. *Evaluating Audit: provider audit in England*. A review of twenty-nine programmes. London: Capse Research; 1995.

9. Tabandeh H, Thompson GM. Auditing ophthalmology audits. *Eye*. 1995; **9**(Suppl.): 1–5.

10. McKay J, Bowie P, Lough M. Variations in the ability of general medical practitioners to apply two methods of audit: a five year study of assessment by peer review. *J Eval Clin Pract*. 2006; **12**: 622–9.

11. Holden JD. Systematic review of published multi-practice audits from British general practice. *J Eval Clin Pract*. 2004; **10**(2): 247–72.

12. Ivers N, Jamtvedt G, Flottorp S, *et al*. Audit and feedback: effects on professional practice and patient outcomes. *Cochrane Summaries*. 2012 July. Available at: http://summaries.cochrane.org/CD000259/audit-and-feedback-effects-on-professional-practice-and-patient-outcomes#sthash.pBWWYf9x.dpuf (accessed 10 November 2013).

13. Scott I. What are the most effective strategies for improving quality and safety of health care? *Intern Med J*. 2009; **39**(6): 389–400.

14. Shaw CD. Criterion based audit. *BMJ*. 1990; **300**(6725): 649–51.

15. Lough JRM, McKay J, Murray TS. Audit and summative assessment: a criterion-referenced marking schedule. *Br J Gen Pract*. 1995; **45**: 607–9.

16. Donabedian A. Advantages and limitations of explicit criteria for assessing the quality of health care. *Milbank Mem Fund Q Health Soc*. 1981; **59**(1): 99–105.

17. Donabedian A. Evaluating the quality of medical care. *Milbank Q*. 2005; **83**(4): 691–729.

18. General Medical Council. *Good Medical Practice*. London: GMC; 2005.

19. Bowie P, Cooke S, Lo P, *et al*. The assessment of criterion audit cycles by external peer review: when is an audit not an audit? *J Eval Clin Pract*. 2007; **13**(3): 352–7.

CHAPTER 33

Care bundles

Carl de Wet & Paul Bowie

It is well known that a significant minority of patients do not receive all the evidence-based care recommended for their health conditions. It is thought that the quality and safety of care can be improved significantly by reducing this observed variation. The 'care bundle' approach is one method that may be particularly useful to achieve the aims of improving the reliability of evidence-based care delivery and hence clinical outcomes.[1-3] Consequently, care bundles are now being implemented in many acute hospitals and, more recently, have been piloted in general practice.

This chapter begins by answering two related questions:

1. What is a care bundle?
2. What is known about the care bundle method from existing evidence and experiences?

The application of the care bundle method in the general practice setting is then described, using practical examples. Additionally, the findings of a recent pilot study are reported and the potential of the method in this setting is discussed.

WHAT IS A CARE BUNDLE?

A care bundle is simply a small number of healthcare interventions grouped together that normally have a synergistic relationship that has an impact on clinical outcome for patients.[4] Bundles usually contain three to six components, which may include clinical interventions such as care processes, procedures or diagnostic tests, but are not deemed suitable to act as comprehensive lists of all possible care. Selection of appropriate bundle components is based on best evidence and/or local considerations and may change with time and experience.[5,6] Every individual component in the bundle should be recognised as an intervention that is routinely delivered or considered for every patient within a specified period of time. Compliance with a care bundle and its components is measured on an 'all or nothing' basis.

There are many similarities between the care bundle and the criterion-based audit method. In fact, a simple way to conceptualise a care bundle is to imagine it as a group of audit criteria. However, there are also a number of key differences.

- The care bundle method typically focuses on specific clinical areas or conditions, while the focus of audit is typically on specific processes of care.
- The care bundle involves a composite 'all or nothing' compliance measure, while criterion audits typically report singular compliance measures for individual criteria.
- The compliance with individual bundle elements determines the overall (or composite) bundle compliance, whereas the performance achieved for any given audit criterion does not affect the result of any other criterion (assuming multiple criteria were specified).
- With the care bundle method, compliance data is first aggregated at the individual patient level before considering compliance for the selected patient group, while with the criterion audit method the data are aggregated to the group level.

WHAT IS KNOWN ABOUT CARE BUNDLES FROM EXISTING EVIDENCE AND EXPERIENCES?

Rationale for the care bundle method

Wide variation in the provision of evidence-based care is recognised as a fundamental issue in all healthcare systems worldwide. The consequences of such variation often impacts negatively on patients in terms of healthcare quality, safety, experiences and increased financial costs associated with suboptimal clinical practices (including additional treatments and litigation).[7,8]

It is widely accepted that there is a need to minimise unnecessary variation to improve the reliability of best practice care provision and the associated financial costs.[8-10] Practising evidence-based medicine by implementing clinical care guidelines is strongly promoted to assist clinical decision-making and optimise management of patients, but it does not necessarily ensure that patients who should receive all appropriate care actually do so.[11-14]

Around 50% of hospital patients may receive the full recommended care and treatments that their clinical condition merits. The difference between the highest- and lowest-performing healthcare systems suggests that there is 'an enormous gap' in evidence-based (or recommended) care provision.[7,15] In primary care settings, evidence of wide variation has also been found between individual healthcare providers.[16-19]

Secondary care evidence and experience

Specific care bundles have been implemented in a range of secondary care settings, such as paediatric and adult intensive care units (ICU), medical and surgical wards and accident and emergency departments in North America and the United Kingdom (UK).[20,21] Reported clinical outcomes have included: significant reductions in healthcare-acquired infections; lower condition-specific and all-cause mortality; reduced readmission rates of elderly patients; and decreased length of ICU stay and number of ventilation days.[1,22–24] Although higher compliance rates with bundles is associated with improved outcomes,[25] these are difficult to sustain because of organisational and human–system performance factors which often results in rates below 50%.[26–28]

In UK secondary care settings, reported compliance with a variety of clinical care bundles ranges from 19% to 52%.[26,27] Low compliance rates have important safety implications, as a positive and significant association has been found between compliance rates and clinical outcomes such as mortality.[21,22,26] However, a similar association has not yet been shown for primary care. Typically, compliance with individual components tends to be high, while compliance with the overall bundle is typically low. Regular audit and timely feedback, strong leadership and improving clinician engagement can increase compliance.

Reducing variation in quality can decrease costs if the care 'gap' is large, but costs increase as the gap narrows until there is a net expense.[29] Evaluation of care bundle implementation in some secondary care settings has found them to be cost-effective.[30] However, implementing interventions requires initial financial and resource investment. For example, McNeill et al.[28] found that only 20/265 (12%) of acute medicine units in the UK had the minimum facilities to comply with the 'surviving sepsis care bundle'. Aligning care bundles with larger quality improvement initiatives and providing related training appear to be key factors that influence their success and impact.[22]

A STEP-BY-STEP GUIDE FOR APPLYING THE CARE BUNDLE METHOD IN GENERAL PRACTICE

The care bundle method is especially useful for practice teams, but individual healthcare professionals can also use it. The six sequential steps to implement (deliver) a care bundle are shown in Figure 33.1. The steps are discussed in detail here and are illustrated by clinical examples.

Step 1: Choose a topic

Some clinical topics already have suggested care bundles (*see* Box 33.1). If general practice teams decide to choose one of these, they should still consider whether it needs to be adapted for their own purposes. Alternatively, identify and bundle a number of evidence-based interventions that are applicable to a specific patient group, disease and/or setting.

EXAMPLE

The Welcome Practice team wants to further improve the care of their patients with type 2 diabetes mellitus (DM). They decide the care bundle method would be suitable for their setting and purpose.

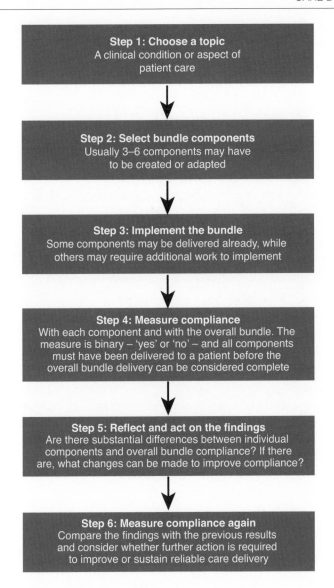

FIGURE 33.1 The six steps of the care bundle process

BOX 33.1 Examples of clinical care bundles†

Secondary prevention of coronary heart disease care bundle

This bundle should be delivered to all patients on the disease register, within appropriate time intervals.*

- *Blood pressure* should be checked and controlled to <150/90**
- *Total cholesterol* should be checked and controlled to <5 mmol/L**
- An appropriate *anticoagulant* should be prescribed regularly, unless a clear contraindication or previous adverse drug reaction has been recorded**

- A licensed *beta blocker* should be prescribed regularly, unless a clear contraindication or previous adverse drug reaction has been recorded**
- An *ACE inhibitor or Angiotensin II antagonist* should be prescribed regularly, unless a clear contraindication or previous adverse drug reaction has been recorded
- Patients should be offered the *seasonal flu vaccination*

* Some bundle components may have to be delivered frequently (every few weeks or months), depending on individual patient requirements. The time interval for delivery of medication-related bundle components is 1 to 3 months. Other components only have to be delivered once a year, hence the suggested annual bundle compliance measure.

** If a patient had been considered for the intervention but had been judged unsuitable for legitimate clinical reasons or had declined the intervention, it should be taken as 'delivered'.

Diabetes mellitus care bundle

This bundle should be delivered to all patients on the disease register, within appropriate time intervals.
- *Blood pressure* should be checked and controlled to <145/85
- *Total cholesterol* should be checked and controlled to <5 mmol/L
- A body mass index should be recorded in the medical record
- An evaluation (presence/absence) of peripheral pulses should be recorded in the medical record
- Neuropathy testing should be performed and the outcome documented in the medical record
- The HbA_{1c} should be <8 (or equivalent according to reference rage of local laboratory)
- Patients should be offered the *seasonal flu vaccination*

Chronic obstructive pulmonary disease care bundle

This bundle should be delivered to all patients on the disease register at least annually.
- Patients' FEV_1 (forced expiratory volume in the first second) should be measured and recorded
- A clinical team member should undertake a general review of the patients' care. This should include a validated *functional assessment* – for example, with the Medical Research Council dyspnoea score, an inhaler technique check and education about potential signs of an exacerbation, and the appropriate ways in which they should access care if this happens.
- Patients should be offered the *seasonal flu vaccination*

† Adapted from de Wet *et al.*[31]

Step 2: Select bundle components

Bundle components can be adapted or developed for most clinical conditions using the selection criteria in Box 33.2.

BOX 33.2 **Criteria for selecting care bundle components**

- A care bundle should relate to a specific clinical condition.
- A care bundle should have a minimum of three components.
- Care bundle components should describe a specific, measurable action.
- Delivery of every component should be possible for the practice team.
- Bundle components should be relevant to all patients with that condition.
- Components must be repeatable, rather than 'one-off' actions.
- Components should not duplicate or be a necessary part of each other.

EXAMPLE

The Welcome Practice team selects the following six components for their DM care bundle.

1. Patients should have their body mass index measured and recorded
2. Patients should have peripheral pulses examined and recorded
3. Neuropathy testing should be performed
4. A urine specimen should be tested for proteinuria
5. A fasting total serum cholesterol test should be requested and the result recorded
6. A HbA_{1c} should be requested and the result recorded in patients' records.

They agree that the bundle should be delivered to every patient with diabetes mellitus every 6 months, and that *practice compliance* with the bundle will be measured twice a year.

Step 3: Implement the bundle

It is important to differentiate between delivering the care bundle and measuring compliance with it. Measuring bundle compliance is very similar to criterion audit. The time intervals for bundle delivery and bundle measurement do not have to be the same. However, measurement intervals always have to be longer than delivery intervals.

In many cases the bundle components will describe care processes that are already being delivered by the team. If the component describes a new action, it is necessary to plan how it can best be implemented. Discuss the proposed bundle with the clinical team who will be responsible for delivering care and checking for agreement and understanding of how it will be implemented.

> **EXAMPLE**
>
> The Welcome Practice team feels confident that they are already delivering all six components of the DM care bundle. They have a dedicated diabetic clinic once a month that is led by the practice nurse.

Step 4: Measure compliance

Compliance with the overall bundle and individual components should be measured regularly. It may be helpful to consider the bundle as a series of simple yet rigorous 'checkpoints'. Each checkpoint requires a yes or no answer ('all or nothing'). A common, initial compliance standard for overall bundle is 80%, rising to 95% after successful implementation. When stated in this way, compliance can be measured using a criterion audit approach – *see* example, p. 301.

Step 5: Reflect and act on the findings

Practice teams analysing the data should compare their compliance with the standard they set. Useful questions to ask include: Which bundle component(s) had the lowest compliance? Can this be explained? How can the compliance be increased? What systems and resources are required? Is it possible to link the bundle to a clinical outcome?

> **EXAMPLE**
>
> Analysis of the first data collection shows that compliance with each component is high (85%–90%) but overall compliance is low (50%). The practice team develops a 'tick sheet' and agree to use this as a memory aid while delivering the bundle during the next 6 months.

Step 6: Measure compliance again

After any necessary changes to implementation of the bundle have been made in practice, compliance should be measured again. The team then asks whether compliance increased and increased sufficiently. How will compliance be sustained? (*See* example, p. 302.)

EXAMPLE

The team agrees the following audit criterion: 'DM patients should receive every component in the DM bundle'.

They set a standard of: '>80% of DM patients should receive every component in the DM bundle'.

They conduct their first data collection, comprising of a random sample of 20 patients from the DM register. A member of staff records whether each bundle component is present or whether it has been considered. Only if every component is present can overall compliance be assumed. A copy of their data and results is shown here.

The Welcome Practice
Diabetes Mellitus Care Bundle
15/06/2011

| Patient identifier | Bundle components | | | | | | Overall compliance |
	BMI measure	Pedal pulses screen	Neuropathy screen	Urinalysis	Cholesterol check	HbA1$_c$ check	
1001	Yes	No	No	No	No	No	No
1002	Yes	Yes	Yes	Yes	Yes	Yes	Yes
1003	Yes	Yes	Yes	Yes	No	No	No
1004	No	Yes	Yes	Yes	Yes	Yes	No
1005	Yes	Yes	Yes	No	Yes	Yes	No
1006	Yes	Yes	Yes	Yes	Yes	Yes	Yes
1007	Yes	Yes	Yes	Yes	Yes	Yes	Yes
1008	Yes	Yes	Yes	Yes	Yes	Yes	Yes
1009	Yes	Yes	Yes	Yes	Yes	Yes	Yes
1010	Yes	Yes	Yes	Yes	Yes	Yes	Yes
1011	No	Yes	Yes	Yes	Yes	Yes	No
1012	Yes	No	Yes	Yes	Yes	Yes	No
1013	Yes	No	Yes	Yes	Yes	Yes	No
1014	Yes	Yes	Yes	Yes	No	Yes	No
1015	Yes	Yes	Yes	Yes	Yes	Yes	Yes
1016	Yes	Yes	Yes	Yes	Yes	Yes	Yes
1017	Yes	Yes	Yes	Yes	Yes	Yes	Yes
1018	Yes	Yes	No	Yes	Yes	Yes	No
1019	Yes	Yes	Yes	No	Yes	Yes	No
1020	Yes	Yes	Yes	Yes	Yes	Yes	Yes
Total (n)	18	17	18	18	17	18	10
Total (%)	90	85	90	90	85	90	50

n = number of patients
Yes = component delivered to patient; No = component not delivered to patient

EXAMPLE

The practice measure component and bundle compliance again after 3 months – the results are shown here.

The Welcome Practice
Diabetes Mellitus Care Bundle
16/09/2011

Patient identifier	Bundle components						Overall compliance
	BMI measure	Pedal pulses screen	Neuropathy screen	Urinalysis	Cholesterol check	HbA1$_c$ check	
1001	Yes	Yes	Yes	Yes	Yes	Yes	Yes
1002	Yes	Yes	Yes	Yes	Yes	Yes	Yes
1003	Yes	Yes	Yes	Yes	Yes	Yes	Yes
1004	No	No	No	No	No	No	No
1005	Yes	Yes	Yes	Yes	Yes	Yes	Yes
1006	Yes	Yes	Yes	Yes	Yes	Yes	Yes
1007	Yes	Yes	Yes	Yes	Yes	Yes	Yes
1008	Yes	Yes	Yes	Yes	Yes	Yes	Yes
1009	Yes	Yes	Yes	Yes	Yes	Yes	Yes
1010	Yes	Yes	Yes	Yes	Yes	Yes	Yes
1011	No	No	No	No	Yes	Yes	No
1012	Yes	Yes	Yes	Yes	Yes	Yes	Yes
1013	Yes	No	Yes	Yes	Yes	Yes	No
1014	Yes	Yes	Yes	Yes	Yes	Yes	Yes
1015	Yes	Yes	Yes	Yes	Yes	Yes	Yes
1016	Yes	Yes	Yes	Yes	Yes	Yes	Yes
1017	Yes	Yes	Yes	Yes	Yes	Yes	Yes
1018	Yes	Yes	Yes	Yes	Yes	Yes	Yes
1019	Yes	Yes	Yes	Yes	Yes	Yes	Yes
1020	Yes	Yes	Yes	Yes	Yes	Yes	Yes
Total (n)	18	17	18	18	19	19	17
Total (%)	90	85	90	90	95	95	85

n = number of patients
Yes = component delivered to patient; No = component not delivered to patient

Compliance with individual components has improved and is now acceptable (85%–95%). The overall bundle compliance has increased markedly from 50% to 85% and fulfils their standard. Patient no. 1004 is the conspicuous exception but on review they determine he had been sent three written invitations to attend the clinic.

EXPERIENCE OF THE CARE BUNDLE METHOD IN GENERAL PRACTICE

Findings from a pilot study

A recent small study was the first known attempt to use the care bundle method to measure the composite reliability of delivered care for specific clinical conditions in UK general practice.[31] Five clinical conditions were considered suitable topics for care bundles:

1. secondary prevention of coronary heart disease
2. stroke and transient ischaemic attack
3. chronic kidney disease
4. chronic obstructive pulmonary disease
5. DM.

Each care bundle had between three and eight components, which were developed from Quality and Outcomes Framework (QOF) indicators.

A retrospective audit was undertaken in a convenience sample of nine general medical practices with a combined patient population of 56 948 in the west of Scotland. Compliance with individual QOF-based care bundle components was high, but overall ('all or nothing') compliance was substantially lower. For example, the practices' compliance with the specified DM care bundle's individual components ranged from 82.9% (DM24) to 98.5% (DM15), yet overall care bundle compliance was substantially lower, at 58.4% (range: 50.3%–65.2%). In other words, 58.4% of all eligible patients received all the care specified by the bundle and 41.6% of patients did not receive one or more care components.

The 'gap' between component and care bundle compliance

There are at least four possible reasons for the observed 'gap' between individual component and overall bundle compliance. First, some components are easier to deliver than others. Second, care bundle compliance will always have a value equal to or lower than that of the indicator with the lowest performance – consequently there will always be a gap, although it is unknown whether or when the size of the 'gap' becomes of clinical significance. Third, the 'gap' will usually increase exponentially with the rise in the number of bundle components. Finally, natural variation is inherent in all healthcare systems and will be affected by the effectiveness and efficiencies of local processes and efforts.

The Quality and Outcomes Framework and care bundles

The QOF has been described as the most ambitious, comprehensive and large 'pay for performance' scheme and quality measure in international healthcare and a 'natural experiment in progress'.[32] There are a number of valid concerns about the QOF that could similarly be raised about the care bundle method, with no clear answers at present.[32-36] For example: QOF can cause a 'street lamp effect' – that is, neglect of healthcare activity and clinical conditions that do not attract financial incentives; it can create a depersonalising 'box-ticking culture'; it is vulnerable to data distortion and potential gaming; the Framework promotes simplicity over complexity and measurability over meaningfulness.

Implementing care bundles in general practice

The care bundle method may help to better differentiate the care quality of practices, given that their current QOF scores are now broadly comparable. To implement the bundle a number of challenges would have to be overcome first, though. For example: resistance from practices who are financially disadvantaged by 'lower' measures than the current thresholds; accounting for 'natural' variation so that practices are not unfairly penalised; existing information technology systems would have to be redesigned; a full evaluation to identify both impact and unintended consequences (e.g. a proportion of patients may end up receiving 'no care') would be necessary. If this new measure is considered desirable, it would also have to be promoted and incentivised. Known incentives that facilitate increased practice participation and may be considered include financial payments, staff training and providing technical support.[37,38]

CONCLUSION

The care bundle method may provide a more reliable measure of care quality in general practice than existing methods such as QOF data, which focuses on compliance with individual indicators rather than individual patients. Applying this approach may enable practice teams to better direct improvement efforts. However, the method's acceptability, feasibility and potential impact on clinical outcomes would first have to be explored.

REFERENCES

1. Marwick C, Davey P. Care bundles: the holy grail of infectious risk management in hospital? *Curr Opin Infect Dis.* 2009; **22**(4): 364–9.
2. Resar R, Pronovost P, Haraden C, *et al.* Using a bundle approach to improve ventilator care processes and reduce ventilator-associated pneumonia. *Jt Comm J Qual Patient Saf.* 2005; **31**(5): 243–8.
3. Hitchen L. England launches scheme to encourage use of 'care bundles'. *BMJ.* 2008; **336**(7639): 294–5.
4. Haraden C. *What is a Bundle?* Cambridge, MA: Institute for Healthcare Improvement; 2011. Available at: www.ihi.org/resources/Pages/ImprovementStories/WhatIsaBundle. aspx (accessed 7 March 2014).
5. Pronovost PJ, Berenholtz SM, Ngo K, *et al.* Developing and pilot testing quality indicators in the intensive care unit. *J Crit Care.* 2003; **18**(3): 145–55.
6. Wip C, Napolitano L. Bundles to prevent ventilator-associated pneumonia: how valuable are they? *Curr Opin Infect Dis.* 2009; **22**(2): 159–66.
7. Hines S, Joshi MS. Variation in quality of care within health systems. *Jt Comm J Qual Patient Saf.* 2008; **34**(6): 326–32.
8. Moore CL, McMullen MJ, Woolford SW, *et al.* Clinical process variation: effect on quality and cost of care. *Am J Manag Care.* 2010; **16**(5): 385–92.

9. Jacobs B, Duncan JR. Improving quality and patient safety by minimizing unnecessary variation. *J Vasc Interv Radiol*. 2009; **20**(2): 157–63.

10. Selby JV, Schmittdiel JA, Lee J, *et al*. Meaningful variation in performance: what does variation in quality tell us about improving quality? *Med Care*. 2010; **48**(2): 133–9.

11. Sackett DL, Rosenberg WM, Gray JA, *et al*. Evidence based medicine: what it is and what it isn't. *BMJ*. 1996; **312**(7023): 71–2.

12. Cinel I, Dellinger RP. Guidelines for severe infections: are they useful? *Curr Opin Crit Care*. 2006; **12**(5): 483–8.

13. Cabana MD, Rand CS, Powe NR, *et al*. Why don't physicians follow clinical practice guidelines? A framework for improvement. *JAMA*. 1999; **282**(15): 1458–65.

14. Woolf SH, Grol R, Hutchinson A, *et al*. Clinical guidelines: potential benefits, limitations, and harms of clinical guidelines. *BMJ*. 1999; **318**(7182): 527–30.

15. Resar RK. Making noncatastrophic health care processes reliable: learning to walk before running in creating high-reliability organizations. *Health Serv Res*. 2006; **41**(4 Pt. 2): 1677–89.

16. Holmboe ES, Weng W, Arnold GK, *et al*. The comprehensive care project: measuring physician performance in ambulatory practice. *Health Serv Res*. 2010; **45**(6 Pt. 2): 1912–33.

17. Tsimtsiou Z, Ashworth M, Jones R. Variations in anxiolytic and hypnotic prescribing by GPs: a cross-sectional analysis using data from the UK Quality and Outcomes Framework. *Br J Gen Pract*. 2009; **59**(563): e191–8.

18. Morrison J, Anderson MJ, Sutton M, *et al*. Factors influencing variation in prescribing of antidepressants by general practices in Scotland. *Br J Gen Pract*. 2009; **59**(559): e25–31.

19. Wang KY, Seed P, Schofield P, *et al*. Which practices are high antibiotic prescribers? A cross-sectional analysis. *Br J Gen Pract*. 2009; **59**(567): e315–20.

20. Crunden E, Boyce C, Woodman H, *et al*. An evaluation of the impact of the ventilator care bundle. *Nurs Crit Care*. 2005; **10**(5): 242–6.

21. Carter C. Implementing the severe sepsis care bundles outside the ICU by outreach. *Nurs Crit Care*. 2007; **12**(5): 225–30.

22. Robb E, Jarman B, Suntharalingam G, *et al*. Using care bundles to reduce in-hospital mortality: quantitative survey. *BMJ*. 2010; **340**: 1234.

23. Koehler BE, Richter KM, Youngblood L, *et al*. Reduction of 30-day postdischarge hospital readmission or emergency department (ED) visit rates in high-risk elderly medical patients through delivery of a targeted care bundle. *J Hosp Med*. 2009; **4**(4): 211–18.

24. Duffin C. Introduction of 'care bundles' reduces patient mortality rates by 15 per cent. *Nurs Manage (London)*. 2010; **17**(2): 7.

25. Guerin K, Wagner J, Rains K, *et al*. Reduction in central line-associated bloodstream infections by implementation of a postinsertion care bundle. *Am J Infect Control*. 2010; **38**(6): 430–3.

26. Gao F, Melody T, Daniels DF, *et al*. The impact of compliance with 6-hour and 24-hour sepsis bundles on hospital mortality in patients with severe sepsis: a prospective observational study. *Crit Care*. 2005; **9**(6): R764–70.

27. Baldwin LN, Smith SA, Fender V, *et al*. An audit of compliance with the sepsis resuscitation care bundle in patients admitted to A&E with severe sepsis or septic shock. *Int Emerg Nurs*. 2008; **16**(4): 250–6.

28. McNeill G, Dixon M, Jenkins P. Can acute medicine units in the UK comply with the Surviving Sepsis Campaign's six-hour care bundle? *Clin Med.* 2008; **8**(2): 163–5.

29. Peabody JW, Florentino J, Shimkhada R, *et al.* Quality variation and its impact on costs and satisfaction: evidence from the QIDS study. *Med Care.* 2010; **48**(1): 25–30.

30. Halton KA, Cook D, Paterson DL, *et al.* Cost-effectiveness of a central venous catheter care bundle. *PLoS One.* 2010; **5**(9): pii: e12815.

31. de Wet C, McKay J, Bowie P. Combining QOF data with the care bundle approach may provide a more meaningful measure of quality in general practice. *BMC Health Serv Res.* 2012; **12**: 351.

32. Gillam S, Siriwardena AN. The quality and outcomes framework: triumph of technical rationality, challenge for individual care? *Qual Prim Care.* 2010; **18**(2): 81–3.

33. Steel N, Willems S. Research learning from the UK Quality and Outcomes Framework: a review of existing research. *Qual Prim Care.* 2010; **18**(2): 117–25.

34. Williams PH, de Lusignan S. Does a higher 'quality points' score mean better care in stroke? An audit of general practice medical records. *Inform Prim Care.* 2006; **14**(1): 29–40.

35. Subramanian DN, Hopayian K. An audit of the first year of screening for depression in patients with diabetes and ischaemic heart disease under the Quality and Outcomes Framework. *Qual Prim Care.* 2008; **16**(5): 341–4.

36. Ashworth M, Kordowicz M. Quality and Outcomes Framework: smoke and mirrors? *Qual Prim Care.* 2010; **18**(2): 127–31.

37. Walker S, Mason AR, Claxton K, *et al.* Value for money and the Quality and Outcomes Framework in primary care in the UK NHS. *Br J Gen Pract.* 2010; **60**(574): e213–20.

38. Halladay JR, Stearns SC, Wroth T, *et al.* Cost to primary care practices of responding to payer requests for quality and performance data. *Ann Fam Med.* 2009; **7**(6): 495–503.

CHAPTER 34

The Plan-Do-Study-Act method

Carl de Wet & Paul Bowie

INTRODUCTION

The Plan-Do-Study-Act (PDSA) method has its roots in Japanese car manu-facturing[1] and industrial statistical quality control.[2] Langley *et al.*[3] used PDSA as the central component of their 'Model for Improvement' and were among the first to propose the use of PDSA cycles in healthcare. More recently, the method has been popularised by the Institute of Healthcare Improvement as a key intervention in quality and safety improvement collaboratives.[4] Since then, the PDSA method has been used as a standalone intervention or as a key com-ponent of many different quality improvement (QI) programmes and projects in healthcare settings worldwide.[5-10]

This chapter begins with a summary of the PDSA method, how it is applied in practice and what potential benefits it may offer. The factors that determine the application and effectiveness of the PDSA approach are then discussed in more detail. The influential factors are classified into four main groups:

1. *Method* – duration, number and timing of cycles and characteristics of attempted actions (changes)
2. *Organisation* – size, stability, culture and leadership
3. *Practitioner* – knowledge, skills, motivation, engagement and 'ownership'
4. *Resources* – information technology, 'expert' support, training, time and money.

THE PDSA METHOD

The PDSA method is an improvement tool that can be used by individuals or teams to plan and test multiple, small and incremental changes to their eve-ryday work practices and systems in a structured manner and then evaluate the impact over time to determine whether improvements in work quality are apparent. A single PDSA cycle consists of the four steps 'Plan, Do, Study and Act', which are performed sequentially (*see* Figure 34.1).

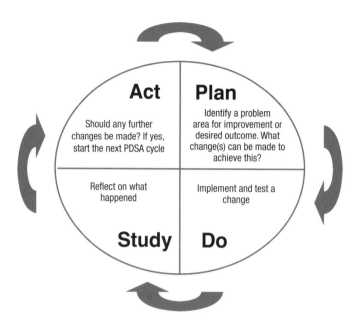

FIGURE 34.1 A single Plan-Do-Study-Act (PDSA) cycle

Most healthcare workers intuitively apply PDSA cycles regularly in their personal and professional lives without being explicitly aware they are doing so. For example, consider a general practitioner who is informed of a new drug that promises superior efficacy in treating patients with a certain disease. She gathers further information about the medication (plan), selects an appropriate patient and prescribes it (do), reviews the patient after a suitable period of time to evaluate the drug's efficacy (study) and decides whether to prescribe it again (act).

Any number of PDSA cycles can be undertaken sequentially, either to try different or adapted change interventions (potential improvements) or to increase the number of patients. Cycles often build on the results of previous efforts so that improvement gains accumulate in an incremental manner. A series of PDSA cycles relating to the same intervention or patient group is sometimes referred to as a 'ramp' (Figure 34.2). Large QI projects often make use of several 'ramps' to achieve their overall aims (Figure 34.3).

The PDSA, criterion audit and care bundle methods

Criterion audit, care bundles and PDSA are three quality improvement methods that may appear similar to healthcare professionals because of their cyclical nature. Criterion audit and care bundles are both methods that can be used to measure clinical performance and quality of care. If performance is found to fall short of a set standard, the individual or team is encouraged to implement change in order to improve care. The PDSA method is one possible method to achieve this aim. It requires measurement as part of this process, which is underpinned by the same considerations as criterion audit and care bundles.

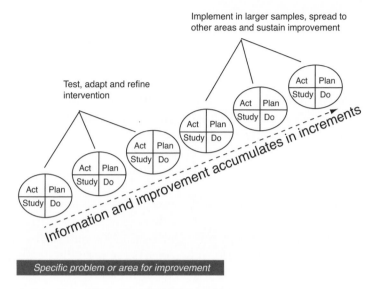

FIGURE 34.2 A 'ramp' of Plan-Do-Study-Act cycles

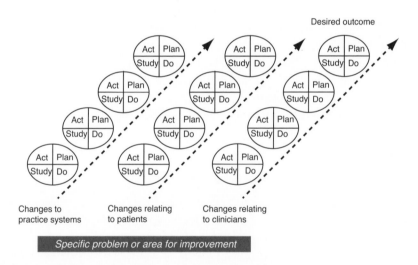

FIGURE 34.3 Multiple Plan-Do-Study-Act cycles and ramps

POTENTIAL BENEFITS OF THE PDSA METHOD

The PDSA method is applied in healthcare to achieve at least one and ideally all three of the following interlinked aims.

1. To *improve* the quality and safety of care processes and clinical outcomes
2. To *sustain* a virtuous cycle of continuous improvement in a specific unit, team or organisation (or at least assure initial improvements are maintained over time)
3. To *spread* the learning and experience from initial, successful efforts to other teams, units and organisations over time, thereby improving their care too.

The PDSA method has a number of potential benefits. Using this approach potentially enables front-line staff to test out planned care or system changes (e.g. introduction of a new checklist protocol for checking refrigerator temperatures and drug expiry dates by a single staff member) in their own local environment without the need for a dramatic large-scale overhaul of the existing work process or system. This increases understanding of the potential feasibility, costs and impact of an intervention before change is implemented on a larger scale, and allows for the opportunity to adapt or abandon the changes if they do not work as planned. As each test (cycle) is small and rapid, the method can provide real-time feedback and is therefore relatively safe and resource efficient.

The PDSA method may also help to overcome initial resistance to change from other practice colleagues who may be sceptical about this need. One or two volunteers trying out suggested changes on a small scale can provide contextual evidence (or otherwise) of potential benefits, which may also help motivate or convince other staff members to accept and adopt changes in practice that have demonstrated improvements.

PRACTICAL APPLICATION OF THE PDSA METHOD

The first step is to define the problem or desired outcome. Next, consider and list all the potential actions or changes to solve the problem or to achieve the desired outcome. Chapters 7 (Task Analysis) and 8 (Process Mapping) may be helpful. Prioritise the actions or changes according to their feasibility and likelihood of success. Implement each action or change in turn, following the steps described in Box 34.1.

BOX 34.1 Practical application of the PDSA method

Plan   Write down the action plan for implementing the change in detail (including who, where, when, what and how). Decide on the best way in which the impact of the change can be measured.

Do   Implement the change and measure the outcome.

Study   Reflect on experiences, findings and their potential implications. *What, if any, was the impact of the change?* Did the change lead to an improvement? What went well and what didn't? Were there unexpected outcomes or factors that introduced variability?

Act   Consider if any further actions are necessary. For example, the 'change' (intervention) may have to be abandoned, adapted and retried or attempted with a larger sample of patients, a different setting or other healthcare workers. If further action is required, it informs the 'plan' stage of the next PDSA cycle. Alternatively, if the change had worked well or is to be abandoned, the next proposed change (intervention) becomes the focus of another PDSA cycle.

Repeat the process until all the proposed actions/changes have been implemented and evaluated, until the problem is solved or the desired outcome has been achieved. A practical example is shown in Box 34.2.

BOX 34.2 Practical example of applying the PDSA method

A general practice realises that patients attending rheumatology, nephrology and endocrinology hospital clinics often have blood tests repeated that had recently been done in primary care. This is inefficient use of time and resources, and may delay management decisions, as results are not immediately available to consultants. They therefore decide to implement an improvement project using the PDSA method with the aim to reduce unnecessary duplication of blood tests in secondary care. The team identifies a number of potential changes that may help them achieve their aim and agree a plan to implement and evaluate the suggested changes.

The first PDSA 'ramp' relates to *patients*. In the first PDSA cycle the practice phlebotomist asks three patients to collect copies of their results before their next rheumatology appointment from the practice. Their 'study' of the cycle reveals one patient is unable to collect her results. Consequently, patients are offered a choice during the second PDSA cycle to collect their results in person or to have the results posted to them – a change that is judged to be an improvement. The third PDSA cycle tests the option to provide results via email. In the fourth and fifth cycles all three options are offered to more patients and to patients attending different hospital clinics, respectively.

The second PDSA 'ramp' relates to *practice systems*. In the first PDSA cycle the rheumatology clinic is contacted to clarify which additional tests are being requested in secondary care that are not routinely done in primary care. They find the ESR blood test is rarely requested by their practice, because the supply of sample bottles is unreliable. For the second PDSA cycle the practice manager arranges a regular supply of ESR sample bottles. For the third PDSA cycle the general practitioner and rheumatologist co-design a phlebotomy request card. Rather than performing the tests in hospital, patients take the completed card to their next appointment in primary care and the results are then forwarded to the rheumatology clinic. As this 'change' seems to be acceptable and feasible, they extend this option to more patients in a fourth PDSA cycle.

FACTORS THAT DETERMINE THE EFFECTIVENESS OF THE PDSA METHOD

Similar to all other QI methods, the application of PDSA cycles to improve healthcare practices and outcomes should not be viewed as a panacea. A recent systematic review of the relevant published literature found that the reported application of PDSA cycles varied significantly, with many studies using this approach also failing to comply with the basic principles of the method. A key conclusion was that there was much room for improvement in the application and use of the PDSA method.[11]

While there is, therefore, evidence of the potential usefulness and impact of the PDSA method in some healthcare settings, it is unclear why, when, for whom and in what contexts it is effective.[11-16] Or why it sometimes achieves only one or two of its original aims – and even then only to a limited degree. Given the considerable investment of time, financial and human resources in QI initiatives in general, and the PDSA method in particular, there is a compelling imperative to proactively identify and describe those significant factors which may enhance or reduce the effectiveness of this approach in different healthcare settings, including general practice. A further systematic review of the relevant PDSA healthcare literature has sought to identify and explain these specific contextual factors,[*] which will be discussed in more detail.

Group 1: Method

> *The PDSA method is more effective if measurable, evidence-based actions with visible outcomes and many short cycles rapidly following each other are used.*

The PDSA method is more effective if the 'actions' (e.g. changes being implemented and tested during the 'do' stage of the cycle) are clearly defined, non-discretionary and applicable to all patients in all situations.[17] 'Actions' can relate to clinical processes or clinical outcomes. The advantage of process measures is that improvements (if any) can generally be demonstrated in a shorter time frame than with clinical outcomes. The disadvantage of using process measures is that it can be difficult to demonstrate the link between them and clinical benefits in the short term.[6] In turn, this can reduce staff motivation to persist with the change to a process, which may be (wrongly) perceived as being box-ticking.[18,19] The implication is that the PDSA method is more effective, and changes more likely to be sustained, if a clear relationship between process measures and clinical benefits are made evident to staff.

There is no 'right' length of time for a PDSA cycle. Generally, the more time each cycle takes, the greater the likelihood that staff motivation will decrease and the PDSA method will be less effective.[18] However, being overly prescriptive about short cycle time lengths may also limit its potential in some instances.[9] For example, in specific instances the disruption some changes may cause can be minimised by conducting one large, longer cycle.[10] There are many reasons why cycles may take too long, including:

- failing to dissect the overall project aim into many small 'changes' (or steps)
- testing the change on too large a sample of patients
- selecting clinical processes or conditions that present less than once a week
- spending too long collecting or analysing baseline data
- being over-inclusive, with too wide a range of staff groups participating.

---

[*]   de Wet *et al.*, Unpublished.

Once an 'action' has been tested and found to have improved care, the next challenge is to 'normalise' (sustain) it. This can be facilitated by ensuring staff are given feedback regularly and frequently, and that the overall progress towards a shared goal is made visible, while successes, even small ones, are celebrated.[17] For example, in some QI projects a 'data wall' is used to display performance measures to staff and patients and the results are updated regularly.[20] However, high visibility can discourage staff if there is little or no obvious progress to be seen despite their best efforts, especially early on in projects.[21]

Group 2: Organisation

> *The PDSA method is more effective in small, stable organisations (or practices) that have strong and positive safety cultures and active leadership support.*

Applying the PDSA method in small, contained and clearly demarcated clinical areas, units or teams increase its effectiveness for several reasons:
- the effects of changes are more visible to staff
- feedback can be undiluted, focused, relevant and rapid
- a 'critical mass' of staff adopting changes can be achieved quicker.[5,9]

However, if the area, unit or team is very small, changes can be implemented simply as a result of discussion and agreement, with no requirement to test or roll them out gradually, making the PDSA method redundant.[22] The implication, therefore, is that the PDSA method may be more suitable to larger general practices than to single-handed or small surgeries.

The PDSA method's unique strength is that improvement can begin on a very small scale before being 'ramped' up. This makes it potentially more resilient than other QI methods to organisational instability, but certainly not immune. The PDSA method's effectiveness may therefore be reduced through:
- a high rate of staff turnover
- reliance on a small number of 'champions'
- high proportions of part-time staff in the team
- transient patient populations
- applying the method to clinical conditions that do not allow sufficient opportunity for staff to implement, measure and document changes.[23]

There are at least two other major organisational factors that determine the effectiveness of the PDSA method. The first is the degree to which managers (and senior leadership) actively promote and support its implementation.[10] The second is the prevailing culture in the practice, with a strong and positive safety culture potentially enhancing the method's effectiveness (*see* Chapter 36, Measuring Safety Climate).

Group 3: Practitioner

> *The PDSA method is more effective when used by motivated staff with the required knowledge and skills and they actively engage with and accept 'ownership' of the process.*

The PDSA method can only be used effectively if those staff members who have to implement it have the requisite skills and knowledge to do so.[23] For example, process-thinking skills are necessary, as is the ability to collect and present reliable data and identify valid measures. While some may naturally possess or have acquired these skills and knowledge, others may find it difficult to learn and, even if they receive sufficient training, may need more time to consolidate their learning by applying the method in practice.[24,25]

Possessing the necessary knowledge and skills is not enough, though. Staff need to be highly motivated and actively engaged with the process and to perceive a sense of personal 'ownership' in order to continue to use this approach.[10,26] In some QI projects the act of participation itself is enough to create a sense of ownership among staff, but levels of staff engagement vary widely and it is difficult to predict or achieve.[10] In fact, resistance from some staff groups, particularly clinicians, is one of the major barriers to the effectiveness of the PDSA method.[10] Resistance may be increased if staff are concerned about potential loss of clinical judgement and control, or if they perceive the proposed changes as already being performed or are of dubious value.[27]

Resistance can be reduced or overcome if participation is voluntary and by focusing on 'early adopters'.[17] Allowing staff to decide on change ideas helps to increase 'ownership' but it can slow down improvement, because lessons learned elsewhere (e.g. in another practice in the same geographical area) have to be re-learned.[7]

Group 4: Resources

> *The PDSA method is more effective if adequate resources (training, time, support, information technology and money) are provided.*

Given the many competing demands for staff time in primary care, it can be very challenging to persuade practices and team members of the importance of QI. The reality is that the PDSA method usually *does* require considerable additional staff time, especially at the start of a project.[6] If available time is at a premium, adding additional work may lead staff to prioritise certain tasks over others (the so-called 'street lamp effect'), or complete tasks in a superficial manner or perform tasks in their own time.[23] This is unfortunate, because in some instances the 'extra' initial work may help to increase efficiency and reduce workload once it becomes integrated into 'normal' care.[25]

Financial incentives are, therefore, often required to help overcome initial practice and staff resistance to QI and to ensure active, ongoing engagement.[28] This should include a commensurate financial reimbursement to offset the required time for staff training, implementation of the PDSA method and the monitoring of its impact.[5,10]

Information technology is critical for the successful integration of most improvements into routine care,[28] but it has to be newly created in some instances, which may require additional (potentially expensive) resources for maintenance.[5]

Finally, the evidence suggests that training staff to use the PDSA method effectively is generally considered to be essential.[25] Financial costs can be reduced by providing online educational resources, but evaluations of QI programmes have found that staff prefer face-to-face training.[7] After initial training, ongoing support from QI 'experts' generally increases the effectiveness of the PDA method. This may be because 'experts' can increase staff motivation for QI and effectively promote the evidence-base for interventions. They may also be able to share 'best practice' tips from personal experience and are often able to supply ready-to-use PDSA templates and further training.[10,24]

CONCLUSION

The PDSA method is widely promoted and used as a QI tool, but substantial variations have been found in its effectiveness as a method to improve healthcare quality and safety, and to sustain and spread improvement. This chapter described a number of important contextual and socio-cultural factors that determine how and why application of the PDSA method by clinicians and others may or may not lead to successful improvements in the quality and safety of patient care. The findings will have a pragmatic value for QI practitioners, educators and front-line staff. For policymakers and QI programme leaders, the evidence presented should provide them with more informed insights about the potential suitability (or otherwise) of the PDSA method in specific healthcare settings and contexts, including primary care, so as to ensure its optimal application and maximum effectiveness.

REFERENCES

1. Deming WE. *Out of the Crisis*. Cambridge, MA: MIT Press; 1986.
2. Shewhart WA. *Statistical Method from the Viewpoint of Quality Control*. Deming ED, editor. New York, NY: Dover Publications; 1986 (first published 1939).
3. Langley GJ, Moen RD, Nolan KM, *et al*. *The Improvement Guide*. 2nd ed. San Francisco, CA: Jossey-Bass; 2009.
4. Institute for Healthcare Improvement. *Science of Improvement: testing changes*. Available at: www.ihi.org/resources/Pages/HowtoImprove/ScienceofImprovement TestingChanges.aspx (accessed 26 November 2013).
5. Meredith LS, Mendel P, Pearson M, *et al*. Implementation and maintenance of quality

improvement for treating depression in primary care. *Psychiatr Serv.* 2006; **57**(1): 48–55.

6. Franx G, Meeuwissen JA, Sinnema H, *et al.* Quality improvement in depression care in the Netherlands: the depression breakthrough collaborative. *Int J Integr Care.* 2009; **9**: e84.

7. Gould DA, Lynn J, Halper D, *et al.* The New York City Palliative Care Quality Improvement Collaborative. *Jt Comm J Qual Patient Saf.* 2007; **33**(6): 307–16.

8. Nolan E, VanRiper S, Talsma A, *et al.* Rapid-cycle improvement in quality of care for patients hospitalized with acute myocardial infarction or heart failure: moving from a culture of missed opportunity to a system of accountability. *J Cardiovasc Manag.* 2005; **16**(1): 14–19.

9. Varkey P, Sathananthan A, Scheifer A, *et al.* Using quality-improvement techniques to enhance patient education and counselling of diagnosis and management. *Qual Prim Care.* 2009; **17**(3): 205–13.

10. Leape LL Kabcenell AI, Gandhi TK, *et al.* Reducing adverse drug effects: lessons from a breakthrough series collaborative. *Jt Comm J Qual Improv.* 2000; **26**(6): 321–31.

11. Taylor MJ, McNicholas C, Nicolay C, *et al.* Systematic review of the application of the Plan-Do-Study-Act method to improve quality in healthcare. *BMJ Qual Saf.* Epub 2013 Sep 11. Available at: http://qualitysafety.bmj.com/content/early/2013/09/11/bmjqs-2013-001862.full.pdf+html (accessed 26 November 2013).

12. Grol R, Berwick D, Wensing M. On the trail of quality and safety in health care. *BMJ.* 2008; **336**: 74–6.

13. Schouten LMT, Hulscher MELJ, van Everdingen JJE, *et al.* Evidence for the impact of quality improvement collaboratives: a systematic review. *BMJ.* 2008; **336**: 1491–4.

14. Auerbach AD, Landefeld CS, Shojania KG. The tension between needing to improve care and knowing how to do it. *N Engl J Med.* 2007; **357**(6): 608–13.

15. Walshe K. Understanding what works – and why – in quality improvement: the need for theory driven evaluation. *Int J Qual Health Care.* 2007; **19**(2): 57–9.

16. Mittman BS. Creating the evidence base for quality improvement collaboratives. *Ann Intern Med.* 2004; **140**(11): 897–900.

17. Pulcini C, Crofts S, Campbell D, *et al.* Design, measurement, and evaluation of an education strategy in the hospital setting to contact antimicrobial resistance: theoretical considerations and a practical example. *Dis Manage Health Out.* 2007; **15**: 151–63.

18. Benn J, Burnett S, Parand A, *et al.* Perceptions of the impact of a large-scale collaborative improvement programme: experience in the UK safer patients initiative. *J Eval Clin Pract.* 2009; **15**(3): 524–40.

19. Vos L, Duckers MLA, Wagner C, *et al.* Applying the quality improvement collaborative method to process design: a multiple case study. *Implementation Science.* 2010; **5**: 19.

20. Krimsky WS, Mroz IB, McIlwaine JK, *et al.* A model for increasing patient safety in the intensive care unit: increasing the implementation rates of proven safety measures. *Qual Saf Health Care.* 2009; **18**(1): 74–80.

21. Warburton RN. Preliminary outcomes and cost-benefit analysis of a community hospital emergency department screening and referral program for patients aged 75 or more. *Int J Health Care.* 2005; **18**(6–7): 474–84.

22. Geboers H, Grol R, van den Bosch W, *et al.* A model for continuous quality improvement in small scale practices. *Qual Health Care.* 1999; **8**(1): 43–8.

23. Macintosh-Murray A. Challenges of collaborative improvement in continuing care. *Healthc Q.* 2007; **10**(2): 49–57.
24. Leape LL, Rogers G, Hanna D, *et al.* Developing and implementing new safe practices: voluntary adoption through statewide collaboratives. *Qual Saf Health Care.* 2006; **15**(4): 289–95.
25. Fremont AM, Joyce G, Anaya HD, *et al.* An HIV collaborative in the VHA: do advanced HIT and one-day sessions change the collaborative experience? *Jt Comm J Qual Patient Saf.* 2006; **32**: 324–36.
26. Gitomer RS. Improving access, quality of care, and patient satisfaction in a general internal medicine practice. *J Clin Outcomes Manage.* 2005; **12**(5): 245–9.
27. Nicholls S, Cullen R, Halligan A. Clinical Governance . . . after the review: What next? Agreement and implementation. *Br J Clin Gov.* 2001; **6**(2): 129–35.
28. Green CJ, Fortin P, Maclure M, *et al.* Information system support as critical success factor for chronic disease management: necessary but not sufficient. *Int J Med Inform.* 2006; **75**(12): 818–28.

CHAPTER 35

The trigger review method

Carl de Wet, Moya Kelly, John McKay & Paul Bowie

INTRODUCTION

In general practice, safety incidents are typically reported by patients, identified directly by clinicians or highlighted by colleagues as part of routine practice. However, some incident types are not detected so easily. Systematically reviewing clinical records for previously undetected incidents and potential threats using the trigger review method (TRM) can provide care teams with a whole new perspective on patient safety.[1] It also offers valuable opportunities to take pre-emptive action before harm can occur or pinpoint learning needs where patient safety may have been avoidably compromised.

The terms 'trigger review method' or 'trigger tool' may be new or unfamiliar to some, but it is not a new approach to learning or improvement. The underlying principle – essentially an adaptation of case note audit review – will be familiar to most clinicians. The TRM is a structured approach to screening clinical records for undetected patient safety incidents (PSIs).[1-4] It was adapted from approaches in other healthcare sectors in 2007 and subsequently developed and validated in Scottish general practices.[1-4] The TRM was tested as part of the Health Foundation–funded Safety and Improvement in Primary Care Pilot Programme in around 60 general practices in four territorial health boards in Scotland.[5,6] The programme evaluation suggested that TRM has important educational and improvement value by enabling previously undetected threats to patients to be uncovered in clinical records, thereby providing the general practitioner (GP) team with a new perspective on how to make patient care safer.[5]

The potential utility of the TRM continues to evolve and expand, while its uptake in general practice is rapidly increasing. For example, from a healthcare policy and implementation perspective, it was agreed during 2012 that TRM evidence could be submitted as a Quality Improvement Activity as part of GP Appraisal in Scotland.[7] The TRM is one of the three key components of the Scottish Government's Patient Safety Programme for Primary Care (SPSP-PC) that was launched nationally in March 2013,[8] while the Royal College of General Practitioners (RCGP) has included the method as one potential evidence source for revalidation purposes.[9] Since April 2013, all Scottish general practices (approximately 1000) are also financially incentivised through the Quality and Outcomes Framework (QOF) to routinely apply the TRM and report their findings.

PRACTICAL APPLICATION OF THE TRIGGER REVIEW METHOD

The TRM allows primary care clinicians (GPs, GP trainees and practice nurses) to review small samples of patient records for previously undetected PSIs in a structured, focused, rapid and active manner.

- *Structured*: clinical reviewers consider each of the five sections of a primary care record in turn (*see* Table 35.1).
- *Focused*: a specific search for predefined 'triggers' is conducted. Triggers are prompts or 'signs' in the record that *may* indicate the occurrence of PSIs (*see* Table 35.1).
- *Rapid*: a maximum of 20 minutes is allocated per record and only a pre-specified period in each record is reviewed (usually 3 calendar months).
- *Active*: clinical reviewers are encouraged to reconstruct each patient journey and should probe, analyse and critically appraise the record for evidence of PSIs and latent risks hidden in it.

TABLE 35.1 The five sections of any primary care record and predefined triggers

Section of the record	Trigger (must be present during the review period)
1 Clinical encounters (face to face, telephone or house calls)	Three or more clinical encounters in any given 7-day period
2 Medication	'Repeat' medication item discontinued
	Optional triggers:
	• acute prescription of non-steroidal anti-inflammatory drugs
	• acute prescription of opiates
3 Clinical codes	A clinical read code for an adverse drug event and/or allergy was added
	Any new 'high priority' clinical code added
4 Correspondence (referrals, clinic letters, discharge summaries, reports)	Any out-of-hours healthcare contact (out-of-hours service or accident and emergency)
	Emergency hospital admission for 1 day or longer
5 Investigations (imaging, laboratory)	Haemoglobin ≤10.0 g/dL
	Optional triggers:
	• INR >5 or <1.7
	• AST/ALT >100 IU/L

Clinical reviewers are encouraged to record their findings, reflections and actions on a Trigger Review Summary Report (TRSR). The TRSR is a two-page pro forma for collecting and summarising data on the number of detected 'triggers', the details of any PSIs uncovered, any learning needs identified and actions that were or should be taken as a result of the review process.

The TRSR includes the National Patient Safety Agency's definition of a PSI: 'any unintended or unexpected incident which could have or did lead to harm for one or more patients receiving NHS care'.[10] This is useful because, from a clinical risk and patient-centred perspective, it reminds the reviewer that the TRM's key focus is on detecting a circumstance where harm occurred (physically or psychologically and regardless of severity) or could have happened but was prevented (a near miss) or could happen at some point in the future (a latent risk).

The three steps of the TRM are:
1. planning and preparation
2. review of records
3. reflection and action.

1. PLANNING AND PREPARATION

One of the first steps is to define the specific patient population or medical condition from which a small random sample of clinical records will be sampled for review. Although *any* patient population or medical condition could conceivably be selected, the records of frail elderly patients and those with multiple co-morbidities and polypharmacy are more likely to contain evidence of PSIs and latent risks. Examples of potential high-yield patient sub-populations are shown in Table 35.2. Specific patient population characteristics may suggest

TABLE 35.2 Examples of specific high-risk patient groups who could be selected for review

Group 1: Specific, shared patient characteristics	Group 2: Chronic disease areas	Group 3: High-risk medications
• Nursing home patients	• Chronic obstructive pulmonary disease	• Insulin
• Older than 75 years	• Stroke or transient ischaemic attack	• Morphine
• Last 25 out-of-hours attendees		• Warfarin
• Last 25 hospital referrals	• Cardiovascular disease	• Non-steroidal anti-inflammatory drugs
• Housebound patients	• Diabetes	• Diuretics (×2)
• Last 25 hospital admissions	• Heart failure	• More than five repeat medication items
	• Chronic kidney disease	

Group 4: Combinations of Groups 1–3

For example: patients over 75 years of age, taking five or more medications, who attended in the previous 12 weeks; nursing home patients prescribed non-steroidal anti-inflammatory drugs; patients with heart failure who are prescribed two or more diuretics

Group 5: Choose your own sub-populations

For example, patients discharged after emergency hospital admission (review the period before and after admission); a random selection of any 25 patients registered with the practice

optional triggers. For example, a trigger of 'INR >5' would be suitable for a sample of patients prescribed warfarin.

The next step is to decide the number of clinical records to sample and what period of time is to be reviewed in each record. Practical experience suggests that reviewing three recent consecutive calendar months in each of the 25 records (randomly sampled from the chosen patient population) is feasible for the vast majority of clinicians.

2. REVIEWING RECORDS

Once the sample of records has been identified, a clinical reviewer screens each record, searching for previously validated predefined 'triggers' (*see* Table 35.1) that may point to the existence of an unknown PSI or latent risk to the patient. For example, the reviewer finds an INR >5 (trigger) and, on further examination of the record, detects that the patient was treated for an associated bleed in secondary care. There is no 'correct' number of triggers. Instead, the number of triggers should be decided by balancing available time and resources (fewer triggers) and the number of PSIs to detect (more triggers). In practice, only a few triggers will be 'positive' – for example, lead to the detection of a PSI. On the other hand, one trigger may lead to the detection of more than one PSI.

When PSIs are detected, a brief summary of the event should be recorded on the TRSR. Reviewers are also encouraged to rate the perceived severity and preventability of each detected PSI on a scale from 1 to 4. This dual scoring system was developed in response to the lack of published guidance on how to judge the 'preventability' of detected PSIs and is shown in Table 35.3. This is a critical and often overlooked issue in the patient safety literature. Unfortunately but inevitably, patients will be unavoidably harmed as a result of their interactions with healthcare for a range of highly complex reasons. The key focus from the patient's and the clinician's perspective should be on detecting and learning from those incidents that are judged to be preventable – that is, there is consensus that they should not have occurred if the appropriate preventive strategies had been in place.

TABLE 35.3 Severity and preventability rating scales for detected patient safety incidents

Severity	Scale	Preventability
Any incident with the potential to cause harm	1	Not preventable and originated in secondary care
Mild harm: inconvenience, further follow-up or investigation to ensure no harm occurred	2	Preventable and originated in secondary care *or* not preventable and originated in primary care
Moderate harm: required intervention or duration for longer than a day	3	Potentially preventable and originated in primary care
Prolonged, substantial or permanent harm, including hospitalisation	4	Preventable and originated in primary care

3. REFLECTION AND ACTION

In the third stage of the TRM, reviewers document any clinical actions they performed during the review and indicate which further actions they intend to take on their TRSRs. A selection of possible actions is shown in Box 35.1. They are also encouraged to reflect on their findings and write down any learning points and needs on a professional and practice level.

BOX 35.1 Examples of possible actions that could be performed during and after the review

Possible actions to undertake during the review

- *Coding*: updating, correcting, QOF template completion
- *Prescribing*: issue, amend, review or cancel prescriptions
- *Investigations*: arranging further investigations, repeating investigations or referral to other agencies
- *Communication*: clarification of clinical information with patients or carers, scheduling review appointments, providing patient education.

Possible actions to undertake after the review

- Significant event analysis
- Criterion audit
- Implement change for improvement and how this will be achieved
- Provide feedback to a colleague
- Add TRSR to appraisal documentation
- Submit a formal incident report
- Update or develop a protocol
- Discuss with a GP educational supervisor

Once the TRSR is completed, the reviewer should consider whom they should share the findings with. The ideal forum for sharing the finding is during a practice meeting involving all staff. Finally, the reviewer should consider when they are going to conduct another trigger review. At present, the requirements of the SPSP-PC and QOF are for two reviews during a 12-month period.

EVIDENCE FOR THE TRIGGER REVIEW METHOD

The TRM finds *more* PSIs than all other types of measurement and improvement methods combined.[11] However, the types of safety incidents and risks typically uncovered by the TRM tend to be different in general terms from those highlighted by complaints, significant event analyses and other methods.[11] In an ongoing study of the TRM, 26 clinical reviewers from 12 practices in the west of Scotland returned 46 TRSRs for analysis. The clinical reviewers were GPs (n = 12), practice nurses (n = 11), a community pharmacist (n = 1), GP specialist trainee (n = 1) and a nurse practitioner (n = 1). They reviewed a cumulative 3417 patient months in 1139 medical records and detected 136 PSIs. In a comparable study, 25 GPSTs reviewed 520 unique patient records and found 80 previously undetected PSIs.[12] A few selected examples of detected PSIs are shown in Box 35.2.

BOX 35.2 Selected examples of patient safety incidents detected using the trigger review method

- 'Patient's hospital discharge letter stated aspirin & clopidogrel were both indefinite. Clopidogrel should have been for only 12 weeks.'
- 'Patient prescribed citalopram when already on sertraline.'
- 'New essential thrombocytosis diagnosed. On looking through notes, platelets had been raised for two years or so. Referred.'
- 'A 70 year old patient on aspirin and clopidogrel with no gastroprotection. Emergency admission for confusion/falls secondary to hepatic encephalopathy. Encephalopathy secondary to constipation and UTI. Had inpatient upper gastrointestinal haemorrhage secondary to oesophageal ulcer. PPI may have prevented upper GI bleed and low haemoglobin?'
- 'Female (1937) – Nine [courses of] oral steroids in 12 months – no DEXA results in files – only on calcichew.'

The PSIs uncovered by this method (and in Box 35.2) will most likely be familiar to most primary care clinicians – the important issue is that they had remained undetected until the TRM review was undertaken. The majority of detected incidents are of low to moderate severity or are 'near misses' but still provide many opportunities to tackle issues that can be addressed by the practice team or a clinician reviewer. More serious incidents tend to originate in secondary care or are detected through methods other than the TRM.

Perhaps one of the strongest issues arising from application of the TRM is the identification of incidents that can serve as topics for significant event analysis (SEA) and criterion audit – for example, delayed diagnoses, suboptimal therapeutic management, poor disease and drug monitoring, and the appropriate use of information technology. This is particularly helpful given that appraisal and revalidation requires GPs to analyse two significant events per year (with the General Medical Council encouraging these events to be PSIs rather than broader quality-of-care issues).[13] Identification and analysis of these previously undetected PSIs are particularly pertinent to improving the opportunity cost of SEA topics.

The majority of reviewers perform at least one clinical or patient care-related action when performing the review, while the vast majority also indicate their intention to take further actions as a result of the review process (*see* Box 35.3). The most common actions of GP and nurse reviewers is to give feedback about the review findings to colleagues and to 'add to appraisal documentation', while GPSTs are more likely to discuss the findings with an educational supervisor.

The original purpose of the 'trigger tool' approach as applied in secondary care settings was to 'reliably' measure rates of harm detected in the records of specific groups of hospitalised patients over time.[1,3] External reviewers 'objectively' determine and monitor harm rates for individual clinical wards, units and hospitals and share the aggregated results with the care teams. This method of application has two major drawbacks: the first is that front-line staff do not have ownership of the data and the second is that no attempt is made to investigate why the detected incidents occurred or how they may best be prevented in future. From a primary care perspective, measuring harm rates is – at the individual practice level – a potential distraction from the arguably greater risk management benefits to be accrued from applying the method to enhance learning and facilitate the improvement of care quality and safety. However, as previously demonstrated it is possible that the TRM can be used to measure harm at the regional and national level if specific feasibility and statistical challenges are overcome (Chapter 5).[14]

EDUCATIONAL VALUE OF THE TRIGGER REVIEW METHOD

The evidence shows that the majority of reviewers are able to identify learning points and learning needs at the professional and practice team level. Individual learning needs often concern chronic disease management, while at the practice level the need for improved communication between primary and secondary care and for more consistent coding and 'protocols' for specific high-risk responsibilities are commonly identified. Selected examples of learning needs and learning points are shown in Box 35.3.

The TRM also has a role to play in specialty training to help prepare GP trainees for the contractual and regulatory demands of independent clinical practice. This is particularly so given the proposal to extend specialty training to a 4-year programme, which will include the need to undertake a quality improvement project with the TRM being a potential method of choice for this purpose.[15] A recent pilot study found that the vast majority of trainees were able to use the TRM to detect preventable PSIs directly related to issues within the practice, particularly in the high-risk elderly patient groups.[12] All participants were able to demonstrate some element of reflection, document potential learning needs and develop improvement action plans. This study suggests that the TRM has potential value in GP patient safety curriculum delivery and preparing trainees for future safety improvement expectations.[9] Further research is now being conducted to determine if the TRM may also serve as a substrate for both formative and workplace case-based discussions and assessments.

In terms of regulatory and educational policy in the United Kingdom, 'safety and quality' is one of four professional domains describing the expected duties and standards of every doctor registered with the General Medical Council.[13] Specifically, registered doctors are expected to

---

BOX 35.3 **Selected examples of learning needs and learning points identified by the trigger review method**

Professional learning needs

- *'How to target heart rate for atrial fibrillation* [management].*'*
- *'I need to review CKD* [chronic kidney disease] *management as I could not remember specific contraindications for ACE-I.'*
- *'Update my diabetic knowledge – online module.'*

Practice team learning needs

- *'Several patients overdue annual reviews – should we check notes and call patients via telephone rather than just letters?'*
- *'*[Need to] *liaise with colleagues who do bloods to ensure the correct tests are carried out and to reduce the need for the patient to return unnecessarily.'*
- *'Should discuss and agree how to prioritise* [clinical] *read codes.'*

Learning points

- *'Personally, the trigger review of patient notes did change my mind-set and I look for certain triggers now as part of my practice. You tend to memorise certain triggers and look out for them with all patients, it tends to become imbedded into practice.'*
- *'Awareness of need to ensure warfarin is stopped pre-op where appropriate.'*
- *'That whilst as a practice we are fallible we do have reasonable processes in place. The missed increase in bisoprolol was a concatenation of events between primary and secondary care at the discharge interface. This is a fraught area.'*

---

take part in systems of quality assurance and quality improvement to promote patient safety by: (a) participating in regular reviews and audit of the standards and performance of . . . work . . . taking steps to remedy any deficiencies [and] (b) regularly reflecting on the standards of practice and care you provide.[13]

The TRM is perfectly aligned with this expectation and given the evidence outlined can play an important role in helping to achieve this standard.

ACCEPTABILITY AND FEASIBILITY

Clinical reviewers require a basic level of training to ensure that they understand the key principles of the TRM and how to apply it most effectively in their practices. Training typically requires a minimum of 1 hour and only rarely exceeds 2 hours. It is mainly the available resources and the preferences of new reviewers that determine the choice of training method. A range of training methods and materials have been developed and tested by NHS Education for Scotland, including the following.

- *One-to-one or small group training*: the novice reviewer(s) sit at a computer workstation, preferably in their own practice premises, with a colleague who is experienced in the method and apply the TRM to a small selection of 'real life' electronic patient records. Key principles are demonstrated and feedback is given on performance.
- *Practical guides and case studies*: novice reviewer(s) can familiarise themselves with the TRM by reading about its basic premise then practising on simulated medical records and comparing their findings with the provided solutions.
- *Collaborative learning events and larger groups*: novice reviewer(s) attend a dedicated TRM workshop training session. After a brief presentation by an experienced reviewer participants are given the opportunity to independently conduct a trigger review of a pre-prepared simulated full patient record (which contained 'planted' evidence of PSI scenarios) and then discuss this in a group work session. There are also opportunities for discussion, clarification and feedback. This is in keeping with other quality improvement techniques such as criterion audit and SEA, which can be taught by both clinicians and non-clinicians in large group settings and then applied at the individual and practice-based levels.

The vast majority of teams and reviewers perceive the TRM as at least as useful as other quality improvement methods and recognise its potential to complement existing tools such as SEA and clinical audit. The first time the TRM is used, a clinician reviewer requires, on average, about 2 hours of protected time to complete all three stages and the TRSR – although this may range from around 1 hour to a maximum of 4 hours. Reviewers typically find that subsequent reviews take less time. A selection of reviewer comments about the TRM is shown in Box 35.4.

BOX 35.4 Selected reviewer comments about the trigger review method

'It has been a fantastic tool . . . the trigger tool is probably one of the most important things that we are looking at in the safety improvement in primary care.'

'[It was useful in] finding things before they have gone drastically wrong.'

'I began to get a real handle on how it fitted in to the big scheme of things and how it could be a really useful tool in the practice.'

'[We identified] one or two huge near misses that would never have otherwise been unveiled to anybody ever but had very significant learning.'

SUMMARY POINTS

- The TRM allows trained clinicians to review random samples of their patient records in an active, rapid, focused and structured manner in order to detect PSIs.
- The practical application involves three steps: (1) planning and preparation, (2) reviewing records and (3) reflection and action.
- The main benefits of the TRM are its educational value and its potential for improving the quality and safety of care.
- The vast majority of teams and reviewers perceive the TRM as acceptable and feasible.

FURTHER READING

The TRM educational materials and 'guide sheets' developed over the past few years are freely available to NHS Scotland staff, to enable them to adapt and use these resources to suit their own contexts. To view these materials or for more information, please visit:

- www.healthcareimprovementscotland.org/our_work/patient_safety/spsp_primary_care_resources/trigger_tool.aspx

REFERENCES

1. Woloshynowych M, Neale G, Vincent C. Case record review of adverse events: a new approach. *Qual Saf Health Care.* 2003; **12**(6): 411–15.
2. de Wet C, Bowie P. Screening electronic patient records to detect preventable harm: a trigger tool for primary care. *Qual Prim Care.* 2011; **19**(2): 115–25.
3. Griffin FA, Resar RK. *IHI Global Trigger Tool for Measuring Adverse Events.* IHI Innovation Series. Cambridge, MA: Institute for Healthcare Improvement; 2007.
4. de Wet C, Bowie P. The preliminary development and testing of a global trigger tool to detect error and patient harm in primary-care records. *Postgrad Med J.* 2009; **85**(1002): 176–80.
5. Bowie P, Halley L, Gillies J, *et al.* Searching primary care records for predefined triggers may expose latent risks and adverse events. *Clin Risk.* 2012; **18**(Jan): 13–18.
6. Health Foundation. *Safety Improvement in Primary Care.* Available at: www.health.org.uk/news-and-events/newsletter/safety-improvement-in-primary-care/ (accessed 2 January 2013).
7. Scottish Executive Health Department; Royal College of General Practitioners in Scotland; NHS Education for Scotland; *et al. GP Appraisal Scheme: a brief guide.* Edinburgh: Scottish Executive Health Department; 2003.
8. Scottish Government. *Delivering Quality in Primary Care National Action Plan: implementing the Healthcare Quality Strategy for NHS Scotland.* Edinburgh: Scottish Government; 2010.
9. Royal College of General Practitioners. *RCGP Curriculum 2010. Statement 2.02: the contextual statement on patient safety and quality of care.* London: RCGP; 2012.
10. National Patient Safety Agency. *What is a Patient Safety Incident?* Available at: www.

npsa.nhs.uk/nrls/reporting/what-is-a-patient-safety-incident/ (accessed 2 January 2013).

11. Olsen S, Neal G, Schwab K, *et al.* Hospital staff should use more than one method to detect adverse events and potential adverse events: incident reporting, pharmacist surveillance and local real-time record review may all have a place. *Qual Saf Health Care.* 2007; **16**(91): 40–4.

12. McKay J, de Wet C, Kelly M, *et al.* Applying the trigger review method after a brief educational intervention: potential for teaching and improving the safety of GP specialty training? *BMC Med Educ.* 2013; **13**: 117. Available at: www.biomedcentral.com/1472-6920/13/117 (accessed 19 November 2013).

13. General Medical Council. *Good Medical Practice 2012*. London: GMC; 2011.

14. de Wet C, Johnson P, O'Donnell C, *et al.* Can we quantify harm in primary care records? An assessment of precision and power using computer simulation. *BMC Res Methodol.* 2013; **13**: 39. Available at: www.biomedcentral.com/1471-2288/13/39 (accessed 1 November 2013).

15. Jaques H. RCGP wins bid to extend GP training to four years. *BMJ Careers.* 2012 Apr 20. Available at: http://careers.bmj.com/careers/advice/view-article.html?id=20007125 (accessed 1 January 2013).

CHAPTER 36

Measuring safety climate

Carl de Wet & Paul Bowie

INTRODUCTION

Similar to safety-critical industries worldwide, building a strong and just culture is a prerequisite in any healthcare organisation to enable safety performance to be critically examined within a non-threatening, positive learning environment.[1-3] To achieve this key aim in primary care, clinicians, managers and support staff need to be aware of the prevailing safety culture in their own general practices. Only then can they begin to adequately reflect upon, understand, compare and then improve local safety culture and related behaviours and practices among the team and in the wider organisation. However, to reliably measure, monitor and improve upon this over time requires a pragmatic and accessible method that generates rapid, formative and comparative feedback on team-based perceptions of safety culture features.

Starting in 2007, NHS Education for Scotland (NES) began a 3-year process of designing, developing, testing and then implementing a team-based questionnaire (SafeQuest) to measure perceptions of safety climate in a range of Scottish general practices.[4] At that stage, it was the first known attempt to innovate and create such a measure for primary healthcare. The developed questionnaire was then further tested as part of the UK Health Foundation–funded Safety and Improvement in Primary Care (SIPC) Pilot Programme in around 60 general practices in four health authority regions in Scotland.[5]

Based largely on the positive experiences in the SIPC programme, the measurement of team-based safety climate perceptions using the SafeQuest system was included as a key intervention in the Scottish Patient Safety Programme for Primary Care.[6] Since April 2013, all Scottish general practices (approximately 1000) are now financially incentivised through the Quality and Outcomes Framework to complete the questionnaire, meet as a group to discuss and act upon the survey findings, and then submit a summary report of the improvement outcomes to the local health authority.

This chapter describes the practicalities of how primary care teams can assess or measure the prevailing safety climate using different available methods, but with a particular focus on the NES-developed SafeQuest approach. The benefits of safety climate measurement and how to make the most of related survey findings are highlighted, together with the key lessons captured from the literature and recent experiences with SafeQuest in general practice in Scotland.

PRACTICAL STEPS TO MEASURING SAFETY CLIMATE

Safety climate instruments (or questionnaires) are used to measure the values, attitudes, norms, behaviours and perceptions of individual members of a workforce, normally in high-risk industries such as petrochemical, nuclear power and aviation organisations, and increasingly also in healthcare in the past decade.[7] In this way, the implicit and shared understandings about *'the way we do things around here'* can be rendered visible to the team in the first instance, but also potentially to others such as safety managers and clinical leaders in the organisation. Typically, the four main 'steps' to measure the safety climate of a general practice team would be similar to those shown in Figure 36.1.

Step 1: Select a suitable instrument
A suitable instrument is one that is valid and reliable, acceptable and feasible and is specifically developed (or adapted) for the general practice context

Step 2: Invite everyone in the practice team to participate
The rationale for measuring or assessing the team's safety climate should be explained and their support should be obtained

Step 3: Collect and aggregate data
Individual participant responses are collected anonymously, aggregated to the required level (staff group, practice, regional or national) and a report of the main findings is compiled

Step 4: Disseminate and discuss the results
The report is shared with the team, including (ideally) those who did not participate. The team meets to discuss and reflect on the findings, agree any actions to improve their safety culture (directly or indirectly) and write up a summary of the meeting

FIGURE 36.1 Practical steps to measure safety climate

Step 1. Selecting a suitable instrument

There are two main groups of instruments that can be used to measure team-based safety climate perceptions: typological and dimensional. A team can use *typological* instruments to label (or 'diagnose') their practice culture by comparing it with a pre-specified classification (or framework) of culture types, normally during a facilitated group meeting. Two examples of typological instruments are Westrum's framework and the Manchester Patient Safety Framework (MaPSaF).[8-10] MaPSaF is a content-validated instrument that was developed for use initially in primary care organisations, including the National Health Service-managed part of the service, but now also for other areas of healthcare. It specifies five levels of increasingly mature safety culture, from which the team forms a consensus on the one that best fits their practice conditions: Pathological, Reactive, Bureaucratic, Proactive or Generative (*see* Box 36.1). It is highly unlikely that there are many general practices or healthcare organisations that have truly achieved D or E levels of safety culture maturity using this framework. The MaPSaF approach, similar to other methods, can be used in a number of different ways; for example:

- to facilitate reflection on patient safety culture
- to stimulate discussion about the strengths and weaknesses of the patient safety culture
- to reveal any differences in perception between staff groups
- to help understand how a more mature safety culture might look
- to help evaluate any specific intervention needed to change the patient safety culture.

BOX 36.1 MaPSaF's five levels of safety culture

A. **Pathological**: organisations with a prevailing attitude of 'why waste our time on safety' and, as such, there is little or no investment in improving safety.

B. **Reactive**: organisations that only think about safety after an incident has occurred.

C. **Bureaucratic**: organisations that are very paper-based and where safety involves ticking boxes to prove to auditors and assessors that they are focused on safety.

D. **Proactive**: organisations that place a high value on improving safety actively invest in continuous safety improvements and reward staff who raise safety-related issues.

E. **Generative**: the nirvana of all safety organisations, in which safety is an integral part of everything that they do. In a generative organisation, safety is truly in the hearts and minds of everyone, from senior managers to front-line staff.

In contrast, *dimensional* instruments are typically questionnaire based and are periodically administered as self-reported, anonymous staff surveys.[11] Participants indicate their levels of agreement with each of a number of questionnaire items on Likert-type rating scales, which allows numerical ratings of perceived culture measures to be captured at the individual level.[12] Survey participants' individual scores for each questionnaire item (attitudinal statement or related question) are aggregated to provide 'snapshots' of the overall safety climate perceived by the team and also of those related factors that are known to be important workplace indicators of safety performance (e.g. perceived effectiveness of team working, leadership or communication systems). Dimensional instruments are now almost exclusively used in most high-reliability, safety-critical industries and in many healthcare settings worldwide.

There is a vast array of potential survey questionnaires from which healthcare teams can choose, including the Safety Attitudes Questionnaire,[13] the Hospital Survey on Patient Safety Culture[14] and SafeQuest,[4] to name but a few. The available instruments all have differences in content and method, including the numbers of questionnaire items and the types of safety climate factors that they purport to measure.[11,15] This is acceptable in the context that safety climate is underpinned by a set of core variables, which are complemented with factors that are specific to a particular healthcare setting.[15-17] The three 'core' safety climate factors in any healthcare or non-healthcare setting are (1) leadership, (2) communication and (3) safety systems. Of the three, the leadership commitment to safety is arguably the most important.[16,17] The aforementioned development work by NES found two additional factors that should be considered as 'core' for primary care settings: workload and teamwork.[4]

It is important at the outset to consider the following three key criteria when selecting a suitable instrument to measure safety climate.[7,10,17]

1. The instrument should have been specifically developed (or adapted for) all relevant professional and staff groups, the type of organisation it is to be applied in (e.g. primary, secondary or tertiary care) and for the geographical setting it will be used in (e.g. the United States or the United Kingdom). This is important, because safety culture (by its very definition and nature) is strongly determined by social and geographical contextual factors and is, therefore, different from setting to setting. Because of these differences, questionnaire instruments are *not* always directly transferable between settings.
2. The instrument's psychometric properties should have been tested and found to have an acceptable degree of validity and reliability. This is important to ensure that the instrument actually measures what it purports to measure (validity) and that the survey results generated are precise and accurate (reliable).
3. The questionnaire instrument and the implementation process should be professionally acceptable to staff invited to participate and feasible for them to complete and access findings from. This last factor is crucial, as without strong staff engagement, the process is unlikely to be successful.

SafeQuest has been demonstrated to fulfil all three of these essential criteria for the general practice setting.[4] Unlike most other questionnaire development processes, a wide range of clinical and non-clinical front-line staff were involved from the earliest design stages, which informed its potential use by primary care team members in the United Kingdom. SafeQuest is a 30-item

SafeQuest:

Measuring perceptions of safety climate in primary care

Please read each item below and circle the number that best represents the extent to which each statement **applies to or characterises** your practice. Don't take too long over your replies. Your immediate reaction to each item will more likely be accurate than a long, thought-out response.	7. to a very great extent 6. to a great extent 5. to a considerable extent 4. to a moderate extent 3. to a limited extent 2. to a very limited extent 1. not at all						
1. Workload							
a) The performance of team members is impaired by excessive workload.	1	2	3	4	5	6	7
b) Team members always have enough time to complete work tasks safely.	1	2	3	4	5	6	7
c) The level of staffing in the practice is sufficient to manage the workload safely.	1	2	3	4	5	6	7
d) When pressure builds up, team members are expected to work faster even if it means taking short cuts.	1	2	3	4	5	6	7
2. Communication							
a) Team members feel free to question the decisions of those with more authority.	1	2	3	4	5	6	7
b) Team members are comfortable in expressing concerns to the practice leadership about the way things are done in the practice.	1	2	3	4	5	6	7
c) There is open communication between team members across all levels in the practice.	1	2	3	4	5	6	7
d) Team members are kept up to date about practice developments.	1	2	3	4	5	6	7
e) The practice leadership communicates its vision for the development of the practice.	1	2	3	4	5	6	7
3. Leadership							
a) The hierarchy in the practice is a barrier to effective working.	1	2	3	4	5	6	7
b) Highlighting a significant event will likely result in negative repercussions for the person raising it.	1	2	3	4	5	6	7
c) The practice leadership does not deal effectively with problem team members.	1	2	3	4	5	6	7
d) When team members suggest ways to improve how things are done, the practice leadership does not take this seriously.	1	2	3	4	5	6	7
e) There is a low level of trust between practice team members.	1	2	3	4	5	6	7
f) Practice team members frequently disregard rules, protocols and procedures.	1	2	3	4	5	6	7

SafeQuest   www.hf.gpsafetyclimate.com

FIGURE 36.2 Extract from SafeQuest with examples of questionnaire items

validated questionnaire that reliably measures the overall safety climate as well as five safety climate factors: (1) leadership, (2) teamwork, (3) communication, (4) workload and (5) safety systems. A selection of questionnaire items is shown in Figure 36.2 for interest. SafeQuest has been adapted for use in primary care settings in Spain and North America, and similar development work is currently under way in community pharmacy and general dental practice in Scotland.

Limitations of safety climate surveys

Safety climate questionnaires are an efficient way to ask standardised questions of respondents in a concurrent and anonymous manner, but they are potentially limited in a number of ways.[7,11,18–20] Although these types of questionnaires typically provide relatively superficial and simplified survey results, they may not adequately capture the complexity and the deeper underlying aspects of a prevailing safety culture. This is especially true in organisations where there is a perceived 'hidden agenda' by some or all of the workforce in terms of the decision-making and intent at the management or executive level (or equivalents in the primary care context). Organisational cultures are also strongly affected by external influences such as national and regional economic conditions; political, regulatory or accreditation pressures; and by people factors such as the educational, socio-economic or even religious background of the workforce. Safety climate instruments do not necessarily target or uncover these influential cultural issues, many of which can impact directly or indirectly on workplace performance, behaviours and patient safety.

The questionnaire approach is often labelled as a 'quick and dirty' method of collecting attitudinal data from survey participants. However, to generate statistically significant conclusions from these types of surveys requires relatively large population sample sizes. This is reasonably straightforward when aggregating data to the organisational level, but it might not be feasible at the individual practice level, especially for single-handed general practitioners and small care teams.[4] The practical significance of numerical scores also remains unclear. For example, what score can be considered 'adequate' and what is the relation between scores – for example, is a score of 50% really twice as 'good' as 25%? Finally, while some respondents may be 'unconscious' of their surrounding safety culture, most people will express an attitude if prompted. This attitude may be influenced by many factors that are not necessarily relevant or being measured and can therefore potentially bias the findings.

Step 2. Invite all team members to participate

In the case of SafeQuest, the practice manager (or any other team member taking responsibility) begins the safety climate survey by registering the practice online for free access to a range of supporting educational materials and to the survey software (*see* Box 36.2). Next, they enter the email addresses of all potential participants, who are then invited to participate via an automatically generated electronic invitation containing an online link to the survey website.

Completion typically takes 10 minutes and the responses are data-protected to ensure confidentiality. Team members who are yet to respond to the survey invitation are sent electronic reminders at pre-specified intervals, while there is also the option of download, completing and submitting a paper-based copy of the questionnaire.

BOX 36.2 Key features of the SafeQuest Survey Questionnaire System

- SafeQuest was developed after extensive psychometric testing in primary care with a full range of professional and staff groups.
- It is a five-domain, 30-item questionnaire that is accessed via a confidential web-based online survey system.
- A practice manager, or nominated other, quickly registers with the system and enters the email addresses of all potential participants.
- Potential participants are automatically sent an email generated by the system and containing a web link to the questionnaire pages.
- Participants follow the link and complete the questionnaire, which takes between 5 and 10 minutes.
- The practice manager logs back onto the system when satisfied that all or most participants have completed the survey.
- A numerical and graphical report of the main survey findings is then automatically generated and printed for the team to discuss and reflect and act upon.
- The report provides a measure of overall safety climate, mean safety climate scores for each of the five dimensions and scores by professional and staff groups. All of these scores are also compared with the mean scores of those practices that have completed the survey previously.

Step 3. Collect and aggregate data

After a suitable period of time (normally ranging from 1 to 4 weeks) the practice manager selects the option online to conclude the survey. The software package offers the option to automatically generate a safety climate report for the practice by aggregating the scores of the individual team members. The report is generated as a PDF and can be forwarded to a selected email address or saved to a disk or computer. An example of a fictional practice safety climate report is shown in Figure 36.3.

Certain aspects of the report require a minimum of three participants from a given professional or staff group before it will calculate mean scores (to help protect anonymity). The main sections in the report focus on outlining the following.

- Numerical scores (the mean aggregated scores of all participants) for the overall safety climate and the five safety climate factors for the practice. The minimum and maximum scores are 1 and 7, respectively. Higher scores indicate more-positive perceptions and lower scores indicate less-positive perceptions.

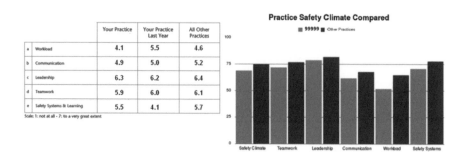

Safety Climate Report

Overall

	Your Practice	Your Practice Last Year	All Other Practices
a Workload	4.1	5.5	4.6
b Communication	4.9	5.0	5.2
c Leadership	6.3	6.2	6.4
d Teamwork	5.9	6.0	6.1
e Safety Systems & Learning	5.5	4.1	5.7

Scale: 1: not at all - 7: to a very great extent

© 2013 NHS Education Scotland

FIGURE 36.3 Example of a safety climate report

- Numerical scores comparing the overall safety climate and the five safety climate factors of different staff groups: (1) 'management' vs. 'non-management' and (2) clinical vs. non-clinical staff.
- Numerical scores comparing the practice's overall safety climate and five safety climate factors with (1) all other practices that have previously completed the survey and (2) previous results from the practice (only if available).
- Aggregated scores for each questionnaire item for interest.

Step 4. Disseminate and discuss the safety climate survey results

It is highly recommended that the findings are shared with everyone in the practice team, including those who did not complete the survey. A dedicated practice meeting is the ideal setting to discuss the report and can be successfully facilitated in less than an hour. The discussion and analytical process is flexible and practice teams can adapt it according to their circumstances, but it should ideally focus on all of the following actions.

- Identify how many team members completed the survey
- Identify one safety climate factor perceived positively
- Identify one safety climate factor perceived less positively
- Compare and contrast the results of different staff groups
- Compare the practice's results with those of other practices
- Compare the practice's results with those from previous surveys (if available)
- Summarise the main discussion and action points

Examples of potential reflective type questions and their rationale are shown in Figure 36.4. Practice teams are encouraged to identify one or two important issues only and resist being distracted by minor or insignificant differences in survey scores.

NHS
Education
for
Scotland

Making the most of your safety climate survey report

Practices often ask what they are supposed to 'do' once they have conducted their safety culture survey and generated their report. While there is no right answer to this question, we recommend sharing the report's findings with everyone in your team, including those who did not complete the survey. A practice meeting is the ideal setting to discuss and reflect on your report.

This guide summarises a process to successfully facilitate a safety culture meeting in your practice in less than an hour. It is completely flexible and you may choose to use all, part, or none of it.

Action	Reflective questions	Potential implications
Identify how many members of your team completed the survey *5 minutes**	What proportion of your team did not complete the survey? Do non-participants have a specific characteristic in common? Why did they not complete the survey?	The more people that complete the survey, the more likely that the results will reflect the perceptions of the whole team. If they do, it makes it more difficult to interpret the rest of the report with confidence Do you need to better promote the survey or reconsider the timing in future?
Identify one safety climate factor that your team perceived as positive (do not consider the scores of other practices) *10 minutes**	Do you think this perception is a true reflection of the reality in your practice? What evidence is there to support this perception? Explore actions (if any) to improve this area further or ensure perceptions of this area remain positive.	Sometimes perceptions and reality do not quite 'match up' This helps your team to identify your current strengths in this specific area
Identify one safety climate factor that your team perceived less positively (do not consider the scores of other practices yet) *5 minutes**	Do you think this perception is a true reflection of the reality in your practice? What evidence is there to support this perception? Explore actions (if any) to improve perceptions of this area.	It may not always be possible or desirable to 'improve'.
Compare the results of the different staff groups in your practice *10 minutes**	Are there differences between staff groups? If yes, does one staff group consistently perceive things more positively (or negatively) than the other? Is the difference in one or more areas? Explore why their perceptions may be different? Can perceptions be aligned?	Focus on the differences in perceptions and not on whether the perceptions of one group is 'right' This may be a good opportunity to allow someone from every staff group to suggest a reason
Compare your results with the results of other practices *5 minutes**	Are the scores (perceptions) comparable or different? If different, how large are the differences? Can you think of reasons why there might be differences?	Small numerical differences are normal and expected. Look out for larger differences in a specific area. Differences do not necessarily imply 'better or worse' or 'right or wrong'.
Compare your results with any previous surveys (if applicable) *10 minutes**	Have perceptions changed over time? Explore why this may be the case?	
Summarise the main discussion points through team consensus *5 minutes**	Are there specific actions you could take to improve the practice safety culture?	

*Suggested times for each point to ensure all sections are discussed. Aim to identify one or two important issues and resist being distracted by minor or insignificant differences in scores.

FIGURE 36.4 Suggested template for a facilitated safety climate meeting

Practice teams are encouraged to document the main findings, discussion points and intended actions (if any) from the meeting on a report template (*see* Figure 36.5). The report findings can be adapted at the individual level and submitted as evidence for appraisal (e.g. as a demonstration of leadership, quality improvement, team working or making care safer) and they are also acceptable for Quality and Outcomes Framework purposes in the Scottish context.

Practice report of a safety climate meeting

General practice name and 5-digit practice code:	The Dowell Practice, 99999
Date survey commenced:	01/02/2013
Date of meeting to discuss results:	10/03/2013
Number of team members present at meeting:	22/28

Action	Findings, reflection and discussion	Next steps
Survey participation	The practice team was notified about the survey during a practice meeting in January. 24/28 (86%) of people invited by the practice manager completed the survey. Of the four who didn't complete it, two were on holiday, one forgot and one person's reason was unclear. The team agreed that, while this was a very good response, it could be even better in the future	The practice manager will send reminder e-mails to everyone after a week. The report will be generated after four weeks (rather than two like this time) to allow those people on holiday a chance to complete the survey.
Safety climate factor perceived as positive	The Leadership (6.5) factor was perceived most positively. The team agreed this reflected reality because the practice manager had been there for 27 years. Also, one of the senior and older GPs has a managerial role in the health board.	The practice leadership is perceived positively. We do not plan any changes.
Safety climate factor perceived less positively	The Workload factor was perceived least positively. The team agreed that workload had been particularly high during the last few months. The main reasons were felt to be seasonal (winter) and the festive period. However, the practice had also started providing services to another local nursing home during the last few months.	One of the GPs will be retiring in the next few months. The practice will audit appointment availability for three months after she retires to inform the partners' decision whether to replace her or not.
Perceptions of different staff groups	The perceptions of the staff groups seem broadly comparable	
Comparison with other practices	The practice perceptions are broadly comparable to others, except for workload. The team discussed this at length again and agreed that this may in fact be an issue	The practice manager will conduct a two week audit of all the work in the practice and report her findings to the partners.
Comparison with previous surveys	The team's perception of workload is much less positive this year. However, perceptions of safety systems are much better. This may be because of the practice's participation in the pilot patient safety programme for primary care	
Summary	The workload in the practice has been a concern for some time. The safety culture survey results seem to suggest that it is a real problem and not just a case of 'everyone' struggling.	

FIGURE 36.5 Example of a safety climate meeting report

POTENTIAL BENEFITS OF MEASURING SAFETY CLIMATE

Measuring safety climate has potential benefits at the individual, practice and regional/national level.[7,17,19] At the level of the individual team member, safety climate surveys may increase awareness of safety and safety-related conditions and behaviours. At the practice team level, safety climate surveys may have application as a diagnostic and educational tool, allowing primary care teams to measure their overall safety climate and identify their relative strengths and weaknesses by comparison with the regional or national aggregate. They can then prioritise, design and implement initiatives to build a stronger safety culture and evaluate their progress through periodic surveys. For example, some participating practices in the SIPC programme reported the following changes as a result of measuring their safety climate with SafeQuest: increasing the frequency of staff meetings, ensuring clinical representation at staff meetings, improving 'two-way' communication and sharing the results of meetings with all staff.[5] A selection of participant quotes is shown verbatim in Box 36.3.

BOX 36.3 Selected quotes on SafeQuest benefits from survey participants

- *'Many of us in the practice staff hadn't really made the link that us failing to communicate in was a threat to patient safety . . . we had a lot of really good stuff came out of it, a lot of very open discussion.'*
- *'[We]* weren't as good as we thought we were.'
- *'[There was a]* mismatch between what the clinical and non clinical staff thought.'
- *'[SafeQuest]* prompted some very open discussion.'
- *'It did sound good, being able to ask questions and get answers straight away from doctors or receiving instructions etc instead of going through a third party.'*
- *'. . . encouraged to speak out if you think something isn't right.'*

A consistent and main finding of the vast majority of safety culture surveys – irrespective of industry or geographical setting – is that respondents grouped as 'management' because of seniority or influence in the organisational hierarchy frequently perceive the prevailing safety climate significantly more positively than those in the 'non-management' group or with less organisational influence.[20-23] These differences in perceptions have potentially serious implications, as the number of safety-related incidents increases with the degree of variation in perception between different staff groups.[24] Determining which group's perceptions are closer to reality can be very difficult and, indeed, unhelpful in practice. While it may be tempting to speculate or attempt to determine which group's perception is closer to reality, it is the degree of variation between the groups that is more important.

In general medical practice, doctors have a multifaceted organisational role as leaders, managers, educators and front-line clinicians. Arguably, this should provide them with sharper insights into the safety of patient care and related practice systems than other staff groups. However, a recent study has found significant differences between 'management' and 'non-management' in general medical practices in the west of Scotland.[20] For a positive and strong safety culture to be built perceptions of all primary care staff groups may therefore first have to be aligned.

From previous SafeQuest research and evaluation, it is clear that practices in Scotland have different overall perceptions of safety climate and of the different safety climate factors. However, the reported safety climate in primary care appears generally to be positive.[20,23] A small minority of practices has significantly less-positive perceptions of safety climate than the main group and it may be that they could be specifically targeted in the future as a priority group for safety interventions. However, this variation within and between teams has also been shown in secondary care studies and should therefore be interpreted with caution.

CONCLUSION

Measuring safety climate is an important first step for primary care teams to help build a strong and positive safety culture. SafeQuest is an example of a valid and reliable questionnaire that may be used for this purpose and has been found to have potential value for some teams as an educational and improvement tool. The very real challenge now is to ensure the active engagement of the whole team in a manner that is feasible and acceptable. While safety climate meetings and reports may be helpful in this regard, it could also be perceived as a box-ticking exercise by some, paradoxically leading to a less 'open' culture. Despite much research effort in the last decade, the concept and role of 'culture' within the healthcare context remains an important yet highly complex and poorly understood notion. There is a pressing need, particularly in primary care, to gain a deeper understanding qualitatively of this area and how it impacts on safe practices, and also to determine, for example, whether it is possible to quantify the association between levels of safety climate perception and specific clinical outcomes – if suitable examples or proxies can be defined.[24]

FURTHER READING

The safety climate educational materials and 'guide sheets' developed by NES are freely available to healthcare staff to adapt and use to suit their own contexts. For more information, please visit: www.healthcareimprovement scotland.org/.

REFERENCES

1. National Patient Safety Agency. *Seven Steps to Patient Safety*. London: NPSA; 2004.
2. Reason J. Human error: models and management. *BMJ*. 2000; **320**(7237): 768–70.
3. Department of Health. *An Organization with a Memory: report of an expert group on learning from adverse events in the NHS*. London: HMSO; 2000.
4. de Wet C, Spence W, Mash R, *et al*. The development and psychometric evaluation of a safety climate measure for primary care. *Qual Saf Health Care*. 2010; **19**(6): 1–8.
5. Health Foundation. *Safety Improvement in Primary Care*. London: Health Foundation. Available at: www.health.org.uk/news-and-events/newsletter/safety-improvement-in-primary-care/ (accessed 30 November 2013).
6. Scottish Government. *Delivering Quality in Primary Care National Action Plan: implementing the Healthcare Quality Strategy for NHS Scotland*. Edinburgh: Scottish Government; 2010.
7. Nieva VF, Sorra J. Safety culture assessment: a tool for improving patient safety in healthcare organizations. *Qual Saf Health Care*. 2003; **12**(Suppl. 2): ii17–23.
8. Westrum R. A typology of organisational cultures. *Qual Saf Health Care*. 2004; **13**(Suppl. 2): i22–7.
9. Parker D, Lawrie M, Hudson P. A framework for understanding the development of organisational safety culture. *Saf Sci*. 2006; **44**: 551–62.
10. Kirk S, Parker D, Claridge T, *et al*. Patient safety culture in primary care: developing a theoretical framework for practical use. *Qual Saf Health Care*. 2007; **16**(4): 313–20.
11. Scott T, Mannion R, Davies H, *et al*. The quantitative measurement of organizational culture in health care: a review of the available instruments. *Health Serv Res*. 2003; **38**(3): 923–45.
12. Guldenmund FW. The use of questionnaires in safety culture research: an evaluation. *Saf Sci*. 2007; **45**(6): 723–43.
13. Sexton JB, Helmreich RL, Neilands TB, *et al*. The safety attitudes questionnaire: psychometric properties, benchmarking data, and emerging research. *BMC Health Serv Res*. 2006; **6**: 44.
14. Sorra JS, Nieva VF. *Hospital Survey on Patient Safety Culture*. Rockville, MD: Agency for Healthcare Research and Quality; 2004.
15. Colla JB, Bracken AC, Kinney LM, *et al*. Measuring patient safety climate: a review of surveys. *Qual Saf Health Care*. 2005; **14**(5): 364–6.
16. Flin R. Measuring safety culture in healthcare: a case for accurate diagnosis. *Saf Sci*. 2007; **45**: 653–67.
17. Flin R, Burns C, Mearns K, *et al*. Measuring safety climate in health care. *Qual Saf Health Care*. 2006; **15**: 109–15.
18. Kho ME, Carbone JM, Lucas J, *et al*. Safety climate survey: reliability of results from a multicenter ICU survey. *Qual Saf Health Care*. 2005; **14**(4): 273–8.
19. Hopkins A. Studying organisational cultures and their effects on safety. *Saf Sci*. 2006; **44**: 875–89.
20. de Wet C, Johnson P, Mash R, *et al*. Measuring perceptions of safety climate in primary care: a cross-sectional study. *J Eval Clin Pract*. 2012; **18**(1): 135–42.
21. Gershon RRM, Karkashian CD, Grosch JW, *et al*. Hospital safety climate and its relationship with safe work practices and workplace exposure incidents. *Am J Infect Control*. 2000; **28**(3): 211–21.

22. Firth-Cozens J. Evaluating the culture of safety. *Qual Saf Health Care.* 2005; **12**(6): 401.

23. Hutchinson A, Cooper KL, Dean JE, *et al.* use of a safety climate questionnaire in UK health care: factor structure, reliability and usability. *Qual Saf Health Care.* 2006; **15**(5): 347–53.

24. Health Foundation. *Evidence Scan: measuring safety culture.* London: Health Foundation; 2011. Available at: www.health.org.uk/public/cms/75/76/313/2600/Measuring%20 safety%20culture.pdf?realName=rclb4B.pdf (accessed 30 November 2013).

CHAPTER 37

Improving out-of-hours care

Nigel Williams & Mike Norbury

BACKGROUND

Unintentional medical harm is recognised as a major problem for healthcare systems in the United Kingdom and internationally, with increasing evidence of preventable harm and suboptimal care in daytime primary care.[1] In response, patient safety programmes from acute hospital settings are now being spread to daytime general practice in Scotland,[2] with adaptations based on experience gained from Health Foundation-supported pilots.[3] However, out-of-hours (OOH) primary care services provide care for more than 70% of the time in each week, yet the safety of care in this setting has received comparatively little or no attention. While there are similarities between daytime and OOH primary care teams and the care they deliver, there are also differences,[4] posing the challenge of determining if improvement interventions in daytime primary care are applicable to this setting.

This chapter describes a project that aimed to examine and improve patient safety in the OOH service of a large Scottish health board by piloting three previously validated improvement methods:

1. structured case note review
2. safety climate assessment
3. a clinical assessment 'care bundle'.

Adult patients presenting to the OOH services with symptoms and signs suggestive of acute asthma were used as the exemplar condition, as this medical condition is relatively common, potentially serious and evidence-based guidance for its assessment and management is readily available.[5] In addition, presenting to OOH with acute asthma is a recognised additional risk factor.

Lothian Unscheduled Care Service (LUCS) provides primary medical services for a population of approximately 850 000 people during the OOH period. The public interface is NHS24, a national service in Scotland, which operates a nurse-led telephone triage system. Patients are referred by NHS24 if deemed appropriate to LUCS for telephone advice, a face-to-face consultation in a primary care centre or for a home visit. The LUCS operates from five bases across Lothian and is mainly staffed by general practitioners (GPs) and emergency nurse practitioners (ENPs), but there is also a small number of community paramedics and non-clinical support staff. The service employs 67 GPs and 36 ENPs, and has contracts with approximately 200 independent contractor GPs for flexible sessional work by mutual agreement. Non-clinical staff includes hub administrators (who coordinate site activity and GP home visits), receptionists and car drivers. All clinical encounters are recorded electronically in the Adastra software package.

STRUCTURED CASE NOTE REVIEW

Prior to the improvement programme, clinical audits performed at the LUCS bases found significant variation between clinicians in terms of examination, assessment and management of adult patients presenting with acute asthma. A structured case note review was therefore undertaken at the start of the programme to measure the baseline rate of performance and to identify undetected harm or suboptimal care.

Case record numbers of all patients attending LUCS bases with consultation codes for acute asthma were identified and collated for the 12-month period from April 2011 to March 2012. From these, a random sample of 100 case records was selected for review. A draft case note review template was developed from evidence-based clinical guidance in conjunction with LUCS associate clinical directors. A final revised template was agreed after a small pilot and stakeholder feedback. Reviewers used the template to screen the records in a structured, rapid and focused manner for evidence of six specific clinical acts of omission or commission that may have or did lead to patient harm. The findings are shown in Table 37.1.

TABLE 37.1 Structured case note review findings (n = 100)

Clinical acts of commission and omission screened for with template	Number of records in which it was detected
Incomplete clinical assessment	72
Nebulised β2-agonist administered without justification	34
Prescribing an inadequate dose of oral steroids	16
Antibiotic treatment without justification	14
Not recording an action plan (safety-netting)	6
Not recording patient's smoking status	50

The findings have a number of important implications for patient care, as follows.

- The high incidence of 'incomplete clinical assessment' provides justification for the development and introduction of the acute asthma clinical assessment 'care bundle'.
- Nebulisation is an expensive and time-consuming method of administrating β2-agonists. For mild and moderate cases of acute asthma, multi-dosing using a spacer and metered-dose inhaler is equally effective and is shown to enhance patient enablement and self-management[6] and it ensures consistency in treatment between the OOH service and daytime primary care.
- An inadequate dose of oral steroids may result in treatment failure, avoidable re-attendance or even hospitalisation.
- Antibiotic treatments without clinical indication represent an unnecessary cost and have the potential to cause preventable harm (antibiotic-associated diarrhoea).
- Enquiring about patients' smoking status and offering them brief cessation advice (if appropriate) is an evidence-based intervention that should be offered to everyone.[7] Recording the smoking status in the medical record may also act as a reminder or prompt to daytime clinicians to also offer cessation advice.
- Recording agreed action plans (safety-netting) for patients with asthma potentially enhances their ability to self-care and potentially assures continuity of their management in daytime general practice.

The experience with the structured case note reviews and the main findings were comparable with previously published accounts of the value of applying the trigger review method in a general practice daytime setting.[8] The method helped to reveal undetected patient harm and instances of suboptimal care that were not detected by clinical audit or incident reporting[9] and it demonstrated the potential improvement and educational value of the programme to staff. While this method cannot and should not be used to 'benchmark' service quality, the quality of care provided by LUCS seems to compare favourably with an ongoing audit of asthma care in UK general practice.[10]

MEASURING SAFETY CLIMATE

A positive safety culture can increase the psychological safety of staff, facilitates learning from patient safety incidents and improves the adoption of discretionary safety attitudes and behaviours.[11] However, while safety culture assessment has been associated with improved clinical outcomes in the acute sector,[12] this association is less certain for primary care settings.[13]

The 'SafeQuest' instrument was chosen to measure perceptions of the safety climate in LUCS, as it has sound psychometric properties, was developed for general practice and is used routinely in this setting.[14] SafeQuest is a self-report questionnaire that individual healthcare staff complete (in confidence) by indicating their levels of agreement with 30 items (statements associated with safety). The individual and team scores are aggregated to measure the overall perception of safety climate of the team (or organisation) as well as five safety climate factors: Leadership, Teamwork, Communication, Workload and Safety Systems. The SafeQuest software allows the team or practice manager to automatically generate a safety climate report.

For this programme, the wording of the cover sheet and some of the questions were amended to better reflect the OOH setting (e.g. 'GP practice' was replaced by 'Primary Care centre'). The changes were minor and felt to be appropriate and acceptable, as there are precedents for adapting safety climate instruments for different settings and to incorporate local terminology.* Feasibility was confirmed by piloting a paper version of the tool at a LUCS base. The SafeQuest instrument was then administered electronically at two LUCS bases in December 2011 and February 2012. All LUCS primary care team members (clinical, non-clinical and managerial) were invited to participate. Participation was promoted through a meeting with the LUCS Clinical Governance lead and staff, electronic reminders and informal encouragement.

Safety climate reports were generated and disseminated to all staff to help facilitate reflection and further discussion. During a dedicated safety climate meeting, the findings of each OOH primary care team were also compared with the 'typical' daytime GP safety climate report and all staff were invited to comment on, and provide feedback about, the potential significance of the observed differences in perceptions. Specifically, the OOH teams' perceptions were lower than those of daytime GP teams for the communication, leadership, teamwork and safety systems domains. Respondents with management roles also perceived the safety climate as being more positive than those considered as non-management.

The reported perceptions arguably reflect the nature of the OOH setting. The OOH teams are even more diverse than in daytime practice and team members literally change from shift to shift. Clinical leaders are also less visible because they are temporally removed from non-management due to working 'normal' office hours while the service is provided OOH. However, the differences in perceptions between staff groups may suggest a real imperative to improve communication about service development, safety initiatives and incident reporting.

One of the key benefits of measuring safety climate is that it can stimulate reflection and discussion in the team about their priorities and potential differences. However, simply administering a survey can have a corollary effect to improve patient safety awareness.

The main learning points that derived from conducting the safety climate survey for LUCS were as follows.

---

* Carl de Wet, 'Adaptation of SafeQuest for use in out of hours primary care settings', email message to authors, 28 September 2011.

- There is a need for management to improve communication and to encourage feedback from front-line staff.
- Lower numerical scores do not necessarily imply poor safety; in fact, a high numerical score may indicate that a team overestimates their susceptibility to latent risks.
- Non-clinical staff can meaningfully contribute to the safety of care and their involvement in improvement initiatives should be encouraged.

ASTHMA ASSESSMENT CARE BUNDLE

A care bundle is simply a number of healthcare interventions grouped together. The rationale is that bundling interventions and implementing them together can improve reliability and patient care outcomes more than the sum of the individual elements.[15] A bundle usually has between three and six components. Each component should ideally be evidence-based, part of a guideline or protocol or widely accepted and established as standard and best care. Every component in the bundle should routinely be delivered or considered for every patient within a specific period of time. Compliance with a care bundle and its components is measured as 'all or nothing'.

A thorough clinical assessment is necessary to determine the severity of an acute asthma attack and to inform the selection of an appropriate management plan. To ensure this happens, an asthma assessment care bundle was developed from Scottish Intercollegiate Guidelines Network guidelines. The six components of the asthma assessment care bundle that should be documented in every patient's record are:

1. heart rate
2. respiratory rate
3. oxygen saturation
4. work of breathing
5. peak flow (measured)
6. peak flow (personal best).

A target of 95% for overall compliance with the bundle was set. In other words, all six components should be documented in the case records in a minimum of 95% of patients with acute asthma.

The acceptability and feasibility of the care bundle was tested and improved by applying the Plan-Do-Study-Act method. This involved starting with small numbers of patients at one base, and revising the process iteratively in response to feedback and results. Once the care bundle method and process was agreed, it was introduced in one LUCS base from October 2011 to February 2012 and the implementation was supported by clinical updates and educational interventions. Performance data were fed back to clinicians using A4-sized run charts – these were updated every 2 weeks and were prominently displayed in every consulting room.

Next, the asthma assessment care bundle was spread to the other four LUCS bases. Compliance rates were calculated every 2 weeks from data extracted from a sample of 40 patient records randomly selected from all the bases. The results included a 'dashboard' of compliance rates with each of the bundle components, the overall compliance for that base and the overall compliance in Lothian. Run charts were annotated with educational interventions, practical changes or feedback from participants. A site lead was appointed for each base with the responsibility to prominently display run charts, update results regularly and as initial contacts for any staff who may request additional information. An example of a 'dashboard' is shown in Figure 37.1.

The initial aim of the programme was to determine 'what works' in an OOH setting, and to identify practical ways to ensure sustainability and spread. The care bundle approach was found to be feasible and acceptable in this programme. However, because interpretation of run charts typically requires a minimum of 15 data points, equating to 30 weeks in the programme, it was not possible to infer whether improvements in compliance would be sustained in the longer term or, if they are, whether there will be a positive association with improved clinical outcomes. Anecdotal feedback suggested good clinical engagement and there was some evidence of transferrable benefit in the form of more structured recording of objective clinical variables for conditions other than acute asthma and improved adherence to evidence-based guidance for acute asthma management. For example, a comparison of a random sample of 60 patient records at the start of the project with a second random sample of 60 patient records when the project was established revealed a reduction in nebuliser use from 52% to 16% ($p < 0.001$).

REFLECTION ABOUT THE PROGRAMME

This programme clearly demonstrated that patient safety and quality improvement methods can be successfully transferred from daytime general practice to the OOH setting. The OOH service may be different to and operationally dispersed compared with GP practice teams, but there are still many similarities in terms of the challenges of engaging clinicians in improvement. This programme demonstrated the value of providing clear, prominent and timely results to help raise awareness of improvement initiatives, motivate staff to become involved and promoted long-term engagement and ownership. Although many GPs work as independent contractors, the service is located within the managed network and clinical policy implementation is more practicable. In addition, standardisation of clinical records, prescribing and outcomes through the Adastra software system makes data retrieval and analysis relatively straightforward.

Some of the suggestions for improvement that emerged from the programme components in general and the safety climate assessment in particular, were:
- induction shifts for new doctors
- promotion of formal handovers between shifts
- introducing staff from bases to one another

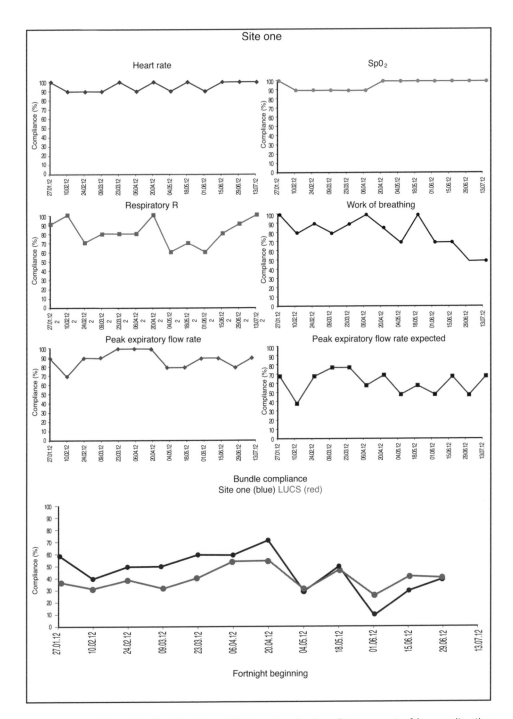

FIGURE 37.1 Example of a 'dashboard' of results displayed at one out-of-hours site; the run charts graphically demonstrate compliance rates with the asthma assessment care bundle overall and with each individual component

- better integration and understanding of clinical and non-clinical roles
- display boards at reception with information about the practitioners on duty
- promotion of incident reporting with improved feedback to staff afterwards.

These suggestions align well with the evidence base for human factors interventions in patient safety.[16]

In general, implementation challenges reflected established models of change management.[17] However, it is interesting to note that quality improvement activity may initially be perceived as scrutiny by service management, and there may also be legitimate concerns about disruption to service delivery that need to be explored carefully. Similarly, practitioners may view improvement activity as a form of performance management and it is therefore essential to consult clinicians at all stages and to ensure that suggestions are considered seriously and feedback given to ensure a sense of ownership.[18]

At a more strategic level, this project illustrates the key role of the OOH primary care service in providing continuity of care and acting as a link between acute hospitals and GP practices. Consideration should be given to promoting informational continuity by routine use of Anticipatory Care Plans and accurate Emergency Care Summaries or by extending access to daytime primary care records to OOH clinicians. Finally, this programme suggests that the OOH service has great potential value as a setting for the initial design, development and piloting of new primary care improvement tools and innovative approaches.

REFERENCES

1. de Wet C, Bowie P. The preliminary development and testing of a global trigger tool to detect error and harm in primary care records. *Postgrad Med J*. 2009; **85**(1002): 176–80.
2. Healthcare Improvement Scotland. *Patient Safety in Primary Care*. Edinburgh: Healthcare Improvement Scotland; 2011. Available at: www.healthcareimprove mentscotland.org/programmes/patient_safety/patient_safety_in_primary_care.aspx (accessed 7 March 2014).
3. Healthcare Improvement Scotland. *Safety Improvement in Primary Care*. Edinburgh: Healthcare Improvement Scotland; 2011. Available at: www.healthcareimprovement scotland.org/our_work/patient_safety/spsp/patient_safety_in_primary_care.aspx (accessed 7 March 2014).
4. O'Malley J. Out-of-hours and primary care: closer and closer apart. *Br J Gen Pract*. 2012; **62**(597): 176–7.
5. British Thoracic Society and Scottish Intercollegiate Guidelines Network. *British Guideline on the Management of Asthma: a national clinical guideline*. Edinburgh: Scottish Intercollegiate Guidelines Network; 2011.
6. Silverman J, Kinnersley P. Calling time on the 10-minute consultation. *Br J Gen Pract*. 2012; **62**(596): 118–19.
7. Mooney H. Doctors are told to make every contact count to reduce costs of poor life-styles. *BMJ*. 2012; **344**: e319.

8. Bowie P, Halley L, Gillies J, *et al*. Searching primary care records for predefined triggers may expose latent risks and adverse events. *Clin Risk*. 2012; **18**(1): 13–18.

9. Dawada P, Jenkins R, Varnam R. *Quality Improvement in General Practice*. London: The King's Fund; 2010.

10. General Practice Airways Group. *UNSAFE: audit of patients presenting with uncontrolled asthma*. 2012. Available at: www.guideline-audit.com/unsafe/index.php (accessed 7 March 2014).

11. Edmondson A. Psychological safety and learning behaviour in work teams. *Admin Sci Q*. 1999; **44**(2): 350–83.

12. Colla J, Bracken A, Kinney L, *et al*. Measuring patient safety climate: a review of surveys. *Qual Saf Health Care*. 2005; **14**(5): 364–6.

13. Hann M, Bower P, Campbell S, *et al*. The association between culture, climate and quality of care in primary health care teams. *Fam Pract*. 2007; **24**(4): 323–9.

14. de Wet C, Spence W, Mash R, *et al*. The development and psychometric evaluation of a safety climate measure for primary care. *Qual Saf Health Care*. 2010; **19**: 578–84.

15. Langley G, Nolan K, Nolan T, *et al*. *The Improvement Guide: a practical approach to enhancing organizational performance*. 2nd ed. San Francisco, CA: Jossey-Bass; 2009.

16. NHS Institute for Innovation and Improvement. *Patient Safety First: implementing human factors in healthcare*. London: NHS III; 2010.

17. Kotter J. Leading change: why transformation efforts fail. *Harv Bus Rev*. 1995 March–April.

18. Kirk S, Parker D, Claridge T, *et al*. Patient safety culture in primary care: developing a theoretical framework for practical use. *Qual Saf Health Care*. 2007; **16**(4); 313–20.

CHAPTER 38

Care improvement: a personal reflection

Andy Crawford

INTRODUCTION

In the last decade, two seminal publications from the Institute of Medicine[1,2] have contributed to a dramatic rise to prominence of the international health-care focus on safety, and how to reduce healthcare associated harm. This has seen the emergence of nationally sponsored improvement programmes, such as the Scottish Patient Safety Programme (SPSP), which set mandatory require-ments on healthcare providers to establish reliability in specific safety critical clinical processes and related outcomes. Given the consequence to patients, this focus on safety has its own justification, but for some it has been the stalking horse of a much larger set of concerns for healthcare quality. This arises from a more challenging realisation that healthcare organisations cannot currently provide a quality of healthcare that meets the requirements of patients or the general public.[3] So, in Scotland we observed SPSP leading eventually to the publication of a national Healthcare Quality Strategy.[4]

Even so, safety still dominates the clinical improvement landscape. It is interesting to ponder what form of practices may have emerged if the quality strategies had grown from a root of clinical effectiveness or a person-centred quality focus. I wonder if learning defences may have kicked in, obscuring the challenge and the possibility of improvement. Perhaps only the moral impera-tive of unintentionally harming patients had the power to generate the now global healthcare improvement movement? Yet, reflecting on this question and the safety imperative reveals a bias away from primary care. The scale, degree and relative ease of measurement of harm in acute care settings potentially distorts our thinking. As the Health Foundation has concluded, 'errors occur in primary care but this has received far less priority'.[5]

Quality strategies also generate a focus on the question of how to improve healthcare. An initial barrier to understanding is separating *change* from *improvement*. It appears healthcare is the embodiment of the Heraclitean phrase *'change is the only constant'.* So within this diversity of activity our sense of which intentions and interventions lead to improvement can be difficult to accurately discern. Not surprisingly, there is a mixed history of approaches and results in applying quality improvement methods.[6,7] When linked to a range of limitations, including a dearth of studies, we find a major gap in 'what is known about how best to improve quality in healthcare'.[6] In relation to improvement and improving safety in primary care this general challenge is described as even more profoundly lacking in clarity or response.[8]

In this potential bias away from primary care contexts, I sensed the need to pay attention to how improvement is and can be developed. Recognising the limitations of experimentally derived knowledge we turn to observation, so reflection on experience becomes an important part of theory building. One of the key areas of reflection is the way different types of improvement thinking are translating into various healthcare settings. In this discussion I wish to reflect on personal experience of improvement using the methods and tools derived from what is described as 'process improvement through reduced variation',[9] including initiatives based in primary care. I consider in particular the methods advocated by the Boston-based Institute of Healthcare Improvement (IHI), which lie at the core of the SPSP approach.[10-12]

As I review other improvement methods, such as the waste reduction of Lean or defect reduction of Six Sigma, I notice an often unresolved question of *how to best perform the current process?* This frames the observation that resolution of any question as to what is the best process, product or service 'cannot be found without some form of experimentation'.[13] For me, therefore, the concept testing of IHI-advocated methods (IHI-AM) can have a specific utility that is not always explicit in other improvement approaches. So I focus on IHI-AM for reasons of choice as well as familiarity.

SPSP AND THE INSTITUTE OF HEALTHCARE IMPROVEMENT ADVOCATED METHODS

SPSP was formally launched in January 2008 and founded on a mix of research and empirical evidence derived from preceding safety programmes in the United States and the United Kingdom. Its initial focus was solely on acute adult care settings but has since seen additional subsets developed, including the attempt at a substantial translation into primary care. Concern remains about the robustness of evaluation but it appears to me that there is a sufficient volume of literature (though often grey) and personal narrative to move beyond the question of efficacy (does this improvement method work at all?), and to consider the question of effectiveness (how well does it work?). So my attention is now on how and why it is effective as I seek to enhance its effectiveness.

I am conscious of a potential arrogance in choosing to provide my own interpretation of the implementation of IHI-AM and its impact. I excuse this in the context of sensemaking, linking personal interpretations and actions[10] with the hope of contributing to a sharing of meaning. Even if you may disagree I hope that my perspective may encourage your own development and deeper application of quality improvement thinking.

I see at the core of the IHI-AM the juxtaposition of two interrelated conceptual devices: the *model for improvement*[12] and the *system for profound knowledge*.[12] This produces a multifocal improvement approach involving a knowledge building methodology that combines localised concept testing with the enumerative study of variation to develop a reliable process. The local focus on process knowledge is then embedded in a broader attentiveness to context, which links systemic thinking and awareness of the psychology of change.

The model for improvement is represented as the Plan-Do-Study-Act (PDSA) cycle, described by Deming[12] as a means of process improvement and generally understood as a simple representation of the scientific method. The PDSA cycle is then grounded by questions of improvement purpose, measurement and improvement concepts – the Model for Improvement.[11]

On holiday in Scotland I once watched a woodcarver in his studio. His attention on the block of wood was total. He reached for a chisel without taking his gaze from the wood as his fingers found the required implement. It was brought into use in an automatic way but as its job was done his eyes came at last onto the tool and a thumb flicked the edge before it was placed back in position on the bench. On reflection I was so struck by where his attention was and how it came to the tool after use. I wondered about our practices, how this related to our use of improvement tools, contrasting with the relative lack of attention after use or reflective thinking about how they actually functioned.

It is recognised that innovation and improvement 'often fails on the application end'.[13] So, using the woodcarver's attitude, I have been keeping notes of my own reflections, along with outputs from conversations with colleagues, building a sense of our experience with improvement tools. Successful use of the Model for Improvement in our local experience appears to be associated with a number of features.

- *Diligent application in a systematic way*, where each question and step in the PDSA cycle is successively and methodically addressed in an iterative learning process. There also appears to be a relationship with the experience of the user and the application, where the most experienced improvers demonstrate the most diligent practice.
- A recognised need to *generate the highest frequency of experiments* on the process. I have observed reluctance to high-paced experimentation in less-experienced users. Part of this situation appears to relate to past experience of improvement. The contrast with the slower methods of clinical audit, for instance, has at times been part of the slow-paced explanation. There is a further feature relating to fear of failure that has emerged as a reason for slow pacing. Although routine experimenters do not plan to fail, they are more accepting of failed experiments and continue to see these as valuable learning opportunities. To test effectively you need to be capable of making

mistakes, of living with failure. My own attitude is that no tests fail. If properly conducted, even when it might not turn out as predicted, there will always be a learning output.

- Interactive team development where *the process is built by involving many people in the testing*. The local improvement leads can often start by undertaking a test on their own. This certainly gets things moving quickly but if this continues the failure to involve others delays progress and appears to limit the quality of the new prototype process. The involvement of many different perspectives in many different circumstances enhances process development but also builds ownership that appears to ease implementation of the final model.

- Improvement arises from forms of *change that occurs in the process*. A common trap observed is misplaced reliance on feedback of the data picture that often descends into a form of intra-team *nagging*. Sharing the data picture is important but its role is not to beat up others on performance. Data is a provocation to thinking on what is happening in the process, to generate changes concepts from which the tests of change are developed.

- Some of the richest examples of well-documented PDSA cycles I have encountered have been from primary care teams. This is an exception and there is a general resistance among clinicians to such effective record keeping. The lack of these records limits expression of the reliable prototype, its history and key design components, which are the basis of communicating the effective working process design to others.

- It is obvious that clinical teams using the model successfully begin to display higher degrees of *process literacy*. In this they are more likely to use process maps to expose the shared appreciation, break down the process into components amenable to tested change (sometimes referred to as segmenting) and think about how the flows of work are connected. Another observed feature of such teams is they avoid the trap of under-justification. There is an occasionally encountered but worrying behaviour where even in conditions of inadequate understanding of the process people launch into testing changes. Using the excuse of it's *just a test* rationale fails to appreciate that without a reasonable sense of aim, of understanding of the cause and effect mechanism in the process, there is no prediction, no theory and ultimately such tests are meaningless gambles.

- The role and interpretive use of data has been a challenge as teams can struggle to understand the shift in thinking linked to interpreting variation displayed on run charts or Shewhart charts. *Process measures should be selected to be diagnostic.* Here I also notice tension between the dominant organisational mode of thinking, which tends to be performance (and assurance) driven, and the diagnostic principle. Organisations often overprescribe aggregated measurement schemes that inhibit flexible diagnostic measurement. It is disheartening to watch teams slavishly capture and report data that long ago became redundant.

- *Reliability becomes absorbed into language as a key quality concept.* Here reliability can indicate that quality is locked into the clinical process in a way that means the process is predictable and meets requirements.

I think there is one final observation I would add to this list: improvement is an activity that, like sports, is best developed through practice and application. On my first encounter the model for improvement appeared so conceptually simple I sense now a personal learning defence dropped into place. There was no way this simple device could contribute to the resolution of apparently intractable healthcare quality challenges. It wasn't until I got *my hands dirty* in the field that I began to appreciate its nuanced elegance. Of course as I worked with process I also increasingly realised how important working with context was too, which brings me naturally to the role of Deming in IHI-AM.

Deming[12] describes the system of profound knowledge in four interrelated parts:
1. appreciation for a system
2. theory of knowledge
3. knowledge about variation
4. psychology.

Systemic thinking is supported by a large literature that strongly suggests its continued relevance to thinking about organisations and improvement. One aspect I would like to draw out is the *central law of improvement*.[11] This law – that the systems output is a consequence of its interconnected design – connects the idea of systems performance and the nature of change required. If a system is normally capable of meeting requirements then a fix or first-order change is appropriate. If the system is not capable of meeting requirements then a redesign to create a new level of improved performance or second-order change is appropriate.

The theory of knowledge relates to an underpinning philosophy and scientific methodology. The philosopher CI Lewis was a pragmatist and is important as the provider of the philosophic cradle from which some of the most significant quality improvement thinking of the twentieth century emerged.[14] Lewis asserts that when we are confronted by the chaos of the universe we try to impose some kind of stable order through which we can distinguish signs of future possibilities. The signs coalesce in our minds as concepts and theories through which we judge our future experience. So we recognise that knowledge is implicitly predictive and without interpretation of experience against those theories there can be no knowledge.[14]

It appears there is an explicitly pragmatic epistemology (or how we generate knowledge) underpinning the IHI-AM that is derived from the philosophical roots in Lewis's writing. This leads to two interesting observations. First, there is the role of perfection and, second, some potential cultural challenges in embedding IHI-AM in primary care.

There is an interesting divergence in how perfection can be perceived, that can appear on the surface to be somewhat contradictory. We have the pursuit of perfection described in a number of quality improvement approaches, notably by researchers observing Lean organisations.[15,16] Womack and Jones[16] state this as bringing 'perfection into clear view so the objective of improvement is visible and real'. It is a statement of constant intent recognising quality improvement as a process not an outcome. However, anti-perfectionism has also appeared in the literature as an important characteristic of quality improvement.[8] I have seen this represented as the critique of design by committee, where groups can spend long periods of time invoking the perfect and idealised process, but as reflected earlier the question of what is best can only be achieved through experimentation. This reminder of the dangers of over-design appears contradictory but is in experience complementary to the perfection principle.

There is recognition that identity and values can affect integration and the adoption of ideas. It is not surprising that the IHI-AM appears as deeply pragmatic, seeing truth as established by the scientific method. It is observed that this is one end of the moralism–pragmatism cultural spectrum.[17] If primary care practitioners derive truth as being validated in more general philosophies or social processes, then those approaches that are so deeply pragmatic are likely to run into adoption problems. In recognising the descriptor *science of improvement* linked to IHI-AM, I have been checking the notion of the scientific identity with various clinical audiences. Interestingly, despite being consumers of research, of the scientific product, no one in primary care has ever identified with the label of scientist. I have, therefore, completely adjusted my pitch when working on improvement ideas with clinical communities.

In thinking about variation it often appears to me that healthcare exhibits the attitude of nineteenth-century manufacturers, in always seeking more 'relaxed specifications'.[9] We offer any number of reasons why harm exists in healthcare that can at times seem to drift towards justification for attitudinal norms that accept prevailing levels of harm and quality. Shifting indicators to match performance rather than shifting performance to match requirement is another potential illustration of this attitude. Yet it is missing the point that in our role of constantly improving the patient care we provide, there is a path to quality through reduced variation. Unfortunately this often frames some fairly difficult attitudes to standardisation, raising issues of concordance to the agreed process by various members of the clinical team. Perhaps it is time to see the agreed standardised process as a shared expression of the best practices, drawing on every available contribution. The best in healthcare needs to be a cooperative or group position rather than a personal one.

The fourth part, psychology, is prone to some trainers replacing it with a variety of alternative, personally derived labels such as human behaviour, sociology or theory of organisational change. It essentially represents the relational context, or human dimension of organisational life. In my experience, this is the vital dimension of any quality improvement approach. The literature on context, culture and social and psychological aspects of organisational life is too large to represent. I would only observe that in drawing this body of knowledge to improvement practice there is one fundamental question that orientates reading and interpretation. How do we make the persistent pursuit of quality an everyday lived experience for each primary care team?

In reflecting on my writing I sense a superficiality, a difficulty in sharing a complex experience. There is a depth to improvement thinking that I cannot represent, so here I am only framing an invitation to learn for yourself. Yet even with this qualification limiting my sense of responsibility, I still feel an obligation to share one final observation. It arises from Morgan's[18] assertion that all theory is incomplete. So if this set of improvement theories is partial, what might be outside the mental map? Process control and systems thinking provide a strong basis for helpful intentions in improving even very complicated, interconnected processes, but they have been observed as inapplicable to the social complexity of human interaction.[19] I know myself as a pragmatist, who can comfortably pursue the benefits of scientific modes of thinking. I also recognise that my rational modes of thinking appear incompatible with the novelty and unknowable causality I experience in aspects of healthcare. Primary care is both an exciting and a challengingly complex place to work. It is exciting because it is challenging. Although it may appear slightly contradictory, part of that challenge for me is finding out how to more fully exploit the benefits of improvement thinking while knowing it is also an incomplete answer.

FURTHER READING

For more information on SPSP and the improvement methods outlined, please visit:

- Scottish Patient Safety Programme: www.scottishpatientsafetyprogramme. scot.nhs.uk/
- NHS Scotland Quality Improvement Hub: www.qihub.scot.nhs.uk/

REFERENCES

1. Institute of Medicine. *Crossing the Quality Chasm: a new health system for the twenty-first century.* Washington, DC: National Academies Press; 2001.
2. Kohn LT, Corrigan JM, Donaldson MS, editors. *To Err is Human: building a safer health system.* Washington, DC: National Academies Press; 1999.
3. Scottish Government. *The Healthcare Quality Strategy for NHS Scotland.* Edinburgh: Scottish Government Health Department; 2010.
4. Bate P, Mendel P, Robert G. *Organizing for Quality: the improvement journeys of leading hospitals in Europe and the United States.* Oxford: Radcliffe Publishing; 2008.
5. Health Foundation. *Evidence Scan: levels of harm in primary care.* London: Health Foundation; 2011.
6. Health Foundation. *Evidence Scan: improvement science.* London: Health Foundation; 2011.
7. Powel AS, Rushmer RK, Davies HTO. *A Systematic Narrative Review of Quality Improvement Models in Healthcare.* Edinburgh: NHS Quality Improvement Scotland; 2009.

8. Dawda P, Jenkins R, Varnam R. *Quality Improvement in General Practice*. London: The King's Fund; 2010.

9. Wheeler DJ, Chambers DS. *Understanding Statistical Process Control*. 2nd ed. Knoxville, TN: SPC Press; 1992.

10. Myers P, Hulks S, Wiggins L. *Organisational Change: perspectives on theory and practice*. Oxford: Oxford University Press; 2012.

11. Langley GJ, Moen R, Nolan KM, *et al.*, editors. *The Improvement Guide: a practical approach to enhancing organizational performance*. 2nd ed. San Francisco, CA: Jossey-Bass; 2009.

12. Deming WE. The New Economics for industry, government, education. Cambridge, MA: MIT Press; 1994.

13. Moen RD, Nolan TW, Provost LP. *Quality Improvement through Planned Experimentation*. 2nd ed. New York, NY: McGraw-Hill; 1998.

14. Lewis CI. *Mind and the World Order: outline of a theory of knowledge*. Mineola, NY: Dover; 1929.

15. Liker J. *The Toyota Way: 14 management principles from the world's greatest manufacturer*. New York, NY: McGraw-Hill; 2004.

16. Womack J, Jones D. *Lean Thinking: banish waste and create wealth in your corporation*. London: The Free Press; 2003.

17. Schein EH. *Organisation Culture and Leadership*. 4th ed. San Francisco, CA: Jossey-Bass; 2010.

18. Morgan G. *Images of Organization*. Thousand Oaks, CA: Sage Publications; 2006.

19. Stacey RD. *Complexity and Management: fad or radical challenge to systems thinking?* London: Routledge; 2000.

Epilogue

Crossing the Quality Chasm: A New Health System for the 21st Century (Institute of Medicine, 2001) remains one of the most significant publications in the field of quality and safety in healthcare. The report identified six separate but linked dimensions of healthcare quality – safe, effective, family-centred, timely, efficient and equal – and proposed that there should be a multi-agency, managed approach to improving outcomes in each of these dimensions of quality in order to transform healthcare and provide reliable, high-quality healthcare on a population basis.

That these proposals are as relevant to the delivery of health and social care in 2014 is in part testimony to the vision of the authors. '*Safe, effective and person-centred care*' have become the essential, underpinning priorities for the Scottish Government's whole-system approach to health and social care integration and reform.

However, it is also pertinent to reflect that the ongoing relevance of the IOM dimensions of healthcare quality and the importance of improvement as a way of working is, in part, due to our failure to successfully tackle and implement the challenges set out in *Crossing the Quality Chasm* in a systematic and sustained manner. Improvement methods are not consistently integrated into normal practice across whole systems, and patient safety is still a major concern with ongoing evidence of the human and financial costs of avoidable and unintended harm in most healthcare systems.

Over the last 20 years, the international patient safety movement has grown exponentially and through scientific approaches to measurement and improvement methodologies many hundreds of thousands of patients have benefited and lives saved. However, much of the focus has been in acute care settings and the improvements have been dependent on managed programmes.

Perhaps, then, the greatest challenges to make the transformation envisaged in *Crossing the Quality Chasm* are, firstly, to spread best practice in improving quality and safety across the whole health and social care system and, secondly, to move from a predominately programmed-based approach to implementing change to one where safety and improvement are normal, integrated components of health and social care planning and delivery – the 'elusive safety culture' referred to by Paul Bowie and Carl de Wet in the Preface to this book.

A further challenge for us in the educational world is to demonstrate the importance and effectiveness of educating the workforce and public in delivering *'safe, effective and person-centred care'* in a measurement- and outcomes-focused improvement world. Educational outcomes are inevitably one step away from clinical improvements and it is therefore difficult to assess the direct impact of education on patient outcomes.

The publication of *Safety and Improvement in Primary Care: The Essential Guide* is both therefore timely and important given that more than 90% of healthcare interventions occur in the community and the current emphasis and drive of Scottish Government Health and Social Care policy is to deliver a sustainable whole-system approach to personalised care, which is arguably a first in international terms.

Editors Paul Bowie and Carl de Wet have assembled an experienced team of clinical practitioners, health service managers and educational researchers to create a book that provides the reader with easy access to the underpinning theory behind improving quality and safety in primary care, linked to practical illustrations and examples of how to implement change in the context of different clinical settings. The resulting book will be equally valuable to students and novices wanting to understand the basics and principles, and experienced clinicians looking to implement improvements in their clinical practice.

The scope and range of different approaches needed to deliver change and improvement in a sustained, whole-system manner are captured in the five sections of the book encompassing the importance of systems-based approaches, people, learning and education, human factors and improvement methodology.

It is only through attention to all of these elements of safety and improvement, combined with the flexibility to tailor the solutions and interventions to different clinical settings and contexts, that we will achieve the transformational changes envisaged in *Crossing the Quality Chasm* and that elusive safety culture.

Philip Cachia
Professor and Postgraduate Dean
NHS Education for Scotland
March 2014

Index

Entries in **bold** denote figures, tables and boxes.

CPD with Radcliffe

You can now use a selection of our books to achieve CPD (Continuing Professional Development) points through directed reading.

We provide a free online form and downloadable certificate for your appraisal portfolio. Look for the CPD logo and register with us at: www.radcliffehealth.com/cpd

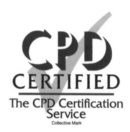